The Hearing Sciences

The Hearing Sciences

Teri A. Hamill
Lloyd L. Price

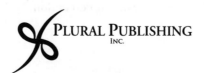

PLURAL PUBLISHING
INC.

PLURAL
PUBLISHING
INC.

5521 Ruffin Road
San Diego, CA 92123

e-mail: info@pluralpublishing.com
Web site: http://www.pluralpublishing.com

49 Bath Street
Abingdon, Oxfordshire OX14 1EA
United Kingdom

ISBN-13: 978-1-59756-199-0
ISBN-10: 1-59756-199-1

Library of Congress Cataloging-in-Publication Data:

    Hamill, Teri.
  The hearing sciences / Teri A. Hamill and Lloyd L. Price.
    p. ; cm.
  Includes bibliographical references and index.
  ISBN-13: 978-1-59756-199-0 (alk. paper)
  ISBN-10: 1-59756-199-1 (alk. paper)
1. Hearing. 2. Sound. 3. Psychoacoustics. 4. Ear—Anatomy. 5. Ear—Physiology.
  [DNLM: 1. Hearing—physiology. 2. Psychoacoustics. 3. Ear—anatomy & histology. 4.
Ear—physiology. 5. Hearing Disorders. 6. Speech Perception. WV 272 H217h 2007] I.
Price, Lloyd L. II. Title.
  QP461.H24 2007
  612.8'5—dc22

               2007046225

Contents

SECTION TWO: INTRODUCTION TO SPEECH ACOUSTICS

SECTION 4: BASIC PSYCHOACOUSTICS

Preface

This text provides resources to guide the student in all areas of hearing science: acoustics, instrumentation, anatomy and physiology and psychoacoustics. It also provides a brief introduction to speech acoustics. The text is intended for undergraduate courses in hearing science. The professor can select from among the introductory chapters as he or she feels appropriate. More advanced chapters are also available, and can be used to supplement doctoral courses in hearing science.

Our goal was to create a very readable text. We endeavored to explain concepts as simply as possible. Also, we believe in redundancy. Although many of the concepts covered in this book are well known to experienced audiologists, we know that does not mean that they are easily understood and remembered the first time they are presented. We intentionally review concepts from earlier introductory chapters as we present more complex ideas in the later chapters.

Although we think the hearing sciences are intrinsically interesting, we know that some students have a strong preference for those aspects that relate directly to patient care. We have included "Clinical Correlates," which show examples of how the hearing sciences relate directly to clinical applications, for those who can use some motivation to master the scientific underpinnings.

Some chapters are introductory, some are intermediary in depth, and a few are advanced. The later introductory chapters require only material from other introductory chapters, and similarly, one can read and understand intermediate chapters without having read any of the advanced chapters. The following is a breakdown of which chapters have which level of information.

ACOUSTICS AND INSTRUMENTATION

Introductory: Chapters 1, 2, 3, 4, 5

Intermediate: Chapters 6, 7

Advanced: Chapter 8

SPEECH ACOUSTICS

Intermediate: Chapters 9, 10

ANATOMY AND PHYSIOLOGY

Introductory: Chapters 11, 12, 13, 16, 18, 20

Intermediate: Chapters 14, 15, 19, 21, 23, 24, 25

Advanced: Chapters 17, 22

PSYCHOACOUSTICS AND SPEECH PERCEPTION

Introductory: Chapters 26

Intermediate: Chapters 27, 29, 31, 32, 35, 36, 37

Advanced: Chapters 28, 30, 33, 34, 38

Some chapters have "prerequisites" - understanding the material in that chapter requires that the reader be familiar with the material covered in earlier chapters. These are listed in the chart below.

Chapter No.	Prerequisite Chapters
1	None
2	None
3	1
4	1
5	1, 2, 3, 4
6	1
7	2, 4, 6
8	1, 2, 3, 6, 7
9	1, 2, 3, 4, 5
10	1, 2, 3, 4 ,5, 9
11	None
12	11
13	1, 2, 3, 4, 5, 11, 12
14	1, 3, 11, 12, 13
15	1, 4, 12, 13, 14
16	1, 3, 11, 12, 13
17	6, 16
18	16
19	18
20	11, 16, 18
21	20
22	1, 3, 4, 7, 16, 17, 18, 19, 20, 21
23	16, 20
24	16
25	12, 16, 20, 24
26	None
27	1, 11, 16, 18
28	26, 27
29	1, 2, 3, 11, 16, 18, 20, 26, 27
30	1, 2, 12, 13, 18, 29
31	1, 11, 16, 18, 29
32	1, 11, 16, 18, 21, 26
33	2, 23, 32
34	21, 32, 33
35	26, 29, 31
36	23, 26, 29, 32
37	1, 3, 29
38	1, 3, 9, 10, 12, 14, 16, 18, 20, 26, 29, 30, 31, 32, 33, 34, 35, 36, 37

Acknowledgments and Dedication

We are thankful for all the students who gave us feedback over the years this text has been in development, and we thank them for their encouragement to publish it. It is to you that we dedicate this book.

Our thanks also to Tom Barron of www.audstudent.com for his assistance in fact-checking issues related to digital signal processing and instrumentation.

The idea for the cover design belongs to Nicole and R. J. Ball and Lisa Diaz. Thank you! The cover art was created by Brian Phillips.

About the Authors

Lloyd L. Price, Ph.D., Professor Emeritus of Audiology, taught undergraduate and graduate student courses in the hearing sciences at Florida State University. When he began teaching an undergraduate hearing science course in 1983, there were no texts suitable at that level. In order to cover the material he deemed important, it was necessary to develop a text, which evolved over a 15-year period. Changes were made as the field advanced and based on student feedback and that from several doctoral students who took copies for use in similar courses when they became faculty members at other universities.

Teri A. Hamill, Ph.D., Professor of Audiology at Nova Southeastern University, teaches Au.D. students at Nova Southeastern University. Dr. Price had been her major professor in her doctoral studies. Her students, particularly those who were not audiology undergraduate majors, complained about having difficulty understanding their graduate texts. When provided with Dr Price's draft, they had the foundation to better understand the graduate texts. Over the next six years, Dr. Hamill added to the text so that it now introduces all of key topics in hearing science: acoustics, speech perception, analog and digital instrumentation, and anatomy and physiology of both the auditory and vestibular systems, as well as psychoacoustics.

Both Drs. Hamill and Price have backgrounds in both clinical audiology and academia. Dr Price worked as a professor for 31 years after having worked clinically for the previous nice years. Dr Hamill is in her 18th year as an academic, having also worked in a hospital setting. Dr. Hamill's knowledge of instrumentation was furthered by having worked with engineers: her post-doctorate in 1987 to 1988 was with Project Phoenix/ Nicolet, which produced a commercially unsuccessful fully digital hearing aid. Her knowledge of digital signal processing also comes from being married to a computer scientist.

Dr. Price is now retired, living in Havana Florida with his wife, Cindy, and their poodle, Katie. They travel, particularly to Europe, frequently. Dr. Hamill lives in Hollywood, Florida with her husband, Tom, and dingo, Dixi (who reliably raises her paw when she hears a tone). The three of them sail their 30-foot Cape Dory as often as work permits.

SECTION ONE

Basic Acoustics and Instrumentation

1

Physical Properties of Sound

Acoustics is the study of sound: what it is, how it is produced, how it travels from place to place, and the effect of objects in its path. A general understanding of some of the principles governing sound is essential for anyone who wishes to understand how we hear. Some concepts of physics are required in order to understand the nature of sound. These basic concepts are described before the material on properties of sound is introduced.

Appendix A of this text has a review of basic math. We hope that this will serve as a useful refresher or reference to help with the mathematical concepts.

ENERGY

Energy is the ability to do work, that is, the force required to move some mass some distance in some amount of time. It is common to express **mass** in kilograms, **distance** in meters, and **time** in seconds.

All matter is made up of particles (atoms, molecules, etc.) and particles have mass. It is the mass of the individual particle and the spacing of the particles (how close they are together) that determine the **density** of a given substance. Obviously, a cubic meter (a cube one meter tall, one meter

wide, and one meter deep) of iron has greater density than a cubic meter of air. Not only do particles of iron have more mass than particles of air, but also the particles of iron are much closer together. As matter has length, width, and height, particle density is three-dimensional and the concept of mass must include a statement of space. The scientific unit for mass, the kilogram, is abbreviated *kg*.

When we speak of **distance** (space), we may be concerned with one, two, or three dimensions. A straight line has one dimension (length) and is measured in meters (m). The line in Figure 1–1A, illustrates a line that is 10 m long. An area has two dimensions (length and width) and is measured in square meters (m²). The area of a surface is

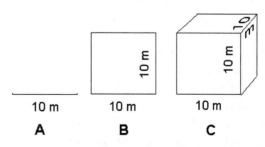

Figure 1–1. Illustrations of one dimension (length) (**A**), two dimensions (area) (**B**), and three dimensions (volume) (**C**).

found by multiplying its length by its width. The square in Figure 1–1B has an area of 100 m² (10 m × 10 m). A volume has three dimensions (length, width, and height) and is measured in cubic meters (m³). The volume is obtained by multiplying length times width times height. In Figure 1–1C, the volume of the cube is 1000 m³ (10 m × 10 m × 10 m).

The unit of **time** is the second, a measure so common as to require no further discussion. The time-related concept of velocity, however, needs some mention. **Velocity** is the rate of movement, that is, how far an object moves in a given amount of time, and in what direction. The average velocity is determined by dividing the distance moved by the time required for the movement. For example, if a mass is moved 100 meters in 5 seconds, its velocity is 100 divided by 5, or 20 meters per second, which is often written as 20 m/sec.

OPPOSING FORCES

If one wishes to move some mass through some distance at some velocity, there is another important group of variables to be considered. These are the opposing forces that limit the motion. Opposing forces take three different forms. First, **friction** or **resistance** is always a factor. When any object (or substance) moves across or through any other substance, friction is present. This friction, or rubbing together, tends to impede or oppose the movement of the object.

A second opposing force to be considered is **inertia**; the tendency for a mass at rest to remain at rest, and a mass in motion to remain in motion. The amount of inertia is related to the amount of mass. The greater the mass, the greater the inertia, and the more force required to change the velocity of the mass, whether the change is from rest to motion or motion to rest.

A third opposing force is related to another fundamental property of all substances, called **elasticity**. If one applies a force to an object it is likely that the object will be deformed to some degree. If the force is removed, the object returns to its original shape. Elasticity, then, can be thought of as springiness, though it is technically defined as the ability to resist changing shape. (Most people think of elasticity as how well an object recovers its shape, but in physics, that definition isn't quite correct.) A very good example of elasticity is a steel spring. The opposition one encounters in stretching the spring is determined by how stiff the spring is—the stiff spring is very elastic (it doesn't want to move, and when moved, as we know, it restores its original shape readily). **Stiffness** is thus related to elasticity. In acoustics, stiffness is often used as a measure of one of the resistive forces that opposes the setting into motion of an object. Elasticity is also the quality of a substance that permits that substance to be compressed (or more correctly, resists its compression). Thus, the compressibility of a substance (for example, air) is also an indication of its elasticity. Air is easy to compress; it's not very elastic and it is not stiff.

UNITS OF MEASUREMENT

Scientists use the meter (m) as the basic unit of measurement of length, and the kilogram (kg) or gram (g) as the primary units for mass. Time is measured in seconds (sec). These are the basic units. Another common unit is that for pressure, which is either called the newton or the dyne. The **newton** (N) is the unit of pressure created by a kilogram of weight divided by a meter of area multiplied by a second squared. Mathematically, that is: $N = kg/m \times sec^2$, or the force required to accelerate a kilogram of weight one meter per second per second. "Per second per second" (sec^2) to a physicist is a description of acceleration. If you haven't had physics, and this concept is foreign to you, you can still understand the basics. Take the palm of your left hand and put it on the fleshy part of your forearm. Press down. During that moment you are compressing your arm, you are applying a force (which we could measure in newtons) and you managed to compress your flesh in a certain distance, which we could measure as a fraction of a meter, and we could also see how fast you are pushing, and how that rate is changing over time (the seconds per second part.) You pressed a given area of your arm, so to be complete, we would also describe the surface area you pressed, in square meters (or in this case, a part of a square meter).

More on pressure of sound energy follows. Before continuing that discussion we need to review the units smaller and larger than a meter, a second, or a gram. As you know, you add a prefix to indicate how much smaller or larger than the basic unit the new unit is. For example, a kilogram is 1000 times larger than a gram, and a milligram is 1/1000 the size. The meanings of the prefixes are listed in Table 1-1. 10,000 is the same as 10^4. If you need a refresher on exponents, one is coming in Chapter 2.

Table 1–1. Common Scientific Units Used in Audiology

kilo—k	10^3	1000
deca—da	10^1	10
centi—c	10^{-2}	0.01
milli—m	10^{-3}	0.001
micro—μ	10^{-6}	0.000 001
nano—n	10^{-9}	0.000 000 001

The units commonly used in audiology and their abbreviations are listed below. Appendix A contains a more complete list.

SOUND ENERGY

Sound is a form of energy. As such, sound is subject to the concepts already discussed. Sound energy cannot exist outside a substance (**medium**) that has mass and stiffness. Although the medium for sound energy is most often air, sound can be generated and transmitted in or through any medium (e.g., sound can travel through water or steel), and the same principles apply. Thus, although this discussion is restricted mainly to sound in air, the discussion applies to all media.

Air, of course, is composed of gas molecules. Nitrogen and oxygen are the most common elements. As you probably remember from basic chemistry, each molecule has a positively charged center, which is orbited by negatively charged electrons. Air molecules will remain spaced out from one another because the negatively charged electron outer surfaces of one molecule repel the negatively charged outer surface of the next molecule, just as two negative poles of magnets repel. Air molecules are always in motion as they struggle to keep distant from each other. The movement is in a random, three-dimensional motion, sometimes called **Brownian motion**.

Air is said to have **pressure**, which is force per unit of area. For example, the meteorologist will speak of high-pressure or low-pressure zones of air. This force is the result of the speed of the random, Brownian movements of air particles (molecules), the mass of the individual molecule, and the number of molecules per unit of volume. As a general rule, the faster the random movement and the higher the density, the greater the force and the higher the pressure. As discussed further in Chapter 2, the magnitude of pressure is measured in pascals (Pa), which are newtons per square meter (N/m²), or in dynes per square centimeter (dynes/cm²). Most of the pre-1980 literature used the dynes/cm² notation whereas much of the more recent writing incorporates the N/m² or Pa notation. One can convert from one to the other since 1 Pa (1 N/m²) equals 10 dynes/cm².

We can now distinguish between the relatively static atmospheric air pressure, which only changes gradually with altitude and weather conditions, and air pressure changes of a much smaller and more rapid nature. It is these small, rapid changes or disturbances in the relatively static atmospheric pressure that we call sound pressure or sound energy. A useful, if not quite accurate, analogy is to compare atmospheric pressure to the water in a lake and the sound pressure to ripples on the lake. The difference between a sound wave and a ripple on water is that the sound wave has a three-dimensional wave front whereas the ripple has a two-dimensional wave front.

A disturbance or pressure change in any given medium is primarily the result of changes in density, that is, in the spacing of particles. Increasing the density means moving the particles closer together (compression) and decreasing the density means moving the particles farther apart (rarefaction). From our previous discussion, we know that the force needed to change density is determined by the mass and stiffness of the medium.

Sound energy in air is a series of compressions and rarefactions in the density of particles of air. A compression is, in fact, a positive pressure change and a rarefaction is a negative pressure change relative to the static atmospheric pressure. This is illustrated graphically in Figure 1–2.

COMPRESSION AND RAREFACTION

These changes in density (compressions and rarefactions shown in Figure 1–2)

are not restricted to a point in space; they travel. That is, when a force is applied to a volume of air particles, the resulting disturbance starts a chain reaction, which spreads in all directions from the point of beginning. Figure 1–3 illustrates this concept. Imagine a solid spot in the center of the figure as a rapidly expanding and contracting ball and the small specks surrounding it as particles of air. As the ball expands it compresses the particles adjacent to it, increasing density and pressure. As it contracts it creates a rarefaction, decreasing density and pressure. Although the two-dimensional figure does not show the third dimension (depth), these compressions and rarefactions travel in all directions from the point of origin.

Let's next think about how the sound energy decreases as it travels outward. There is a certain amount of energy present at the surface of the ball (as determined by the forces which expand and contract the ball) to be transmitted to the air. As the reaction moves away from the source, the available energy is being spread through an ever in-

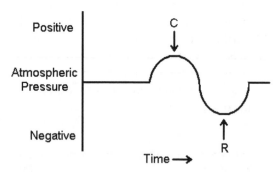

Figure 1–2. An illustration of how the compression (C) and rarefaction (R) of a sound wave is superimposed on atmospheric pressure. If the pressure rises, air molecules are more closely spaced together, a phase of the wave called compression. When the pressure lowers, and the molecules are more spread out, the molecules are rarefied. This figure illustrates a gradual increase then decrease in air pressure over time.

creasing space. The amount of sound energy (per square centimeter, for example) continuously decreases as the point of observation moves away from the source. In Figure 1-3 the amount of sound energy reaching point B is less than the energy reaching point A. The continuously decreasing amplitude of the compression-rarefaction wave (shown by the height of the wave on the right side of Figure 1-3) indicates this.

In order for sound waves to begin, a driving force (something that oscillates or vibrates) is necessary to create the compressions and rarefactions. There are two aspects of this driving force that are important in determining the physical characteristics of the sound wave. They are the rate of vibration (**frequency**) and the magnitude of vibration (**intensity**).

FREQUENCY

One of the more common vibrating sources of sound is the loudspeaker. As the cone of the speaker moves out and in, the air particles in front of the speaker cone are alternately compressed and rarefied. Thus, the frequency of vibration (how many times the cone moves in and out in one second) determines the frequency of the sound wave. Figure 1-4 illustrates this principle. When the cone of the speaker goes through one complete cycle (i.e., compression and back to the starting point followed by rarefaction and back to the starting point), a sound

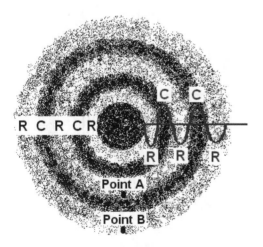

Figure 1-3. If the solid center of the figure were continually expanding and contracting, the expansion phases would compress the adjacent particles of air and the contraction phases would spread out the adjacent particles producing alternating compressions (C) and rarefactions (R) of the sound wave. As the energy spreads out as it travels from point A to point B, the pressure decreases, as shown by the gradually lowering amplitude of the pressure wave on the right side of the figure.

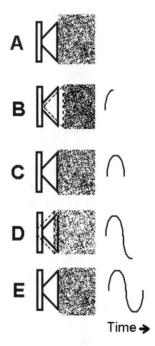

Time →

Figure 1-4. Illustration of how the in and out movement of the cone of a loudspeaker creates a sound wave (a change in the density of the adjacent air molecules). (**A**) The cone at rest; (**B**) the cone moves out producing a compression; (**C**) the cone moves back to rest; (**D**) the cone moves in producing a rarefaction; and (**E**) the cone moves back to rest. The wave to the far right shows the relative air molecule density changing over time.

wave is produced which has one complete cycle. The particles to the right of the speaker cone represent air molecules. The change in the density of the air molecules with the movement of the speaker cone is illustrated. The wave to the far right of the figure illustrates the progressive change in the density of the air molecules over time. The number of cycles that occur in one second (cycles per second or cps) is the frequency of the sound wave. The unit of measure for frequency is the **hertz** (Hz), which is the same as cps. That is, a sound that has 100 cps has a frequency of 100 Hz. The two terms, Hz and cps, can be used interchangeably. The higher the frequency, the higher the pitch of the sound.

Chapter 4 will further describe frequency and the relationship between frequency and the sine wave. The wave shown to the right in Figure 1–4 is a sine wave. (You can either read Chapter 4 next, or after reading Chapters 2 and 3.)

INTENSITY

The magnitudes of the vibration (how far the cone of the speaker in Figure 1–4 moves during its out and in motion) determine the degree to which the density of the air changes, which is related to the sound's loudness. If the cone moves minimally, the density change (sound pressure) is small; if the cone moves through a larger excursion, the density changes increase. The magnitude of the vibration, then, determines the intensity or energy of the sound. As shown in Figure 1–5, frequency and intensity are independent of each other. Note that the cone vibration frequency in Figure 1–5A and 1–5B are different, but the amplitude of vibration is the same, whereas in 1–5B and 1–5C the frequency of vibration is the same, and the amplitude is different.

Note that if one increases the magnitude of vibration without changing the frequen-

cy of vibration, the speaker moves a greater distance in the same amount of time. That means that the velocity (rate of movement) of the speaker cone increases. This, in turn, increases the velocity of the air particles being set into motion by the cone. Thus, the intensity or energy in the sound wave may also be expressed as particle velocity. In summary, a large cone displacement back and forth creates greater pressure change, and a louder sound. So, whereas the speed of vibration relates to pitch, the amplitude of vibration correlates to the sound intensity.

LIMITS OF HUMAN FREQUENCY DETECTION

The human ear is responsive to a wide range of frequencies. It detects and recognizes the sound as a tone from about 20 Hz

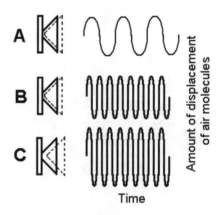

Figure 1–5. Illustrations of how sound frequency and intensity can be varied independently of each other. Waves (**A**) and (**B**) have the same intensity, but different frequencies. Waves (**B**) and (**C**) have the same frequency, but different intensities. The frequency of the wave is illustrated by the number of wave cycles through rarefaction and compression per unit of time. The wave height shows the relative size of the density changes created by the speaker vibration.

to 20,000 Hz. It is inconvenient to talk about (or display graphically) frequency on a linear scale. (In a linear scale, each increment is equal in size.) Therefore, we usually express frequency on an exponential (or logarithmic) scale—each equal distance on the scale represents a doubling of the frequency. Figure 1-6 illustrates this concept. Notice that the scales are equal in length but that a much larger range of frequencies can be displayed on the exponential scale. This exponential frequency scale where frequency is doubled with each given distance change is also called an **octave** scale. In other words, if we go up one octave, we have doubled the frequency; if we go down one octave, we have halved the frequency.

SUMMARY

This chapter has reviewed the basic physics units needed for study of acoustics: grams for mass, meters for distance, and seconds for

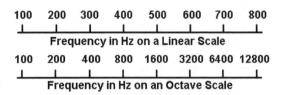

Figure 1–6. Frequency in hertz (Hz) plotted on a linear and on an octave scale (or as we will call it in Chapter 2, an exponential scale: base = 2).

time. We have reviewed the ways of describing units that are increased or decreased in tenfold increments. Sound has been described as a cycling change in atmospheric pressure—air molecules become more closely spaced during compression and less densely packed during rarefaction. The frequency of vibration is related to a sound's pitch, and is measured in Hz. Sound intensity relates to the amount of change in pressure which is created by a speaker cone moving a further distance in and out. Chapter 2 introduces the unit of measurement of intensity—the decibel.

2

Ratios, Logarithms, and Decibels

In this chapter you will learn how to calculate decibels, and learn when different types of decibels are used. If you have forgotten scientific notation, or some of your algebra rules, Appendix A provides a review.

The decibel (dB) is the unit used to express the intensity or pressure of sound. There are three things one must keep in mind when working with decibels. First, the decibel is not an absolute unit; it is a number that comes from taking the **ratio** of two numbers. Second, the decibel system is not linear, it is **exponential** or **logarithmic**. Increasing sound pressure 10 fold creates only a 2 dB increase. Increasing sound pressure 100 times creates a 20 dB increase. And finally, the reference for the logarithmic ratio (the number on the bottom of the ratio) differs depending on the application. This chapter aims to expand and explain these points.

RATIOS

The ratio is an expression of the relationship of one number to another number. It tells us nothing about the actual size of either number. It the value of neither number is known, the ratio tells us only that X is some value of Y. If the value of either X or Y is known (and the ratio is known), then the value of the other can be determined using simple algebra.

The ratio of X to Y is written X:Y or X/Y. (Recall that the numerator is the number on top in a division equation; the denominator is on the bottom.) When the ratios are written in numbers, that is, 20:1, they tell us how many times larger (or smaller) one number is than the other. Any two numbers, where the first is 20 times as large as the second, have a 20/1 ratio. (For example, 20 to 1 and 40 to 2 both have a 20:1 ratio.)

In Chapter 13, we will examine the ratio of the size of the eardrum (tympanic membrane) and the part of the third bone (the stapes, or stirrup) in the middle ear that fits into a "window" into the inner ear. This part of the stapes is called the "footplate." If the area of the eardrum were 64 square millimeters (mm^2) and the area of the footplate of the stapes were 3.2 mm^2; the ratio of the eardrum to the stapes footplate is 64:3.2. Reduced to its lowest common denominator, the ratio is 20:1. Conversely, the area ratio of the footplate of the stapes to the eardrum is 1:20.

EXPONENTS

Positive Exponents

A^n represents a situation where the number represented by A must be multiplied by itself n times. In A^n, A is called the base and n the exponent. We read A^n as "A to the nth power." A^2 is read "A squared," A^3 is read "A cubed," A^4 is "A to the fourth power," and so forth. Examples:

$$Z^3 = Z \text{ times } Z \text{ times } Z$$
$$2^5 = 2 \times 2 \times 2 \times 2 \times 2 = 32$$
$$-5^2 = -5 \times -5 = 25$$
$$-3^3 = -3 \times -3 \times -3 = -27$$

Negative Exponents

A^{-n} is the reciprocal of A^n. Thus, A^{-n} is equal to one over A^n, that is, $1/A^n$. Examples:

$$2^{-4} = 1/2^4 = \tfrac{1}{2} \times \tfrac{1}{2} \times \tfrac{1}{2} \times \tfrac{1}{2} = 1/16$$
$$10^{-2} = 1/10^2 = 1/10 \times 1/10 = 1/100$$

Zero Exponent

Any number (except zero) to the zero power equals one. The only exception is 0^0—there is no such number. If you enter it into your calculator it will read "error." Examples:

$$10^0 = 1$$
$$(-3)^0 = 1$$
$$(a^x)^0 = 1 \text{ (if } a^x \text{ does not equal zero)}$$

LAWS OF EXPONENTS

The following laws must be followed when working with exponents.

Addition

In order to add numbers written as exponents one must first convert to the numbers that the exponents represent. These numbers are then added.

Example: $5^2 + 5^2 = 25 + 25 = 50$

Subtraction

As with addition, in order to subtract numbers written as exponents one must first convert to the numbers that the exponents represent. These numbers are then subtracted. Example:

$$4^4 - 4^2 = 256 - 16 = 240$$

Multiplication, Division, and Exponent of Exponents

These more advanced mathematical concepts are used less often in audiology. These topics are covered in Appendix A, should you wish to review those rules.

SCIENTIFIC NOTATION

When you have very large and very small numbers, for example, ones that you can't type into the calculator, like .00000000000234, or 234,000,000,000,000, you need a convenient way of describing the number (Table 2–1). We can talk about the "**digit term**" or "**significant digits**," the 234 part, and how much bigger or less than zero the number is using scientific notation. The "digit term," 234 in this example, is actually properly written as 2.34. The digit term is one number followed by the decimal, and then the rest of the significant digits (the 34 part in this example.) The **exponent** tells you how much larger or smaller the digit term is than 1. The next step is to count the difference in the decimal places from the number in its original form to the number expressed in this format, where only one number is in front of the decimal. If the original number is smaller than 1, then

Table 2–1. Examples of Numbers Expressed in Scientific Notation

$1,320,000 = 1.32 \times 10^6$
$132,000 = 1.32 \times 10^5$
$13,200 = 1.32 \times 10^4$
$1,320 = 1.32 \times 10^3$
$132 = 1.32 \times 10^2$
$13.2 = 1.32 \times 10^1$
$1.32 = 1.32 \times 10^0$
$0.132 = 1.32 \times 10^{-1}$
$0.0132 = 1.32 \times 10^{-2}$
$0.00132 = 1.32 \times 10^{-3}$
$0.000132 = 1.32 \times 10^{-4}$
$0.0000132 = 1.32 \times 10^{-5}$
$0.00000132 = 1.32 \times 10^{-6}$

the exponent will be negative. The exponent is a positive number if it is larger than 1.0. The exponent is written as the number 10 "raised to a given power."

Returning to the original examples, as we compare .00000000000234 to 2.34, we see that the decimal point is shifted by 12 places, and the number is smaller than 1, so the exponent will be –12. You multiply 2.34 by 10^{-12} to return to .00000000000234. That is:

$$.00000000000234 = 2.34 \times .000000000001$$
$$= 2.34 \times 10^{-12}$$

Another way to think about this is that you would count how many places you have to move the decimal point to get it to be after the 2. As it was 12 places over, that is the same as .000 000 000 001. So, all you need to do when you are faced with a decimal number is count out how many places to the right you need to move the decimal to make sure that the first "significant" (non-zero) digit has the decimal right after it.

And when faced with large numbers, count the other way. See what you need to do to get the decimal after that first significant digit. For example, $234,000,000,000,000 = 2.34 \times 100,000,000,000,000 = 2.34 \times 10^{14}$

Let's explore exponents a bit further. Examine different values of 10^x. Take 1 and add the number of digits noted by the x. For example,

$10^0 = 1.$ Take 1, and don't add any 0's
$10^1 = 10.$ Take 1 and add 1 zero.
$10^2 = 100.$ You get the picture!

When the number in the exponent is negative, it means you need to make the 1 have that many decimal places in front of it.

$$10^{-1} = 0.1$$

You can think of this as how many places over you move the decimal. If you look at the original number (e.g., 0.1) and need to move the decimal to the right to make it 1.0, then you have a negative exponent.

$$10^{-1} = 0.1$$
$$10^{-2} = 0.01$$
$$10^{-5} = 0.00001$$

As you see, in the case of 0.00001, you move the decimal point 5 places to the right to put the decimal at the 1.0 position, so the exponent is 10^{-5}.

Most of us use calculators. To enter numbers in exponents into the calculator, you would type in the digit term, then "exp" (or "ee") and the exponent, either positive or negative. For example, to enter 2.34×10^{14}, type in 2.34 exp 14. Again, some calculators say "ee" instead of "exp."

Try it—for example 5 exp –2 = , and it will show you 0.05 as the answer on some calculators, and 5^{-02} on others. On some calculators you can shift the way it displays the answer by going between scientific and "floating point" notations. That is often a "2nd function" button, for instance on my calculator, I press "2nd" then "SCI" to get it to use the exponential notation, then "2nd" then "FLO" to go back to decimals (floating point numbers).

How would you write the following number in scientific notation?

$$\frac{5}{100,000,000}$$

That is $5/10^8$ and is the same as 5×10^{-8}. You switch the sign when you go from the denominator to the numerator, or the other way around. So, $5/10^{-8}$ is the same as 5×10^8

Adding and Subtracting Numbers in Scientific Notation

If the exponent is the same, life is easy! Just add the part that is getting multiplied by the $10^{exponent}$. Example:

$$.005 + .002 = .007$$
$$\text{and } 5.0 \times 10^{-3} + 2.0 \times 10^{-3} = 7 \times 10^{-3}$$

When the exponents are not the same, for example, $6.0 \times 10^{-3} + 3.0 \times 10^{-4}$, you first have to make them the same exponent, and then you can do the simple addition. In this example, let's make both of the numbers multiply by 10^{-3}. 10^{-4} is smaller than 10^{-3}. When we make 3.0×10^{-4} into a "something times 10^{-3}" we have to shift the decimal on the digit term portion to the left. Therefore 0.3×10^{-3} is the same as 3×10^{-4}. In this example:

$$6.0 \times 10^{-3} + 3.0 \times 10^{-4} =$$
$$6.0 \times 10^{-3} + 0.30 \times 10^{-3} =$$
$$6.3 \times 10^{-3}$$

Subtracting is not much different;

$$5.0 \times 10^{-3} - 2.0 \times 10^{-4} =$$
$$5.0 \times 10^{-3} - .20 \times 10^{-3} =$$
$$4.8 \times 10^{-3}$$

LOGARITHMS ARE BASED ON EXPONENTS

Logarithms of Numbers with Only 1 and 0

If you understand exponents, you'll do fine with logarithms, also called logs. And after you understand the basics, you most likely will be using your calculator.

There are actually two types of logs, natural logs and base 10 logs. We are only going to talk about base 10 logs, which is the "LOG" button on your calculator, so you can ignore the button marked "LN." On your calculator put in the number 1,000 and press the log button. What does it say? (It should say 3, or you need a new calculator.) And if you put in 1000 and hit 2nd SCI to view the number in scientific notation, it would say 10^3, right?

When you are doing a logarithm, you are asking X = "1 × 10 raised to what exponent?"

Let's review:

$10^0 = 1.$ Don't add any 0's.
$10^1 = 10.$ Take 1 and add 1 zero.
$10^2 = 100.$ Take 1, add 2 zeros, and so on.
$10^6 = 1\ 000\ 000$
$10^{-2} = .01$

In finding the log of 1, you are asking "X = 1 × 10 raised to what number?" Get out your calculator and prove to yourself that, in this example, the answer is zero. Type in 1, then log. Do a couple more examples. What is the log of 10 (typically written log10 when you see it in print)? Input this as 10, and then press log on your calculator. Just to solidify the idea, find the log of 100, as well as 1,000,000, and 0.01.

Logarithms of Numbers Other Than 1 and 0

What if you want to know what the log of the number 7 is? (Said another way, 10, raised to what number (multiplied by $1 \times 10^{what\ exponent}$), equals 7?) Well, there are tables for that sort of thing, but the easiest way is to use your calculator. When you try it, you get the answer .845. As 7 is lower than 10, and higher than 1, it makes sense that the answer would be less than 1, but greater than 0.

The logarithm is composed of two parts —the characteristic and the mantissa (Table 2-2). The **characteristic** tells you the general size of the number and is based on the exponent. In the example above, where the log of 7 is 0.845, the characteristic is 0 and the **mantissa** is .845. Although you can easily figure out the characteristic, you need a log table or a calculator to figure out the mantissa.

Why Are Logs Important?

You need an understanding of logs in order to understand decibels. Sound pressures (or powers) can range from very small numbers to very large numbers. A very soft sound has a pressure of 20 μPa, and a very loud sound might be 20,000,000 μPa, which is a million times bigger. It is very difficult to work with numbers that have such a large range. Yet the log of 1,000,000 is 6—a much more manageable number. By turning these sound pressure values into logarithmic/exponential types of numbers, we get this manageable range of numbers.

Another reason for using logarithms is that the ear responds logarithmically. Changing the pressure 10 fold creates about the same intensity increase (approximately four times louder) across the whole range—from very low pressures to very high pressures. If we didn't use logs, then the units wouldn't make sense. We would not want to explain to a parent that at one frequency, hearing changed by 0.5 dynes and that's a lot, but at this other frequency, where the hearing was worse to begin with, it changed by 20 dynes and that isn't significant at all. By dealing with logs and decibels, life makes more sense. However, the tradeoff is that you need to have some understanding of logarithms and antilogs.

Antilogs

When you have a number, and want to know "that was the log of what?" do an antilog. So, if the log of 7 = .845, then the antilog of .845 is 7. Find this on your calculator as "2nd function key" then "log," and it might not surprise you that this is the button marked 10^x.

The Log of X Times Y

If you have to do a log of two numbers that are multiplied by each other, you are actually adding two logarithms. For example:

Table 2–2. A Series of Numbers Showing How the Decimal Point Determines the Characteristic, or First Number, of the Logarithm

log 0.0003 = –4.4771
log 0.003 = –3.4771
log 0.03 = –2.4771
log 0.3 = –1.4771
log 3 = 0.4771
log 30 = 1.4771
log 300 = 2.4771
log 3000 = 3.4771
log 30,000 = 4.4771

Log (5.45 × 1,000,000) is the same as Log 5.45 + Log 1,000,000.

To add logs, you solve each part, and then add. So here, log 5.45 = 0.736, and of course, the log of 1,000,000 is 6, so the answer is 6.736. On a calculator, you could choose to enter 5.45 exp (or ee) 6 = , then press log, or 5,450,000 then press log.

Log of (X Divided by Y)

The laws of math are such that when you take the log of two numbers, one divided by the other, you subtract, so

$$Log (4/8) = \log 4 - \log 8 = .602 - .903 = -.301$$

Of course 4/8 = ½, so it won't surprise you that the log of .5 is also -.301.

Hints on Using the Calculator

The complete number you wish to take the log of must be entered into the calculator before hitting "log." If you were entering log 1/2, you should type in 1/2 =, then press log, then = again. If you type in 1/2 log = you are asking for 1/(log2). With your typical scientific calculator, logs, antilogs, and raising values to an exponent will come "first" in order of operation on your calculator, before multiplication and division.

Recently "algebraic" calculators have entered the market. They have a different way to input the information. If you have purchased one of these calculators, you will need to read the instruction manual to figure out how that form of logic works.

Did you know your Windows operating system has a scientific calculator?

This can be accessed through this menu sequence: Start—Programs—Accessories— Calculator—View—Scientific. If you have the shortcut to the calculator function on your keyboard, then you only need change the "View" to "Scientific."

Obtaining the Log of a Number That Is Raised to a Power

There are many times you will want to know the log of a number that is already expressed as a power. Typically, that power will be 2—a squared number. For example, what is the log of 3^2? That is the same as the exponent times the log of the original number. That is, $\log 3^2 = 2 \times \log 3$.

Try it and see—if you had first done the 3 × 3 to obtain 9, and taken log 9 you would get .954. If you take log 3 you get .477, and multiply that by 2 and you are right back to .954.

This is going to be important, because sound pressure measurements units are always going to be pressure per square area. This is easily handled.

THE DECIBEL

Sound power is the energy transferred, or "work" done, over time. If we are describing a sound's power, the unit is the watt per meter squared. We could describe the same sound in terms of how much pressure that sound exerts, in which case the unit is most often the pascal or newton per square meter. As described above, it's not very convenient to work in the absolute power or pressure units, because there is such a very large range between the smallest power/pressure that creates an audible sound and the largest tolerable sound. We get around this problem by describing the sound in decibels, which is the logarithm of the ratio of the power or pressure measured, divided by a reference power or pressure.

Power

A common reference point for sound power measures is 10^{-12} w/m² (0.000000000001 watts per square meter). Thus, the **intensity level (IL)** of any acoustic stimulus is measured from this starting point. This 10^{-12} w/m² is roughly equivalent to the weakest sound that the human ear can detect. The strongest acoustic power that the human ear can tolerate without discomfort is about 1 w/m², which is 1,000,000,000,000 times greater than 10^{-12} w/m², a very large range of intensity.

Expressing this number in decibels makes it easy to handle such a large range. The first step taken to simplify this tremendously cumbersome range is to express intensity as a ratio on an exponential scale. Let's take the example of the number 1 w/m². The ratio of (1 w/m² / 10^{-12} w/m²) in exponents is 10^{12}. If we now understand (a) that our power units are expressed as a ratio (not an absolute value), and (b) that this ratio is exponential (not linear), we can state that our range of hearing is from 0 to 12 units. Scientists who developed this scale called these units **bels** in honor of Alexander Graham Bell. Thus, the ear can handle a power range of 0 to 12 **bels**. However, one must keep in mind that 0 bels does not represent the absence of sound. It represents a 1:1 ratio, that is, the situation where the comparison power equals the reference power; in this case 10^{-12} w/m². (The number of bels = log $10^{-12}/10^{-12}$ = log 1 = 0. This also means that 10^{-12} w/m² is 0 bels different from 10^{-12} w/m².)

The bel proved to be too large a unit to work with (a change of 1 bel changes a sound intensity ten fold), and it was decided to divide each bel into 10 subunits. Thus the **decibel** (or 1/10 bel) was created. The decibel (dB) range of the ear is then 10 × (0 to 12) or 0 to 120. Table 2–3 shows the range of energy that the ear can respond to on a linear scale, the bel scale, and the decibel scale.

Because we do not usually work with the bel, we must modify the formula for use with the decibels. As each bel represents 10 decibels, all that is required is that we multiply the bel formula by 10:

$$\text{dB intensity level} = 10 \log I_1/I_2$$

When the term **intensity level** (IL) is used, I_1 is the intensity measured and I_2 is always 10^{-12} w/m². Thus, the IL of a sound is 10 times the logarithmic ratio of the power of that sound to 10^{-12} w/m².

Doubling Power

There is one particular decibel calculation that merits note. When you have one sound generating source, and then turn on a second source, you have doubled the

Table 2–3. Power Expressed in Linear, Bel, and Decibel Scale

Linear Ratio	Bel	Decibel
1:1	0	0
10:1	1	10
100:1	2	20
1000:1	3	30
10,000:1	4	40
100,000:1	5	50
1,000,000:1	6	60
10,000,000:1	7	70
100,000,000:1	8	80
1,000,000,000:1	9	90
10,000,000,000:1	10	100
100,000,000,000:1	11	110
1,000,000,000,000:1	12	120

power of the sound source. **Doubling power** creates a 3 dB increase in the sound intensity. Why? You now have twice as much power, a ratio of 2:1; 10 log 2/1 is equal to 3 dB.

Pressure

Although power is often used to describe amplifier output, energy transmission, and so on, acoustic measures are generally made in units of pressure rather than power. We measure the amount of sound pressure the sound exerts, for example, on the surface of a microphone.

Pressure and power are related; the conversion from power to pressure is not difficult. We need only two facts: (a) the square of the pressure ratio of two sounds is proportional to the power ratio of the same two sounds, and (b) the pressure which is equivalent to 10^{-12} w/m^2 of power is 20 micropascals (μPa) or 0.0002 dynes per square centimeter (d/cm^2). The older unit of measure, the **dyne per square centimeter** (d/cm^2) has been replaced by **pascals** (Pa) or **newtons per square meter** (N/m^2) as the preferred unit for sound pressure (1 N/m^2) = 1 Pa. However, as 20 μN/m^2 equals 20 μPa, which equals 0.0002 d/cm^2, any one of the three can be used as the reference for **sound pressure level** (SPL). In this text, we use the pascal notation.

Let's return to the first point. The square of the pressure ratio is proportional to the power ratio: $10 \log I_1/I_2 = 10 \log (P_1/P_2)^2$. Thus, the decibel formula for a power ratio can be converted to a decibel formula for the equivalent pressure ratio by squaring the logarithm of the pressure ratio. This is accomplished as follows:

Power: dB IL = $10 \log I_1/I_2$, and

Pressure: dB SPL = $10 \log (P_1/P_2)^2$, and as a logarithm is an exponent, we square it by multiplying by 2, and

dB SPL = $2 \times 10 \log P_1/P_2$, or
dB SPL = $20 \log P_1/P_2$

Note that P1/P2 represents the pressure ratio, not the power ratio.

Just as **intensity level** (IL) has a specific meaning in power measures; **sound pressure level** (SPL) has a specific meaning in pressure measures. The SPL of a sound in decibels is 20 times the logarithmic ratio of the pressure in that sound to 20 μPa, that is, dB SPL = $20 \log P_1/P_2$, when $P_2 = 20$ μPa.

The power formula and pressure formulas are equivalent. Thus, pressure and power decibels are equivalent: 0 dB IL = 0 dB SPL, 50 dB IL = 50 dB SPL, 80 dB IL = 80 dB SPL, and so forth.

Doubling Power Does Not Double Pressure

A common source of confusion results from the fact that if one doubles the power ratio, the increase is 3 dB (dB = 10 log 2/1 = 10 log 2 = 10 × 0.3010 = 3 dB). Remember, the **square** of the pressure ratio is equivalent to the power ratio. Therefore, doubling the power ratio is not equivalent to doubling the pressure ratio. If you doubled pressure (20 log 2/1) you would get a 6 dB increase. Many students conclude falsely from this that 3 dB of power equals 6 dB of pressure. *This is not so!* When you double power, you have increased the pressure by 1.414 times (the square root of 2); 20 log 1.414 = 3 dB.

Doubling the Distance from the Source

Whereas doubling the power, by turning on two sound sources, creates a 3 dB increase in either power or pressure, a different relationship exists when we double the distance from the sound source. For example, if we measure the pressure of a sound at

2 feet from the source, then measure again at 4 feet from the source, then we have doubled the distance from the sound source. Sound radiates out like the surface of a ball —the farther out you go, the surface area expands. With each doubling of distance from the sound source, the area that encompasses the same amount of radiation of the pressure wave becomes four times as large (Figure 2-1). As you have the same power, now divided into a four times larger area, the power per one area is one-quarter the original. Using the dB IL formula, you can see that 10 log 1/4 = 6 dB. That is, you have lost 6 dB of intensity with each **doubling of distance**. This is called the **inverse square law,** which states that the loss of sound intensity is equal to the inverse of square of the distance from the original measurement. So, if you went out 4 times the original distance from the sound source, you have 4 squared, or one 16th of the original power in each unit of area. You can put this into the power formula: 10 log 1/16 = -12 to see that the power is down 12 dB from the original. An easier method is to use the pressure

formula and just use the distance as the ratio. Use the formula:

dB SPL change = 20 log original distance of measurement/new distance of measurement

Doubling the distance gives you 20 log 1/2 (which equals -6 dB); increasing the distance from one to four feet is 20 log 1/4 (-12 dB).

Practice at Calculating Sound Pressure Levels

How loud is a sound that creates a pressure of 616 µPa? Remember that the pressure formula is dB SPL = 20 log P_1/P_2 where the reference pressure (P_2) is 20 µN/m². We take the measured pressure, 616 µPa, and make that P_1.

$$dB \ SPL = 20 \log 616 \ \mu Pa/ 20 \ \mu Pa$$
$$= 20 \log 30.8$$
$$= 20 \times 1.488$$
$$= 29.76$$

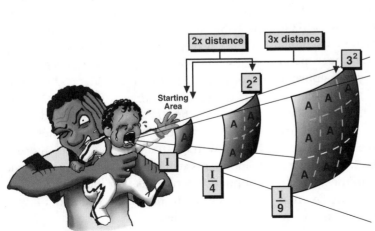

Figure 2–1. As you double the distance from the sound source from the initial (I) measurement area, the area of measurement for the same angle of sound increases fourfold. The intensity per unit area is one-fourth as great. Tripling the distance causes a nine times greater area, and the sound intensity per unit of area is now one-ninth of the original value. Reprinted with permission from *Speech and Voice Science,* by A. Behrman, p. 39. Copyright 2007 Plural Publishing, Inc.

Practice at Calculating Intensity Levels

The process of calculating the intensity level is similar, but the formula is dB IL = 10 log I_1/I_2 and I_2 is 10^{-12} watts/m². As our example, let's assume that a source is producing 100 watts/m².

dB IL = 10 log 100 watts/m² / 1 × 10^{-12}
watts/m²
= 10 log 1 × 10^{14}
= 10 × 14
= 140

Please note that just because your stereo receiver may be rated as 100 watts "per channel" (per speaker) does not mean it is necessarily going to produce 100 watts at the output. As you probably have stereos of at least 100 watts, a bit more thought helps here lest you believe you can crank your stereo up to a full 140 dB SPL. The first issue is that the stereo internally has a certain wattage, but the unit for the decibel is watts per meter². Intuitively, you probably can understand that sending a given power to a small speaker (such as for an iPod) creates a louder sound in the ear than you would hear if you send that same power to a stereo speaker, which is located a meter away. The first issue is the size of the cone (vibrating part) of the speaker. You would need to consider the surface area of each speaker in converting to watts/m². In the above example, the speaker area would have to be 1 meter squared for this to be even a gross approximation of the level.

If you have speakers that could produce 140 dB SPL (remember, SPL and IL are the same), that would be the amount produced right at the speaker. Let's assume that amount exists 1 cm away from the speaker. Remember from the inverse square law that the sound measured will decrease as you in-

crease distance from the speaker. If you are 1 meter away (100 cm—about 4 feet), a factor of 100 times the distance from the measurement at 1 cm, the intensity will be decreased by a factor equal to the square of that—10,000. Put that into your 10 log formula (remember, power is lost with distance as the pressure wave spreads out) and you see that you are down 40 dB already. The iPod speaker is closer to the eardrum, perhaps about 2 cm away, so that creates less loss from distance. Having ventured down this road, there is a danger that the reader might think that sounds will be inherently louder and more damaging through an ear level speaker. The listener in any situation is adjusting to a desired loudness level at the eardrum, so the distance from eardrum to speaker affects how loud the sound is at the speaker—the listener can adjust either speaker system to be equally loud. Additionally, the personally worn earphone is powered by a lower wattage amplifier.

There is another problem with assuming that the 100-watt per channel stereo with a 1-meter surface area can produce 140 dB SPL. That assumes that you have speakers that are perfectly efficient, and do not create any power loss. Even if that were the case, the speaker itself may not permit a 140 dB SPL output. If the speaker were capable of producing 100 watts of output at the speaker without "blowing out" the internal speaker cone, the speaker itself would probably not accurately produce that level. The waveform would probably have its peaks "chopped off," which is called **peak clipping**. The sound would be distorted, and limited in loudness. Figure 2–2 illustrates peak clipping. That doesn't mean that there is no value to having an amplifier with higher wattage than needed. The internal components will not create this sort of peak clipping distortion as you increase the level, which might happen if you had a lower wattage amplifier.

A.

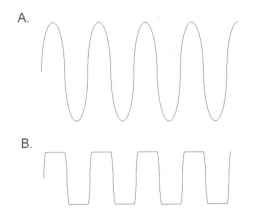

B.

Figure 2–2. A. The original sine wave. **B.** A peak clipped sine wave.

Relative Powers and Pressures

It should be re-emphasized that the decibel is an expression of the logarithm of a ratio. Like other ratios, the decibel has no absolute value. For example, if the power or pressure of a stimulus is increased by 20 dB, this only tells us something about the relationship between the present stimulus level and the previous stimulus level. It does not tell us anything about the absolute power or pressure of either stimulus, or the actual amount of increase in power or pressure. The decibel is a statement of relativity, that is, the value of **A** relative to **B**. Thus, it can be used for discussing **relative** powers neither of which are 10^{-12} w/m^2. For example, 10 watts is approximately 7 dB greater than 2 watts. This is determined as follows:

$$dB = 10 \log I_1/I_2 = 10 \log 10/2 = 10 \log 5$$
$$= 10 \times 0.6990$$
$$= 6.99 \text{ dB}$$

As I_2 is not 10^{-12} w/m^2, our 7 dB difference is not 7 dB IL. Ten watts is 7 dB greater than (relative to) 2 watts. Note that this is "greater than"—not dB IL. (10 watts/m^2 is 130 dB IL; prove it to yourself.)

The decibel is also used for **relative** pressure measures. Thus, it is useful in describing relationships other than SPL. For example, we can ask the question, "How many dB is pressure **A** more than (or less than) pressure **B**?" This question is, of course, unanswerable unless we know the values of **A** and **B**. However, if we know that pressure **A** is 1200 μPa and pressure **B** is 300 μPa, then:

$$dB = 20 \log A/B = 20 \log 1200/300$$
$$= 20 \log 4$$
$$= 20 \times 0.602 = 12.04 \text{ dB.}$$

That is, 1200 μPa is 12 dB relative to 300 μPa or, 300 μPa is –12 dB relative to 1200 μPa. Again, neither the +12 nor the -12 are SPL. In order to determine SPL, the reference pressure would have to be 20 μPa. For example, the SPL of pressure **A** is:

$$dB \ SPL = 20 \log 1200/20 = 20 \log 60$$
$$= 20 \times 1.7782 = 35.56 \text{ dB.}$$

The SPL of pressure **B** is:

$$dB \ SPL = 20 \log 300/20 = 20 \log 15$$
$$= 20 \log \times 1.1761 = 23.52 \text{ dB.}$$

The difference between pressure **A** and pressure **B** is:

$$35.56 \text{ dB SPL} - 23.52 \text{ dB SPL} = 12.04 \text{ dB.}$$

Adding Decibels

Sometimes you may want to know how much sound is produced when two sound generators are operating at the same time. To determine this, you need to add the power of the two sources, and determine how loud the combined power is. Note that you add powers—not pressures.

If you know the power output of each source, the calculations are easy. For example, if one source produced .02 watts and the other produced .05 watts, the two together (assume they are located right next to each other) are producing .07 watts. To put that into decibels, you use the 10 log formula.

$$dB\ IL = 10 \log .07\ watts/m^2/ 1 \times 10^{-12}\ watts/m^2$$
$$= 10 \log 7*10^{10}\ watts/m^2$$
$$= 10 * 10.84$$
$$= 108.4\ dB$$

Often you are not told the wattage, but perhaps know the sound pressure level of the two sources, measured at the same location, when each single source is on independently. In that case, the first step is a straightforward one. By definition, the SPL level and IL levels are the same, so note each source in dB IL. The next step is to find out what the intensity level (in watts/m²) is for each of the two sounds. For example, one sound source is 80 dB SPL, and therefore 80 dB IL. The other source is 90 dB SPL (and 90 dB IL). The 80 dB IL sound is produced by a power equal to "b" watts/m².

$$80\ dB\ IL = 10 \log b\ watts/m^2/ 1 \times 10^{-12}\ watts/m^2$$
$$8\ dB\ IL = 1 \log b\ watts/m^2/ 1 \times 10^{-12}\ watts/m^2$$
$$Antilog\ 8\ dB\ IL = \log b\ watts/m^2/ 1 \times 10^{-12}\ watts/m^2$$
$$10^8 = b\ watts/m^2/ 10^{-12}\ watts/m^2$$

Multiply each side of the equation by 10^{-12} watts/m² to get

$$10^{-4} = b\ watts/m^2$$

Now find the intensity "c" of the 90 dB IL sound source.

$$90\ dB\ IL = 10 \log c\ watts/m^2/ 1 \times 10^{-12}\ watts/m^2$$
$$9\ dB\ IL = 1 \log c\ watts/m^2/ 1 \times 10^{-12}\ watts/m^2$$

$$Antilog\ 9\ dB\ IL = \log c\ watts/m^2/ 1 \times 10^{-12}\ watts/m^2$$
$$10^9 = c\ watts/m^2/ 10^{-12}\ watts/m^2$$

Multiply each side of the equation by 10^{-12} watts/m² to get

$$10^{-3} = c\ watts/m^2$$

Add the two wattages together. (Hint: On your calculator, you will probably enter that as 1 exp –3, which may be entered as 1 exp 3 then use the change sign key. Then add in 1 exp –4. Alternatively, use your knowledge of scientific notation to deduce that in decimal form, that is .001 and .0001, which adds to .0011)

The final step is to convert to dB IL and therefore back to dB SPL.

$$dB\ IL = 10 \log .0011/1 \times 10^{-12}$$
$$dB\ IL = 10 \log 1.1 \times 10^9$$
$$dB\ IL = 90.4$$
$$= 90.4\ dB\ SPL$$

SUMMARY

There is a very large range of either sound power or sound pressures between audible and painfully loud. The decibel scale was created to transform these large ranges of numbers into a more manageable scale.

When calculating decibels sound pressure level, we measure the pressure, and compare it to a reference pressure—20 µPa. We take the ratio of the two, and then take the logarithm of that number. When multiplied by 20, we have the sound pressure in dB SPL.

Turning on a second, equally powerful sound source doubles the power. But as power increase is equal to the square of the pressure increase, the pressure has increased not by a factor of two, but by the square root of two—1.414. Both the power and the pressure increase 3 dB.

The inverse square law tells us that to calculate the drop in sound pressure level as you increase the distance from the first measurement point, you take the ratio of the new measurement distance divided by the old measurement difference, take the log of that ratio, and multiply by 20. That is: dB SPL change = 20 log original distance of measurement/new distance of measurement.

Knowledge of what logarithms are, and what scientific notation means, helps to de-mystify decibel calculations. Remembering the underlying concepts will help the student in more advanced courses in instrumentation and in psychoacoustics.

REFERENCE

Behrman, A. (2007). *Speech and voice sciences.* San Diego, CA: Plural Publishing.

3

FURTHER EXAMINATION
OF PROPERTIES OF SOUND

Chapter 1 covered the basic principles of how vibrations are characterized in terms of frequency and intensity. Chapter 2 discussed how decibels are calculated. This chapter details some of the other ways to describe the characteristics of sound, beginning with a discussion of how quickly sound travels. The different types of decibels are described, with a review of dB IL and dB SPL and the introduction of two other types of decibels used in hearing testing: dB HL and dB SL.

SPEED OF SOUND TRANSMISSION

Chapter 1 mentioned "particle velocity"—how rapidly molecules move in meters per second. **Velocity** refers not just to how fast the molecules move (their speed), but also the direction of movement of the molecules. **Speed** is a simpler and more common concept that does not specify direction of sound travel.

How fast sound travels is the next topic of discussion. Stated more formally, how rapidly does a sound wave disturbance go through a medium from point A to point B? Velocity and **speed of sound travel** are both affected by the medium the sound

must travel through (e.g., air or solids). The density and the elasticity of the medium affect speed of sound; therefore, it will be different for different media. Table 3–1 gives some examples. Note that in air the speed of sound is about 343 meters per second (1126 ft/sec, which we round to 1100 ft/sec). The exact speed in air will vary somewhat due to temperature, altitude, and humidity conditions. However, the speed of sound travel is not affected by the frequency or intensity of the sound. All sounds travel through air at the same 343 meters/sec.

Speed of sound (s) is proportional to the square root of the elasticity (E) of the medium divided by the density (ρ). The formula written out is:

$$s = \sqrt{\frac{E}{\rho}}$$

Table 3–1. Approximate Speed of Sound in a Number of Different Media

Air	343 meters/sec	1,126 ft/sec
Water	1500 meters/sec	4,921 ft/sec
Rubber	1600 meters/sec	5,250 ft/sec
Steel	5800 meters/sec	19,000 ft/sec

As mentioned in Chapter 1, elasticity is the ability of a medium to resist being deformed or bent. In the equation above, elasticity is the numerator of the equation (top part of the number being divided), so the more elastic the medium, the more rapid the speed of sound travel. Solids have very high elasticity, and thus high speed of sound travel. Density increases will decrease the speed of sound travel, as that variable (ρ) is in the denominator of the equation. So, although one might think that a dense solid, like metal, would have a slow speed of sound travel, the high elasticity of the medium more than compensates, and as shown in Table 3–1, the speed of sound is faster through solids and other elastic media.

WAVELENGTH

Next, we define wavelength. The Greek letter lambda (λ) is used as the abbreviation for wavelength. If we know the speed of sound and we know the frequency of the sound, we can determine the length of each individual wave in the sound by dividing the speed by the frequency:

$$\text{Wavelength } (\lambda) = \text{Speed of Sound } (c) / \text{Frequency } (f).$$

Stated another way, we can calculate how far individual maximum compression cycles will be spaced apart from each other through this calculation. Figure 3–1A il-

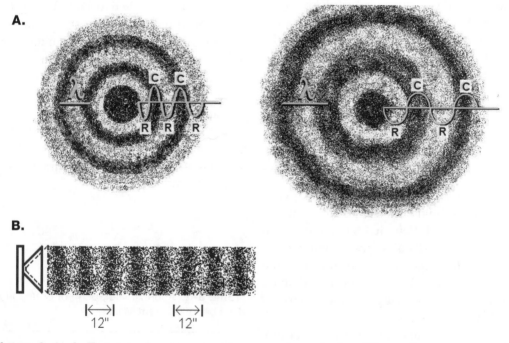

Figure 3–1. A. Two sound sources are shown, each producing different frequency sounds. The wavelength is the spacing between consecutive compression or rarefaction cycles. The higher the frequency *(left)*, the shorter the wavelength. **B.** In this illustration, the speaker is producing a sound with a wavelength of 12 inches (1 ft), which is produced by a 1100-Hz tone.

lustrates the concept that the location of maximum compression is spaced a certain distance apart, which is related to the frequency of the sound. Illustrated slightly differently in Figure 3–1B, we see that the wavelength of this particular sound is 1 ft. The frequency can be solved by the equation:

Frequency (*f*) = Speed of Sound (*c*) / Wavelength (λ)

In this illustration, frequency is 1100 ft per sec/1 foot, or 1100 Hz.

Although wavelength has been defined as the spacing between two compression cycles, it is also the spacing between two points in maximum rarefaction.

PERIOD

It takes some period of time for the cone of the speaker to cycle through movement out, back to the position of rest, through its farthest inward phase, and back to the position of rest. The time that this requires is aptly called **period.** Formally stated, the time required for one complete cycle of rarefaction/compression is the period, which is measured either in seconds, or more commonly, milliseconds. The symbol *T* (for time) is often used to indicate period.

Period (seconds per cycle) is the reciprocal of frequency (cycles per second). To obtain period in milliseconds, multiply by 1000 as there are 1000 milliseconds in one second. For example, to determine the period of 500 Hz in milliseconds, we use the following formula.

$$T = \frac{1}{\text{frequency in Hz}} \times \frac{1000 \text{ msec}}{\text{Sec}}$$

$$T = \frac{1}{500 \text{ cycles/sec}} \times \frac{1000 \text{ msec}}{\text{Sec}}$$

$$= \frac{2 \text{ msec}}{\text{cycle}}$$

RELATIONSHIP OF PERIOD AND WAVELENGTH

Sine waves are discussed in greater detail in Chapter 4. Figure 3–2 shows the wave pattern that comes from **simple harmonic motion**, that is, the smoothest form of back and forth oscillation of an object, such as a tuning fork or speaker cone. When the object is vibrating in simple harmonic mo-

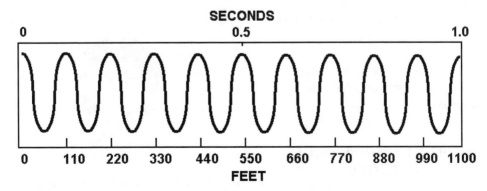

Figure 3–2. A 10-Hz tone plotted against time and distance. As the time is one second and the tone has 10 cycles each second, each cycle takes one-tenth of a second (has a period of 100 msec) and has a wavelength that is one-tenth of 1100 feet long (110 feet).

tion, a **pure tone** is produced, meaning that there is just one simple frequency to the vibration—the motion pattern repeats that many times per second.

In Figure 3–2, we have depicted a sound sine wave of 10 Hz and placed it simultaneously on a distance and time scale to show the interrelationship of period and wavelength. Recall that period is the time required to complete a wave cycle, whereas wavelength is the distance between cycles of a wave in space. The single wave can represent both concepts if we relabel the *x*-axis.

In the example in Figure 3–2, the frequency is 10 Hz. The sound wave displacement will travel a distance of 1100 feet in 1 second (the speed of sound of air). By definition, a 10-Hz sound has 10 cycles in 1 second. As Figure 3–2 shows, we have 10 complete cycles occurring in one second, with the sound traveling 1100 feet in that second. Each wave covers one-tenth of 1100 feet, or 110 feet. (Wavelength = Speed of Sound/Frequency =1100/10 = 110 feet.)

If the frequency had been:

(a) 100 Hz;   Wavelength = 1100/100 = 11 feet,

(b) 1000 Hz;   Wavelength = 1100/1000 = 1.1 feet,

(c) 10,000 Hz; Wavelength = 1100/10,000 = 0.11 feet, and so on.

As speed of sound is the same regardless of frequency, higher frequencies have shorter wavelengths.

SOUND TRANSMISSION EFFECTS

Diffraction and Reflection

Whether sound wraps around a barrier (is **diffracted**) or is **reflected** off the barrier depends on the wavelength of the sound relative to the size of the barrier. If the sound wave has a wavelength that is longer than the barrier, then sound will wrap around the barrier (Figure 3–3B). When the wavelength is shorter than the barrier, the sound wave reflects (Figure 3–3A).

The human head is about 6 to 8 inches wide. Let's assume a person's head is 0.6 ft wide. Sounds that have a frequency above 1800 Hz and that are presented directly to one ear will tend to bounce off the head, rather than wrapping around it. This is calculated by finding the frequency that has a wavelength of 0.6 feet, using the formula:

Frequency of a sound with a given wavelength (f) = Speed of Sound (c)/ Wavelength (λ)

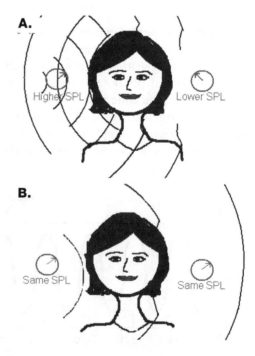

Figure 3–3. When the wavelength of the sound is longer than the barrier, sound wraps around the object. **A.** The human head is a barrier to sounds with frequencies above about 1800 Hz. **B.** The loss of sound energy at the opposite ear is called a head shadow.

f = 1100 ft/sec / 0.6 ft/cycle

f = 1800 cycles/sec

Sounds above 1800 Hz would be less intense on the other side of the head. The **head shadow** is the name for this phenomenon, which will not occur for low-frequency sounds. The difference in intensity between ears provides humans with a cue for localizing high-frequency sounds such as a whistle, but not low-frequency sounds, like a fog horn. Chapter 37 describes how the time at which the sound arrives at the two ears provides the cue for localizing low-frequency sounds.

Sound Absorption, Transmission Loss, and Reverberation Time

When sound waves approach a barrier, such as a wall, some of the sound will be **reflected**, and some will be **absorbed**. For example, a hard wall absorbs less sound than a wall made of acoustic tiles, or one with a drape in front of it. The ratio of sound absorbed to sound reflected gives the **coefficient of absorption**, which will vary depending on the frequency of the sound. For example, drapery material and carpets are better at absorbing high-frequency sound than low-frequency sound.

If you want to keep sound out of a room, you want a wall with a high **transmission loss.** Transmission loss is calculated by determining the fraction of the sound energy transmitted, then putting it into the formula:

Transmission loss in dB = 10 log 1/fraction transmitted.

For example, if half the sound energy is lost as it crosses through a wall, the transmission loss is 10 log 1/½, or 10 log 2, which is 3 dB.

A barrier that has an absorbing layer followed by a reflecting one will have a high transmission loss. The sound that goes through the absorbing layer tends to reflect off the reflecting barrier, and then some of that reflected sound will be absorbed. The absorption is actually the sound energy being transferred into heat.

When you speak inside a sound room (inaccurately called a sound-proof booth—no room is totally sound proof), you may note that your voice seems dull or flat. A room that absorbs a higher percentage of the sound energy rather than reflecting it seems unnatural. However, that type of acoustic environment is good for speech understanding, because the echoed sound does not mask (cover up) other sounds. A highly reverberant classroom, for example, would be undesirable. The degree to which sound echoes in a room can be measured and described in terms of the room's **reverberation time**. Formally, that is the time it takes for a sound to die down by 60 dB.

Sound Propagation Through Holes

When a sound wave propagates through a hole in a barrier, it is as if the hole becomes the new sound source. The sound will radiate outward from that hole, as shown in Figure 3–4.

The Doppler Effect

You may have experienced a change in the sound of an approaching train, plane, or other vehicle as it passes you. As the train becomes closer, the pitch gets higher, but after it passes, the pitch shifts lower. This is related to changes in the wavelength of the sound (Figure 3–5). The approaching object partially over-runs its own wavelength.

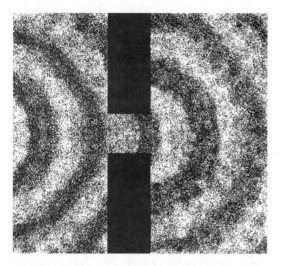

Figure 3–4. When sound travels through a hole in an object with high transmission loss, the hole acts as a new sound source, and the sound waves radiate out from the hole.

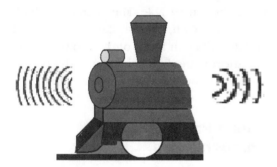

Figure 3–5. The wavelength of the sound of a train is shorter in front of the approaching object, which is perceived as a higher pitch sound. After the passing of the traveling sound generator, the wavelengths become spaced farther apart, with the perception of a lower pitch sound.

The wavelengths are more closely spaced, because as each subsequent compression wave is produced, the train has moved closer to the earlier compression wave. Once the object has passed, the subsequent compression waves are spaced farther apart. The earlier compression waves are "left be-

hind," and the wavelength increases. Wavelength changes are perceived as changes in the sound pitch, as the frequency is inversely related to the sound's wavelength.

Sonic Booms and Thunder

Figure 3–5 illustrates increasingly tightly spaced compression cycles of the sound wave as the train approaches. An airplane also creates a sound pressure wave in front of it. When the plane travels at a speed approaching the speed of sound, the airplane has a barrier in front of it—a segment of compressed air. Going even faster than that compression wave requires extra energy, and the piercing of that wall of sound creates an explosive sound. A plane or train traveling at or above the speed of sound creates a series of these shock waves, or **sonic booms**.

Thunder is another related phenomenon. When super-heated lightning plasma expands the nearby air, it expands outward. The air molecules collide with the cooler nearby air molecules, which creates a shock wave and the resulting sound of the thunder. The time lag between seeing lightning and hearing thunder can be used to estimate how far you are from the lightning. As sound travels at approximately 1100 ft/sec, and one mile equals 5280 feet, it takes about 5 seconds to travel 1 mile.

Air Density Affects Wavelength

You now know that the density of the medium affects the speed at which sound travels. Cool air is denser—there are more air molecules in a given space. That creates a higher pressure. As defined previously, the speed of sound is

$$s = \sqrt{\frac{E}{\rho}}$$

where E is the elasticity and ρ is the density, which is affected by air pressure. So, the higher the pressure, the lower the speed of sound. That means that the wavelengths of a given sound will be closer together when it is cold. The differences are not large, but there is one time when you may notice the effect—when there is a thermal inversion. During the weather phenomenon know as a thermal inversion, there is warm air trapped above cooler air. Most often, the opposite is true. Sunlight warms the ground, and that warm ground warms the air near the surface. Therefore, the sound wavelengths will be slightly farther apart on the ground and more closely spaced above (Figure 3–6A). The wave front points away from the earth. In contrast (Figure 3–6B), if the warmer air is above, the sound waves point downward. Sound seems to "travel farther" on those days, though it is actually that the energy is concentrating near ground level.

A.

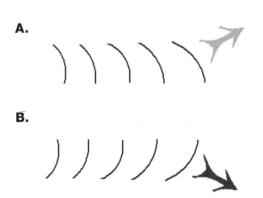

B.

Figure 3–6. Illustration of how wavelength can be different at ground level and above. **A.** The air is colder above the ground, causing wavelengths to be wider spaced at ground level, therefore the wave front moves upward. **B.** When there is a thermal inversion and the warm air is on top, the wave bends down toward earth.

TYPES OF DECIBEL SCALES

Review of dB SPL and dB IL

We have already presented some information on intensity while discussing the decibel in Chapter 2. We now elaborate somewhat on that discussion and relate it to the different types of decibels: dB IL, dB SPL, dB HL, and dB SL.

Although the unit of measure of frequency (Hz or cps) is a straightforward concept, the unit of measure for intensity is not. As we have already seen, the decibel (dB), in fact, is not an absolute unit of measure (such as dyne, pascal, or newton), but is the description of the relationship or ratio of the sound measured and a reference. As discussed in Chapter 2, to further complicate the matter, the decibel is not a simple ratio statement; it is an exponential or logarithmic ratio. This logarithmic ratio can be used to express the sound pressure level (SPL) of a sound; that is, the sound pressure can be compared to the internationally accepted reference sound pressure of 20 μPa. The formula used is dB SPL = 20 log P_1 / 20 μPa, where P_1 is the measured pressure.

Decibels intensity level, dB IL, use a different reference and a different multiplier. Recall that the formula is 10 log I_1 /10^{-12} watts/m². Both dB IL and dB SPL can be used to describe the absolute intensity of the sound—how much more intensity or pressure the sound has than the standard reference (i.e., 20 μPa or 10^{-12} watts/m²).

dB Increase

The decibel notation can also be used for expressing the relationship between any two sound pressures, that is, for expressing how much more intense one sound is relative to any other. Both in describing the relative loudness of two sounds, or when describing the absolute intensity or pressure, we are describing the ratio of two numbers (e.g., for dB SPL, how much more pressure there is relative to 20 μPa). For this reason, if you read "dB" without a reference (such as dB SPL), then the writer is either incorrect, or the writer means that a certain sound pressure (or power) ratio change has occurred. Recall from Chapter 2, for example, that doubling the power gives a 3 dB increase in sound power. It is accurate to say "the sound *was turned up* 3 dB." In the section above, it is acceptable to refer to the time required for the sound to die down by 60 dB, because we have an implied reference—we are describing the amount of sound attenuation. However, it is not proper to say the sound "*is* 3 dB loud," or "*is* 60 dB loud." In those cases you would have to state the type of dB, such as 3 dB SPL, which would mean 3 dB louder than a sound with pressure of 20 μPa (or the same sound described as having a power in watts/m².)

dB HL and dB SL

In addition to the SPL reference for decibels, two other reference levels are common. These are decibels **hearing level (dB HL)** and decibels **sensation level (dB SL)**. The SPL notation is used when we are measuring the physical intensity of a sound, that is, stating how much sound energy is present irrespective of whether anyone or anything can or does hear it. Frequently, however, we wish to make statements or observations concerning how a sound compares with the softest sound the "average normal hearing person" can just barely hear. In other words, we may want to describe whether a given individual's hearing is normal or abnormal; and if abnormal, by how many decibels. When we use decibels to express this relationship, we are saying that the individual differs from

normal by X dB. The starting point (or reference) for making this measure is not 20 μPa, it is the sound pressure that is just barely audible to the average normal listener, and this varies from frequency to frequency. Thus, if a woman's hearing ability is poorer than normal by 50 dB, she has a hearing loss of 50 dB and her **threshold of hearing** is 50 dB HL. Although it may seem counterintuitive, the higher the threshold number, the worse the hearing, and the lower the threshold, the better the hearing. Negative thresholds mean better than average hearing. For example, if a patient's hearing is 10 dB better than normal, the threshold of hearing is -10 dB HL. **Hearing threshold level (dB HTL)** is an older term one may come across. The two terms are used interchangeably, that is, 0 dB HL = 0 dB HTL.

On other occasions, we may wish to express the level of a sound relative to how a given individual hears it, whether or not that individual has normal hearing. In other words, we may wish to provide the individual with a sound at some decibel **sensation level (dB SL)**. To indicate this, we express the level of the sound in reference to the softest sound that the individual in question can hear, that is, his or her threshold. Thus, 30 dB SL means that the sound is 30 decibels above the threshold of the individual who is listening to it, no matter what that person's threshold may be.

In summary, dB SPL means that the starting point is 20 μPa, dB HL means that the starting point is average normal hearing, and dB SL means that the starting point is the individual's threshold. For example, the average normal listener cannot hear a 125-Hz tone until it reaches 45 dB SPL. (Again, the average hearing threshold in dB SPL varies from frequency to frequency, so this example is specific to 125 Hz.) Thus, 45 dB SPL equals 0 dB HL at 125 Hz. Now, if a particular gentleman has a hearing loss of 25 dB at 125 Hz, he will not be able to hear the tone until it reaches 25 dB HL, which is 70 dB SPL. If we wish to let that individual hear the tone at 30 dB above his threshold, we must present the tone at 30 dB SL that is, in his case, 55 dB HL and 100 dB SPL. Figure 3-7 uses the above numbers to illustrate how the SPL, HL, and SL notations can be thought of as different starting points, or zeros, on the same scale.

INTRODUCTION TO THE AUDIOGRAM

The audiogram shows the patient's hearing level at each different frequency, for each ear. The lowest level the patient can hear at each frequency is established. This is called the patient's **threshold** of hearing. The audiogram (Figure 3-8) shows the different frequencies across the top. Intensity is along the side. Unlike most scientific graphs, low intensity is at the top, and high intensity is at the bottom. The worse the hearing, the

higher the threshold in dB HL, the further down the scores.

The audiogram shown in Figure 3-8 reveals the thresholds for the right ear (the O's, often colored red) and the left ear (the X's, traditionally in blue) when tested using earphones. This testing is called **air-conduction testing** because the sound enters the ear by vibration of air molecules. (Chapter 14 will introduce another form of hearing testing, bone conduction.) This patient has poorer hearing in the left ear. Both ears have greater hearing loss in the high frequencies.

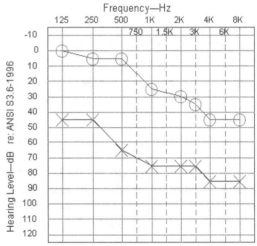

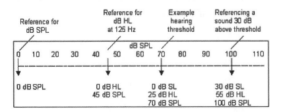

Figure 3–7. An example showing the relationships of SPL, HL, and SL for a 125-Hz tone for an individual who has a 25 dB hearing loss at 125 Hz. The 0 dB SPL references the sound in absolute pressure, but the average audible threshold is 45 dB higher than that—so 0 dB HL equals 45 dB SPL. The patient has 25 dB of hearing loss, so does not hear until 25 dB HL, which is 70 dB SPL. If presented with a 30 dB SL sound (30 dB above this patient's threshold), he is listening to 55 dB HL, which is 100 dB SPL.

Figure 3–8. An audiogram displays the patient's hearing thresholds. The circles show the right ear air-conduction thresholds, the left ear thresholds are the X's. Frequency is on the horizontal axis. Less intense sound is at the top of the graph. The higher the threshold (the larger the dB HL threshold), the more severe the loss is. As the right ear has thresholds that are at lower numbers, the right ear has less hearing loss—this patient is able to detect lower intensity sound in the right ear. Both ears have better hearing in the low frequencies. Audiogram generated with AuDSim software, used and reproduced with permission courtesy of www.audstudent.com.

SUMMARY

Sound will travel through air at the same velocity, regardless of the sound's frequency. However, different frequency sounds have different wavelengths (the distance between the areas where the sound wave is in compression or in rarefaction) and different periods (the time required for the sound wave to cycle from the start of compression to rarefaction back to the start of the compression cycle.)

Sound frequency affects how the sound reacts to different obstacles in its path. If the sound's wavelength is greater than the barrier, the sound diffracts, or wraps around the barrier. Otherwise a sound shadow is created. The sound shadow is more total when the barrier is a wall, but some sound will be transmitted, whereas the rest is either reflected, or absorbed (friction changes the energy to heat.)

We detect pitch based on wavelength. Change in wavelength—from the sound source traveling either to or away from the listener, or as a result of temperature differences at different altitudes—cause changes in the perception of sound.

Decibels IL and SPL describe the absolute power/pressure of the sound wave. This type of measurement is made in acoustics; for example, dB SPL measurements are made with a sound level meter. However, the average normal hearing threshold is at different dB SPL levels at different frequencies, so it is inconvenient to use the dB SPL scale when testing hearing. Instead, dB HL is the decibel of choice. 0 dB HL is the average threshold for normal hearing patients. The higher the threshold (e.g., 90 dB HL), the worse the hearing loss.

One additional type of decibel was described: dB SL. If we know the patient's threshold, and present a stimulus at X dB above that threshold, then we have presented the signal at that many dB sensation level (SL). For example, if the patient with a 90 dB HL threshold at 1000 Hz is presented with a 100 dB HL signal, that signal can also be described as being 10 dB SL.

The patient's hearing thresholds for each ear are measured and plotted on an audiogram, which displays the frequencies from low to high across the top of the chart, and intensity along the vertical axis—with 0 dB HL, the normal hearing threshold, being at the top of the graph.

4

The Sine in Sine Waves and Other Types of Sound Waves

The goal of this chapter is to explain how trigonometry, with its sine, cosine, and tangent, relates to acoustics. We further explore how the vibration of air molecules creates sound, and discuss complex sounds, which occur when two or more different frequency sine waves are combined. Spectral analysis, the technique to determine the frequency and amplitude of the components of a complex sound, is introduced. Common types of complex sound waves and noise are described.

TRIANGLES AND SINES

Before discussing how trigonometry relates to acoustics, we need to define some terms and conventions, and then review basic trigonometry. The "sine" of an angle refers to the relative sizes of sides of a **right triangle**, that is, a triangle with a right angle (a 90-degree angle) in it. The right angle might be marked with a square, as shown in Figure 4-1A. One of the two other angles is the angle of interest. It is typically noted with a curved line with a dash through it. Also, by convention, that angle is drawn on the lower left. The specific degree of the angle may be noted.

The side opposite that angle is quite sensibly called the **opposite** side, and is sometimes called the "height" of the triangle. The side right next to the angle of interest is the **adjacent** side or "base." The remaining side is the **hypotenuse**.

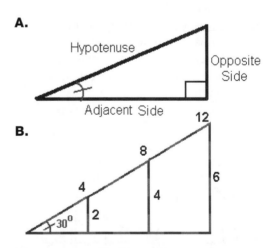

Figure 4–1. A. Shows the common terms used. **B.** There is a constant relationship between the sizes of the sides of a triangle of any given angle. The opposite side length divided by the hypotenuse side length is called the sine of that angle. That ratio is always the same, no matter how large the triangle.

For any given angle, there is a relationship between the sizes of the sides. This is shown in Figure 4–1B. Look at the innermost triangle. The opposite side is 2 units high, and the hypotenuse is 4 units long. As the opposite side grows to 4 units in length, the hypotenuse is 8 units long, and so on. The specific relationship (such as the 1:2 ratio for this 30-degree angle) will vary depending upon the angle.

The ratio of the size of the opposite to the hypotenuse is called the **sine** of the angle. So, in this case, the sine of the 30 degree angle is 2/4, or 0.5. The **cosine** is the ratio of the size of the adjacent side divided by the size of the hypotenuse. The **tangent** is the opposite divided by the adjacent. On your calculator, the buttons are labeled sin, cos, and tan (but you would still pronounce it "sign" and "co-sign" and "tangent").

Of course, the sine value changes with the angle. As shown in Figure 4–2, as the angle gets broader, the size of the hypotenuse gets smaller and smaller, and the sine approaches 1.0. If the "angle" is 90 degrees, then we have a line going straight up. The sine ratio is indeed 1.0 then—the hypotenuse is equal in size to the opposite.

Whereas Figure 4–2 showed the triangles with the opposite side remaining the same length, there are advantages to thinking about the triangles with the hypotenuse remaining at a set size (Figure 4–3). First, if the hypotenuse stays one unit long, then the value of the opposite side equals the sine value. (Remember that the sine of an angle is the opposite divided by the hypotenuse, and anything divided by 1 is that number.) The second advantage is that keeping the hypotenuse the same size helps us see the "circular" nature of the phenomenon, and it lets us think about angles that are larger than 90 degrees.

Figure 4–3 also illustrates that the absolute value of sine of angles that are 180 degrees apart will be the same: the triangles are the same size, just oriented in opposite directions. Because the opposite side of the triangle points downward once the angle is between 180 and 360 degrees, the length

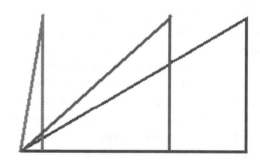

Figure 4–2. As the angle increases, the sine (the ratio of the opposite divided by the hypotenuse) increases.

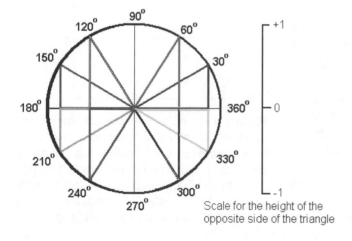

Scale for the height of the opposite side of the triangle

Figure 4–3. The hypotenuse remains one unit long. The size of the opposite angle changes as the angle progresses from 0 degrees though 360 degrees. Recall that the sine of an angle is the opposite height divided by the hypotenuse. Because the hypotenuse is 1.0, the size of the opposite side is equal to the sine of that angle.

of the opposite side is negative, so the sine will be negative. For example, the sine of 30 degrees is 0.5, and the sine of 210 degrees is –0.5. Also, the sine for those angles that are mirror images from 90 degrees are the same. As shown, 30 degrees (which is 60 degrees away from straight up) has the same sine value as does 150 degrees (which is 60 degrees rotated from that 90 degree straight-up angle.)

The phase angle value can be thought of as how far you rotated the hypotenuse. If you started off at 0 degrees—a line to the right, and spun it around the circle back to 360 degrees, then continued rotating counterclockwise another 30 degrees, you have rotated a total of 390 degrees (30 plus 360). Again, you would have that same 0.5-sine wave value as 30 degrees has. You can calculate the sine of any angle; it need not be just from 0 to 360 degrees. Your calculator is able to calculate any angle, even thousands of degrees of rotation.

PLOTTING SINE WAVES

Table 4-1 lists the values of the sines of angles, in 15 degree steps, and Figure 4-4 plots these values. Note how rapidly the sine value increases from 0 to 30 degrees. Amplitude is rapidly changing as we start from 0 degrees, but then the rate of change slows down as the angle nears 90 degrees. The plot of the values of the sine of the angles is a **sine wave,** shown in Figure 4-4.

If you think about the sweeping hypotenuse in the circle in Figure 4-3 as rotating, like the second hand of a clock running in reverse direction, you will see that you could label the x-axis as time just as easily as degrees of **phase**. If the backward moving second hand rotated once in 60 seconds, then we could relabel 90 degrees of phase as 15 seconds, 180 as 30 seconds, and so on, with 360 degrees being 60 seconds.

Table 4-1. The Value of the Sines of Angles

Angle	Sine
0	0
15	0.26
30	0.5
45	0.71
60	0.87
75	0.97
90	1
105	0.97
120	0.87
135	0.71
150	0.5
165	0.26
180	0
195	–0.26
210	–0.5
225	–0.71
240	–0.87
255	–0.97
270	–1
285	–0.97
300	–0.87
315	–0.71
330	–0.5
345	–0.26
360	0

If we wish to know the time at any exact point, it is easily calculated. The first step is to create a fraction that represents the degree of completion of the rotation of the circle. For example, 65 degrees of phase is 65/360, or 0.18 through the complete cycle. Next, multiply that fraction by the time required to make a complete cycle (the **period** of vibration), 60 seconds in this ex-

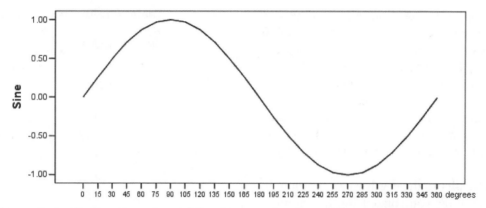

Figure 4–4. Plotting the values of the sine as a function of the angle results in a waveform called a sine wave.

ample. The 65 degree point in the cycle is reached at 10.8 seconds.

SIMPLE HARMONIC MOTION, THE PENDULUM AND THE CIRCLE

At this point, we have explored the relationship between the sine wave and basic trigonometry. Before discussing sound, and how air molecule vibration is related to the sine wave, it is helpful to see how the sine wave relates to the amplitude of vibration of something more easily seen: the pendulum. In Figure 4-5, a pendulum is vibrating. Imagine if the pendulum's shadow could be traced across time—as if a strip chart recorder were below the pendulum, the paper scrolled along under the pendulum so as to record the shadow's location. The tracing would show a sine wave.

Another analogy is in order. Envision a classroom with a large white board along the wall, and your hand outstretched in front of you, grasping a marker in the hand near the white board. Move your hand up and down.

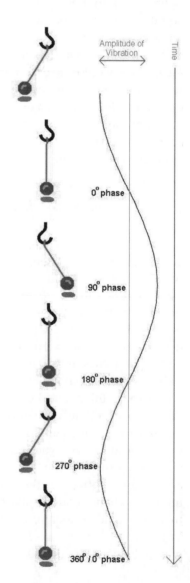

Figure 4–5. A swinging pendulum's shadow, graphed across time, would form a sine wave.

The forces of inertia and momentum will make your hand move more quickly through the middle of the up and down arc, slowing at the top and bottom. Now, walk forward while your hand is still moving up and down, so that you draw a line on the whiteboard as you go. As shown in Figure 4-6, a sine wave results.

MOLECULAR VIBRATION AND THE SINE WAVE

In Chapter 1 we began relating the sine wave and air molecule vibration. We can now explore this in greater detail.

Sound starts with an object vibrating, such as the speaker cone in Figure 1-4. A tuning fork is another object that can be made to vibrate. Striking the tuning fork on another object causes the metal tines to vibrate in and out, with a pendular motion. In Figure 4-7, we have struck a tuning fork, and watch its vibration across time. The air molecules directly adjacent to the tuning fork are also displaced. This type of vibration is called **simple harmonic motion**. It produces a clean musical note sound called a **pure tone**.

In review from Chapter 1, the vibration of an object creates **compression** and **rarefaction** of the adjacent air molecules. The air molecules become more densely packed when the vibrating object comes toward the air molecule. The air molecules are rarefied, spread apart farther, in the partial vacuum that results from the tuning fork creating a small void as it moves the other way. The pressure of the molecules increases and decreases in the same sinusoidal way as we have described in this chapter.

Thus, at 90 degrees of phase of vibration, the tuning fork is farthest from its point of rest and the adjacent air molecules are most densely packed together (maximal compression). At 180 degrees of phase, the

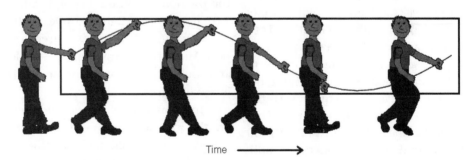

Time →

Figure 4–6. Up and down swinging (vibration) of the arm, recorded over the time taken to walk forward, would create a sine wave.

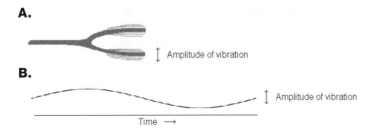

A.

↕ Amplitude of vibration

B.

↕ Amplitude of vibration

Time →

Figure 4–7. A tuning fork also vibrates in simple harmonic motion. Its vibration pattern is a sine wave.

vibration has returned to the starting point, though the tines are now vibrating in the down direction, and normal air molecule density returns. At 270 degrees of phase, the tuning fork has vibrated farthest down. The air molecules above the tuning fork are maximally spread out, that is, rarefied.

The amplitude of the sine wave is related to the size of the vibration. A hard hit to the tuning fork creates farther in/out vibration, and a more intense sound.

Striking a thin, light tuning fork will make the vibrations happen more rapidly than if the tuning fork is heavy. To reiterate, the rate of vibration is related to frequency. The light tuning fork, vibrating more rapidly, has a higher frequency.

HOW WE CALCULATE RELATIVE AMPLITUDE WHEN PHASE IS KNOWN

If you are told the maximum size of a sinusoidal vibration, you can calculate the size of displacement at any given point in time; that is, at any given phase of vibration. Let's take as an example a 1000-Hz tuning fork that is vibrating at a maximum amplitude of 2 units. As we learned in Chapter 3, the period of a sound wave is 1/frequency, so the period (T) is 1/1000 second, or 1 msec. That tells us that the tines vibrate in and out 1000 times per second, and thus once per millisecond. If the tuning fork is at 40 degrees of phase (that is, 40/360 of the way through the vibration cycle), what amplitude of vibration is occurring? To calculate, multiply the maximum amplitude by the sine of that phase angle. On your calculator, find the sine of 40 degrees. (On most calculators, enter 40, then "sin.") Take that number (0.64) and multiply it by the maximum amplitude, 2 in this example, and you discover that the vibration amplitude is 1.28 units.

Sine values for angles with phases between 180 and 360 will show negative amplitude vibration; that is, the vibration is downward.

HOW WE CALCULATE PHASE WHEN TIME AND FREQUENCY ARE KNOWN

In the section on plotting sine waves, you saw how to calculate the time of a given sine wave angle if you knew the period. The next concept is similar. If you know a sound's frequency, and the time since the onset of the vibration cycle, you can calculate phase. We started examining this above with the example of the clock hand rotating backward once per minute. Now let's take a more readily audible frequency of vibration. A 500-Hz tuning fork is vibrating. The time since the beginning of the 2-msec vibration cycle (period of 500 Hz) is 1.87 msec. What is the current phase of vibration? Calculate the fraction of vibration completed. We are 1.87 msec into a 2-msec cycle, or 0.935 of the way through the 360 degrees of vibration. Multiply that fraction by 360 degrees, and you discover that the phase of vibration is 336.6 degrees.

In summary, as period and frequency are the inverse of each other, if given one, you can easily compute the other. If you know the time of the point of vibration, you can calculate the phase at that point in time, or if you know the point in time, you can calculate the phase. As discussed above, if you know the maximum amplitude of the sine wave, you can calculate the amplitude of the sine wave at any given point (described either as time, or as phase).

Working through a few problems will help solidify your understanding. The answers are at the end of this chapter.

1. A sine wave has a frequency of 1000 Hz. What is the period in msec?
2. What is the phase of the sine wave 0.333 msec after the start of the cycle?
3. If this sine wave had a maximum amplitude of three units, what is the amplitude of the vibration at this 0.333-msec point in time?
4. If the 1000-Hz sine wave is at 45 degrees, what is the time since the beginning of the vibration cycle?
5. If the sine wave is 500 Hz and at 45 degrees phase, what is the time since the beginning of the vibration cycle?

COMPLEX SOUND

The simplest sound is one with a single frequency, that is, a **pure tone**. The term "single frequency" does not mean one cycle per second; it means that the oscillations are occurring at only one rate. Thus, 125 Hz is a pure tone; so are 500 Hz, 4000 Hz, 20,000 Hz, and so forth. Pure tones are easy to produce and control electronically and often serve as stimuli when studying or measuring the auditory system. However, most sounds in nature (the human voice, for ex-

ample) are made up of many frequencies occurring simultaneously at varying intensity levels. These are called **complex sounds**. Complex sounds are made up of pure tones mixed together, and the pure tone components of any particular complex sound can be determined.

Summing Pure Tones That Differ Only in Phase or Amplitude

Figure 4–8A shows a single sine wave that has cycled through 360 degrees. The major degrees of phase are noted. In Figure 4–8B, we could say that tone 2 "lags" tone 1 by 90 degrees. That is, tone 2 starts when tone 1 is at 90 degrees of phase. These two waves are not "in phase." In contrast, Figure 4–8C shows two pure tones of different amplitude (1 and 2) that are in phase. When two waves are in phase, the energy in the two waves sum to produce tone 3. That means that if two sine wave generators are producing the same frequency pure tone, at the same phase, the resulting air molecule vibration increases. When two waves are 180 degrees "out of phase" as are tones 1 and 2 in Figure 4–8D, the energies in the two waves

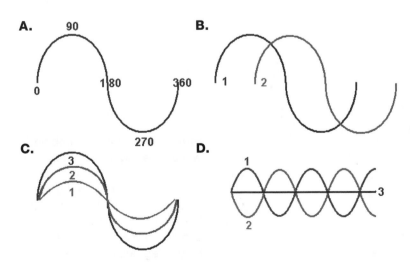

Figure 4–8. A. Illustration of the phases of the pure tone. **B.** Phase relationships between two sine waves where Wave 2 follows or "lags" Wave 1 by 90 degrees. **C.** Waves 1 and 2 sum to be Wave 3. **D.** Waves 1 and 2 cancel when added to form 3, no sound wave.

cancel to produce wave 3 (no tone at all as 1 and 2 totally canceled each other).

If two equal amplitude sine waves, of the same phase, are combined, then the amplitude doubles. As we have just seen, combining two sine waves of the same amplitude that are completely out of phase, cancels out the sound, that is, it sums to nothing. If you add sine waves that are neither completely in nor out of phase, the result is a wave that is somewhere in between being twice as large and being completely canceled. Figure 4–9 illustrates this. You calculate the amplitude of the resulting wave by adding the two wave amplitudes together, at each point in time, as shown in Table 4–2.

Summing Pure Tones That Differ in Frequency

When the combined pure tones are of differing frequencies, the summation wave is a complex wave. It no longer looks like a simple pure tone. Figure 4–10A illustrates this

where waves 1 and 2 combine to form wave 3. All complex sounds are the net result of the summing and canceling effects of different phases, frequencies, and intensities.

A graph that shows the energy present in a sound, as a function of the frequencies making up that sound, shows the sound's **spectrum**. Figure 4–10B shows the spectrum of the sounds illustrated in Figure 4–10A. Each vertical line represents the intensity of the tone at that frequency. Spectrum 1 shows the high energy, low frequency found in wave 1; spectrum 2 shows the low intensity, higher frequency of wave 2; and spectrum 3 the combination of the two.

Figure 4–11 shows the complex sound wave (D) created by mixing three pure tones of different frequencies and amplitudes (A, B, and C). Note how the composite wave (D) tends to follow the lowest frequency (C), and how the higher frequencies (A and B) are superimposed on it.

There is one additional tone combination of particular interest. When two pure tones of equal intensity, but slightly differ-

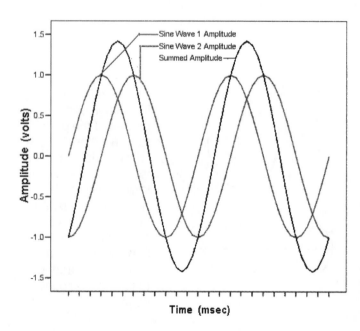

Figure 4–9. When combined waves are slightly out of phase, the amplitude of the summation wave is not twice the amplitude of the original waves as it is when they are in phase. In this figure Wave 2 lags Wave 1 by 90 degrees of phase.

Table 4–2. To Find the Amplitude of the Summation of Two Sine Waves, Simply Add the Amplitude of Each at Each Point in Time

Sine Wave 1 Phase	Sine Wave 2 Amplitude	Sine Wave 1 Phase	Sine Wave 2 Amplitude	Sum of Amplitudes
0	0	270	–1	–1
15	0.26	285	–0.97	–0.71
30	0.5	300	–0.87	–0.37
45	0.71	315	–0.71	0
60	0.87	330	–0.5	0.37
75	0.97	345	–0.26	0.71
90	1	360/0	0	1
105	0.97	15	0.26	1.23
120	0.87	30	0.5	1.37
135	0.71	45	0.71	1.42
150	0.5	60	0.87	1.37
165	0.26	75	0.97	1.23
180	0	90	1	1
195	–0.26	105	0.97	0.71
210	–0.5	120	0.87	0.37
225	–0.71	135	0.71	0
240	–0.87	150	0.5	–0.37
255	–0.97	165	0.26	–0.71
270	–1	180	0	–1
285	–0.97	195	–0.26	–1.23
300	–0.87	210	–0.5	–1.37
315	–0.71	225	–0.71	–1.42
330	–0.5	240	–0.87	–1.37
345	–0.26	255	–0.97	–1.23
360	0	270	–1	–1

ent frequency, combine, the combined tone will have an amplitude envelope that grows to a maximum and then dies down to zero. The difference in frequency between the two tones determines how often the combined tone will cycle up and down in amplitude. In Figure 4-12, the tones are 20 Hz apart (the **simple difference frequency** between 100 Hz and 120 Hz is 20 Hz). The complex tone would increase/decrease in intensity 20 times per second. This is called **beats**—the sound's rhythmic increase and decrease in intensity creates the sensation that you are listening to a single tone, which has a frequency between the two original tones' frequencies that pulses on and off.

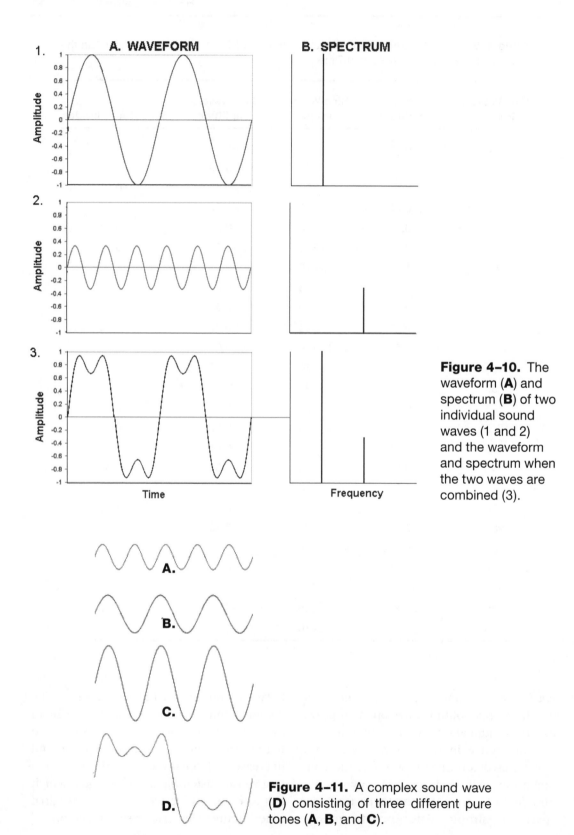

Figure 4–10. The waveform (A) and spectrum (B) of two individual sound waves (1 and 2) and the waveform and spectrum when the two waves are combined (3).

Figure 4–11. A complex sound wave (D) consisting of three different pure tones (A, B, and C).

A.

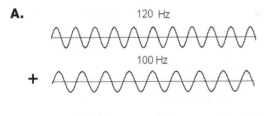

120 Hz

100 Hz

+

B.

Presented simultaneously creates this waveform

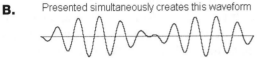

C.

Note the periodicity at 20 Hz, the simple difference frequency.

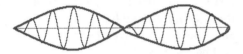

Figure 4–12. A sound that beats on and off is created by combining two tones that are close in frequency. Here, combining 100 Hz and 120 Hz (**A**) creates a complex wave (**B**), which has an envelope (**C**) that pulses on and off at the simple difference frequency of the two tones that were combined.

Harmonics and Distortion

A sine wave sent at a high intensity to a poor quality speaker will no longer have just the single pure tone component—there may be harmonic distortion because the speaker cannot faithfully reproduce the sound wave. The term **harmonics** refers to even multiples of the lowest tone in a complex sound. If the sound is a pure tone, there are no harmonics. However, a pure tone that is transduced by a speaker that creates distortion has harmonics in it—it is no longer pure. If the pure tone that is distorted were 400 Hz, the possible harmonics would be 800, 1200, 1600 Hz, and so forth. If the pure tone were 1000 Hz, the harmonics would be 2000, 3000, 4000 Hz, and so forth. No matter what the **fundamental frequency** (the lowest frequency), harmonics, if present, appear as even multiples of that frequency. (The fun-

damental is equivalent to the first harmonic, so the second harmonic is the fundamental frequency times 2.) If harmonics are present, we no longer have pure tones; we have a complex sound.

Let's state these concepts again, more formally this time. The term **distortion** refers to unintentional changes in a sound due to inaccurate production, transmission, or reproduction. It is due to **nonlinear** and asymmetric vibration. Distortion creates energy not just at the intended, original frequency, but upward to harmonics of the original frequency. When harmonic distortion is present, a pure tone is changed into a complex sound containing the original tone and one or more harmonics of the original.

Distortion is expressed in percent. It is the intensity of the harmonic(s) expressed as a percent of the intensity of the fundamental. For example, 50% distortion is when the intensity of the harmonic is one-half the intensity of the fundamental.

Air Molecule Vibration Pattern for Complex Sounds

When a pure tone is present, the air molecules are vibrating back and forth smoothly. When a complex sound is present, the air molecules are still vibrating back and forth, but the pattern of their movement is more "herky jerky." Consider the sound illustrated in Figure 4–11D. The air molecules would rapidly compress, then begin to rarefy only to compress a bit again, and so forth. The motion of the air molecules will create a similar motion of the eardrum (tympanic membrane).

Fourier's Theorem

The simplest form of vibration is the sine wave. All other signals can be constructed by adding together sine waves of differing frequencies, amplitudes, durations, and phases. That advance in our understanding of sound waves was the work of the French mathematician Jean Baptiste Joseph Fourier. He recognized that any periodic wave could be "broken down" into its component parts, and developed the mathematical method for doing so. That form of spectral analysis is called a **Fourier analysis** (pronounced "foor-ee-a" or in the International Phonetic Alphabet, it would be /fʊr' i e'/).

The sounds we hear everyday, such as speech sounds, contain a complex spectrum. Different people produce sounds slightly differently, so the spectrum will differ from person to person. It makes sense that we test human hearing using pure tones, rather than actual speech sounds, because all speech sounds are not created identically. We can conduct Fourier analysis of speech sounds to analyze the frequencies in them. If we know, for instance, that a patient does not hear high-frequency sounds, we can infer that those speech sounds that contain high frequencies will be inaudible (or unclear, depending upon the amount of loss.)

Fourier analysis is done using computers. Chapter 7 discusses digital signal processing and has more information on Fourier analysis.

Common Types of Tones and Noise

Signal generators often have an option to produce not only sine waves, but specific types of complex waves (Figure 4-13). A **square wave** is one that immediately transitions from full compression to full rarefaction. A **triangular wave** is aptly named, as the compression and rarefaction wave peaks look like triangles. A **sawtooth** wave has an immediate transition from either full compression to full rarefaction or the other way around, then a steady change to the oppo-

site phase, and has the appearance of the teeth of a wood-cutting saw.

All of these complex waves are the result of combining the fundamental frequency with some of the harmonics. The square wave and triangular wave have the odd numbered harmonics contained in them. That is, if the fundamental frequency is 500 Hz, the energy found in the square wave's spectrum will be fundamental frequency (500 Hz), harmonic 3 (1500 Hz), harmonic 5 (3000 Hz), harmonic 7 (4500 Hz), and so forth. (Note that 1000, 2000, 3000 Hz, etc, the even numbered harmonics, are not present.) Sawtooth waves have both even and odd harmonics.

Note the decibel scale in the spectral analysis in Figure 4-13B . Sometimes the absolute intensity of the signal is not as important as the relationship between the intensities of the component frequencies. In this scale, top of the scale is 0 dB, and going down shows negative decibels, that is, the higher frequency harmonics are lower in intensity.

A triangular wave differs from a square wave in the relative intensity of the components. Specifically, the square wave components have 6 dB less intensity for each octave increase. The triangular wave's component frequencies decrease at a rate of 12 dB per octave. Again, these signals only have the odd numbered harmonics. The sawtooth wave has both the even and odd harmonics. The harmonics are 6 dB less intense with each octave increase.

Two common types of noise are white noise and pink noise. Noise does not have a waveform that repeats itself regularly. **White noise**, also called **Gaussian noise**, has equal amounts of energy at each frequency. That is, the spectrum does not show single lines; all frequencies are within the noise, and the amplitude of each frequency is equal. So, on average, over time, there is just as much energy at 1000 Hz as at 1001 Hz or as at 8953 Hz, for that matter. Because of

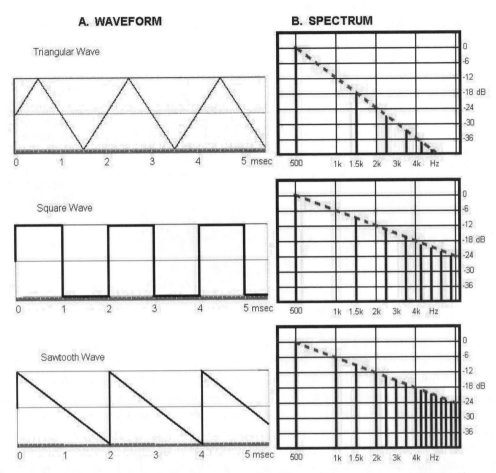

Figure 4–13. Common periodic waves are the triangular, square, and sawtooth waves. Here, each has a 500-Hz fundamental frequency, and thus a period of 2 msec. The signals have different time waveform appearance (**A**) and different frequency spectra (**B**).

the random nature of the noise, at any given time the energy can be a little more or a little less at any given frequency, but if the spectrum of a long segment of noise is observed, then the picture would be of a flat line—no variation in intensity across frequency. **Pink noise** has less high-frequency energy. Its spectrum slopes downward at 3 dB/octave. In other words, there is 3 dB less energy at 2000 Hz than at 1000 Hz. Figure 4-14 shows the spectrum of a brief segment of white and pink noise.

To avoid confusion later, it is helpful at this point to note that the analysis type shown here is frequency-by-frequency. This is called a **level per cycle** analysis. Another way that you can analyze sound is by measuring the total energy within a certain range of frequencies, such as the energy within an octave. That type of analysis, called octave band analysis, is discussed in Chapter 8. The spectrum of white and pink noise measured with octave-band analysis will be different than shown here.

The Click (Transient) Signal

One additional signal is commonly used in hearing science: the **click** or **transient**

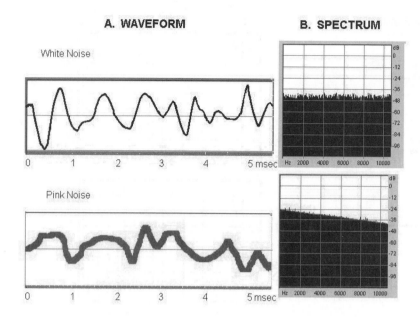

Figure 4–14. The waveform (**A**) and spectrum (**B**) of white and pink noise. The noises cannot readily be identified by their appearance. Pink noise has a 3-dB/octave slope to the spectrum whereas white noise's spectrum is flat.

signal. The sound of a click is similar to what you hear when you tap a pen on a desk or snap your fingers.

A click is a very short duration signal. A mathematician might describe the theoretically ideal click as "infinitely short" in duration; however, in practicality, the signal has to have some duration. A 100-μsec click is an electrical signal that instantly transitions from no voltage to full voltage, stays at that voltage for 100 μsec, then returns to no voltage. Figure 4–15 illustrates this.

The "infinitely short" duration click has a perfectly flat spectrum. Because the click in Figure 4–15 has a 100-μsec duration, it is not completely flat. There are areas where there is less energy—these "nulls" are at 10000 Hz and 20000 Hz. The frequency of the first null is the reciprocal of the click duration. (100 μsec is equal to 0.0001 seconds. 1/0.0001 = 10000 Hz.)

If this click sound were routed to a speaker or earphone, the electrical signal would "tell" the earphone to move instantly outward, causing a compression waveform, hold at that location for 100 μsec, then come back to rest. As Newton's first law of phys-

ics tells us, an object at rest stays at rest, and an object in motion remains in motion. Even though the electrical signal will try to move the earphone diaphragm rapidly, the mass of the earphone will limit its ability to move rapidly. Once that earphone is in motion, it will remain moving—it will overshoot the target. By the time the earphone is recovering from that overshoot, the click duration has ended, and the electrical signal causes the diaphragm of the earphone to return toward the position of rest. The same laws of inertia apply again, and the earphone diaphragm won't stop back at the point of rest, rather it will overshoot. The diaphragm will move outward, causing some rarefaction. The earphone diaphragm has some elasticity to it, which limits how far it will overshoot, and that elasticity will cause the earphone diaphragm to move in the opposite direction. This **ringing** of the earphone may continue another few cycles, depending on the nature of the earphone diaphragm. Figure 4–16 illustrates.

When you send a click into the earphone, the waveform that comes out (Figure 4–16A) is called the **impulse response**

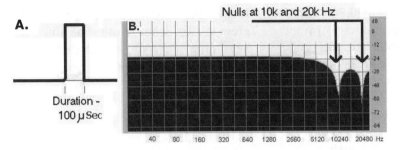

Figure 4–15. A. The electrical waveform of a 100-µsec duration click, or transient, signal. **B.** The spectrum of the sound created by this signal.

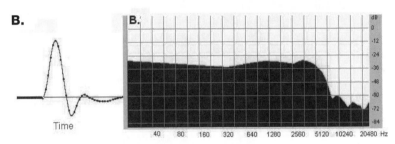

Figure 4–16. A. Time waveform of the click after being sent through an earphone. **B.** The spectrum of the click signal out of the earphone.

of the earphone. The spectrum of the click shows how the earphone has actually filtered the signal. The mass and stiffness characteristics of the earphone allow some frequencies to be transmitted well, whereas others are attenuated.

SUMMARY

Hearing testing is conducted with pure tones, so it is appropriate to understand the nature of this signal. In this chapter we have examined how the sine wave relates to trigonometric functions; we have seen that the back and forth cyclic vibration of a pendulum and a tuning fork create sinusoidal waves. When we hear a sound that vibrates in simple harmonic motion, creating a sine wave, we are listening to a pure tone. Different amplitude/frequency/phase pure tones combined will create complex tones. Complex tones can be separated into their constituent parts in a spectral analysis, typically a digital Fourier analysis, which reveals the component pure tone's amplitudes at specific frequencies. Testing hearing for pure tones then allows us to infer about which types of complex sounds (e.g., which vowels and consonants, which environmental sounds) will not be heard correctly and/or be inaudible.

ANSWERS TO CHAPTER PROBLEMS

1. A sine wave has a frequency of 1000 Hz. What is the period in msec?

    T = 1/ f = 1/1000 second.

    To put into milliseconds:

    T = 1/1000 sec × 1000 msec/sec = 1 msec

2. What is the phase of the sine wave 0.333 msec after the start of the cycle?

    The wave is 0.333 msec into its 1-msec vibration. 0.333/1 = .333

    A complete cycle is 360 degrees; at .333 msec the wave is .333 (1/3) the way through the cycle. 360 degrees × .333 = 120 degrees.

3. If this sine wave had a maximum amplitude of three units, what is the amplitude of the vibration at this 0.333-msec point in time?

The sine of 120 degrees is 0.866. Multiply the maximum amplitude (3) by the sine of the angle (0.866). The amplitude at 120 degrees is approximately 2.6 units

4. If the 1000-Hz sine wave is at 45 degrees, what is the time since the beginning of the vibration cycle?

Period (1 msec) $\times$ 45./360 =
1 msec $\times$ .125 = .125 msec

5. If the sine wave is 500 Hz and at 45 degrees phase, what is the time since the beginning of the vibration cycle?

T = 1/ f = 1/500 second.
To put into milliseconds:
T = 1/500 second $\times$ 1000 msec/sec
= 2 msec
Period (2 msec) $\times$ .125 = .25 msec

5

Impedance, Energy Transfer, and Resonance

This chapter discusses the concept that sound-transmitting media and vibrating objects have a given impedance, that is, resistance to energy flow. The mass and stiffness of the object affect how well it can vibrate as frequency is changed. For example, the "woofer" of a stereo speaker is the large cone. Because it is heavy, it doesn't transmit high frequencies well. The "tweeter," the small, light cone, can easily produce high-frequency sounds, but won't be much help in producing low-frequency sounds. Each speaker has a frequency that it transmits best, based on the mass and stiffness of the cone. That is termed its resonant frequency. In this chapter we examine the concepts of impedance and resonance.

How well a "system" (e.g., vibrating object) transmits any given frequency can be determined if we know the medium's density (related to mass) and elasticity (stiffness). The frequency that creates the least opposition is that system's resonant frequency. We examine this topic and learn how energy transfer is less than complete when sound goes from one medium to another medium if the two media have differing impedances.

We also discuss how the size of a cavity also creates a resonant frequency. The column of air contained in the cavity, like the columns of air in the differing size pipes of a pipe organ, resonate at different frequencies. The longer the tube, the lower the resonant frequency.

IMPEDANCE

As a general concept, **impedance** (symbolized by the letter **Z**) can be thought of as the opposition to the flow of energy. In other words, impedance relates to the opposing forces that act on the particles in a sound wave as the wave passes through a medium, or when the wave is going from one medium into another.

Impedance is a measure of the degree of immobility of particles in a medium set into motion. It can be expressed as: **Z = Force/ Velocity**; that is, the ratio of the force acting on the particles to the resulting velocity of motion of the particles. Stated simply, impedance is how hard it is to obtain a given velocity of molecule motion. As introduced in Chapter 1, **resistance (R)** (from friction) is one form of opposition to motion of the particles. It is produced by the particles rubbing against each other or against surfaces with which they come into contact. The form of opposition produced by the mass (density) and stiffness (elasticity) of the medium is called **reactance (X)**. As we are primarily interested in sound energy, we will discuss **acoustic impedance (Z_A)**.

The frictional component (resistance) opposes all frequencies equally. That is, a 100-Hz tone encounters the same friction as a 1000-Hz tone or a 10000-Hz tone. However, the mass and stiffness components (reactance) vary as a function of (depending on) the frequency of the sound. As frequency goes from low to high, reactance due to mass (**mass reactance**, X_M) increases whereas reactance due to stiffness (**stiffness reactance**, X_S) decreases. Another way to say this is that a heavy system, like a massive tuning fork, transmits low frequencies, but doesn't transmit high frequencies well. A stiff system (like a taught rubber band) doesn't transmit low frequencies well, but will vibrate at a high frequency. The mass in a system inhibits high-frequency sound transmission; the stiffness inhibits low-frequency sound transmission.

The effects of stiffness and mass on impeding vibration are said to be in opposite directions or 180 degrees out of phase. This takes a little explanation. Think about a vibrating weight/spring arrangement (Figure 5-1). Inertia dictates that once a mass is in motion, it wants to remain in motion. As shown at the top of Figure 5-1, the oscillating weight on the spring is influenced by the inertia of the mass to continue moving to the right once it is in motion. The force from the stiffness of the spring works to the opposite effect. The more the spring is stretched out, the stronger the restoring force. In the middle of this figure we see that again, the force from mass and stiffness reactance factors are working in opposition to each other. Their maximum forces are 180 degrees out of phase.

Air molecule motion is similar to the mass and the spring. The air molecule has mass and thus inertia. The force created by the electrons on the outside of the air molecules forces the molecules apart—it resists their extreme movement, acting like the spring. The forces of mass and stiffness working in a system are both in play, but the forces, again, are 180 degrees out of phase.

As mass and stiffness are out of phase, the total reactance is the *difference* between X_M and X_S. The relation of friction, mass and stiffness in producing total impedance is:

$$Z_A = \sqrt{R^2 + (2\pi fm - s/2\pi f)^2}$$

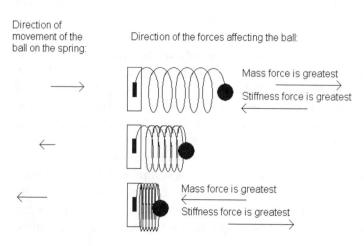

Direction of movement of the ball on the spring:

Direction of the forces affecting the ball:

Mass force is greatest

Stiffness force is greatest

Mass force is greatest

Stiffness force is greatest

Figure 5–1. The inertia of a mass forces a moving object to continue moving in the same direction. The stiffness factor, represented by the coiled spring, has the opposite effect. It has the greatest restoring force just as the mass inertia effect is the strongest. For this reason, the mass and stiffness components of a vibrating system are 180 degrees out of phase.

where Z_A = **acoustic impedance**, **R** = re-sistance, π = 3.1416, **f** = frequency of the sound, **m** = **mass**, and **s** = **stiffness**. The unit of measure of impedance is the **ohm.** Note that resistance is not multiplied by frequency. As previously mentioned, the force from friction (resistance) is the same at all frequencies. Mass is multiplied by frequency, so for a given mass, the higher the frequency, the bigger the impedance from that mass. Stiffness is multiplied by the reciprocal of frequency (1/frequency), so the higher the frequency, the less the stiffness reactance.

The equation above can be simplified a bit to make it easier to understand the underlying concepts. We can say:

$$Z_A = \sqrt{R^2 + (X_m - X_s)^2}$$

X_m is **mass reactance** and X_s is **stiffness reactance**, that is, the parts of impedance that are affected by the mass and stiffness of the system, respectively. Notice that stiffness is subtracted from mass. If mass and stiffness reactance were equal, there would be no reactance factor left, and impedance would come only from the resistance.

Remember the Pythagorean theorem? It states that the sum of the square of the two sides of a right angle equals the square of the hypotenuse: $a^2 + b^2 = c^2$. If you take the square root of both sides of the equation you have

$$c = \sqrt{a^2 + b^2}.$$

Note the similarity to the equation for impedance. For this reason, it makes sense to use a figure like Figure 5–2 to illustrate total impedance.

You will seldom need to calculate the exact impedance. What is far more important to understand are the general concepts. Both mass and stiffness affect total impedance. A system vibrates best when the frequency is the one that makes the mass and stiffness components balance out. At that frequency, there is just resistance left. The frequency where mass and stiffness "balance out" is the **resonant frequency**. We will return to this concept in the section on impedance of systems.

Impedance of a Medium

Another related concept is that different media, with different densities and elasticity, will have different acoustic impedances. One can determine the acoustic impedance of a medium by finding the square root of the product of density and elasticity:

$$Z_A = \sqrt{\text{density} \times \text{elasticity}}$$

This concept will be more than just a passing concern. Chapter 13 will describe how this relates to auditory physiology. Sounds that we hear are transmitted from the air to the fluid-filled inner ear. For this reason, let's examine the impedance differences between air and seawater, because seawater has a density similar to that of the fluids in the inner ear.

Example 1: The density of air is about 0.0012 grams/cm^3 and the elasticity is about 1.42×10^6 dynes/cm^2.

$$\text{Thus: } Z_A = \sqrt{0.0012 \times (1.42 \times 10^6)}$$
$$= \sqrt{1704}$$
$$= 41.28 \text{ ohms.}$$

Example 2: The density of seawater is about 1.024 grams/cm^3 and the elasticity is about 2.53×10^{10} dynes/cm^2.

$$\text{Thus: } Z_A = \sqrt{1.024 \, (2.53 \times 10^{10})}$$
$$= \sqrt{25,907,200,000}$$
$$= 160,957 \text{ ohms.}$$

This shows that sea water is about 4000 times greater impedance than air. The exact ratio is 3899:1.

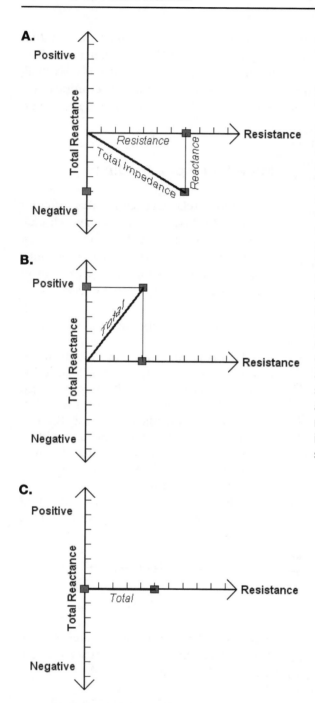

Figure 5–2. Impedance is equal to the square root of the resistance squared plus the total reactance (mass reactance minus stiffness reactance) squared. **A.** A hypothetical system has 1 ohm of mass reactance and 5 ohms of stiffness reactance. The total reactance (mass minus stiffness) is –4 ohms. This same hypothetical system has 7 ohms of resistance. The total resistance is equal to the square root of $-4^2 + 7^2$ (that is, the square root of 65), which is 8.06. The length of the total impedance line is 8.06 ohms. Note that impedance is a positive number even though the reactance was negative. **B.** As a second example, a system has 11 ohms of mass reactance and 6 ohms of stiffness reactance, giving a total reactance of 5 ohms. The system has 4 ohms of resistance, so the total impedance is 6.4 ohms. **C.** This hypothetical system has 12 ohms of mass reactance and 12 ohms of stiffness reactance, so mass minus stiffness equals zero. The impedance value is the same as the resistance value.

ENERGY TRANSFER

A major concern with acoustic impedance is the problem of sound energy transfer when sound goes from one medium to another; for example, going from air to seawater. The degree to which energy flows from the "sending" medium to the "receiving" medium is determined by the ratio of the impedances of the two media. If the impedance of the sending and receiving media are the same, energy flows freely from one to the other. No energy is lost. However, if the impedance of the two are different, an **impedance mismatch** occurs; some proportion of the energy will be transmitted to the receiving medium and some proportion will be reflected back from the juncture of the two media to the sending media. The relationship can be expressed as:

$$T = 4r \div (r + 1)^2$$

where **T** is the proportion of the energy transmitted and **r** is the impedance ratio between the two media.

Example 1: If sound energy traveling through a medium whose impedance is 200 ohms reaches a juncture with a second medium whose impedance is 100 ohms, the ratio is 2:1 and:

$$T = 4r / (r + 1)^2$$
$$= 4 (2) / (2 + 1)^2$$
$$= 8 / 9$$
$$= 0.89$$

that is, 89% of the energy enters the receiving medium and 11% is reflected back into the sending medium.

Example 2: If the energy traveling through a medium whose impedance is 1000 ohms reaches a juncture with a second medium whose impedance is 100 ohms, the ratio is 10:1 and:

$$T = 4r / (r + 1)^2$$
$$= 4 (10) / (10 + 1)^2$$
$$= 40 / 121$$
$$= 0.33$$

that is, 33% of the energy enters the receiving medium and 67% is reflected back into the sending medium.

It is clear that with a very large mismatch, a very small proportion of the en-

ergy is transmitted. It should also be noted that the effects are the same whether going from high to low impedance or from low to high impedance, that is, a 10:1 ratio produces the same energy "loss" as a 1:10 ratio. The term **energy loss** is applied to the proportion of the energy not transmitted. There is, of course, no actual energy lost; it is either reflected back or converted to heat.

However, the reflected energy can be thought of as energy lost when passing from one medium to another. This loss may be expressed in decibels by multiplying 10 times the logarithm of the energy transmission ratio.

In example 1 above, the energy transmission ratio is 1:0.89; that is, for each unit of energy in the sending medium, 0.89 units enter the receiving medium. Converting the energy loss to decibels:

$$dB = 10 \log 1.0/0.89$$
$$= 10 \log 1.124$$
$$= 10 \times 0.05$$
$$= 0.51 \text{ dB}.$$

In example 2 above, the energy transmission ratio is 1:0.33. Converting the energy loss to decibels:

$$dB = 10 \log 1.0/0.33$$
$$= 10 \log 3.03$$
$$= 10 \times 0.4814$$
$$= 4.8 \text{ dB}.$$

Thus a 2:1 impedance mismatch gives 0.5 dB of energy loss, and a 10:1 impedance mismatch gives a 4.8 dB of energy loss.

Example 3: Now let us examine what happens with a large impedance mismatch when a sound in the air strikes the surface of seawater. Remember, air has an impedance of 41.5 ohms whereas seawater has an impedance of 161,000 ohms. Thus, the impedance ratio is 160,957/41.28, or 3899, and:

$$T = 4r / (r + 1)2$$
$$= 4 \times 3899 / (3899 + 1)2$$
$$= 15,596 / 15,210,000$$
$$= 0.001$$

That is, only 1/1000 of the energy in air actually enters the seawater. For every 1000 units of energy in the air, only one unit is transferred to the seawater. This means that 99.9% of the sound energy is reflected back into the air. To put this into the decibel formula for energy loss:

$$dB = 10 \log 1000/1$$
$$= 10 \log 1000$$
$$= 10 \times 3.000$$
$$= 30 \text{ dB.}$$

Thus, the sound energy going from air to seawater encounters a 30 dB loss of energy.

Again, this calculation is more than just of passing interest in the study of audiology. As discussed in the physiology of the middle ear (Chapter 13), sound energy must pass from air to fluids in the inner ear. There will be a loss of 30 dB due to the impedance mismatch between these two media (air and cochlear fluids).

opposition decreases as the frequency of the sound is raised. We also know that the reactance due to mass (X_M) provides opposition to the flow of sound energy and that the opposition increases as frequency is raised. Furthermore, we have learned that X_S and X_M act 180 degrees out of phase, meaning that the total opposition due to reactance is the difference between the two.

Figure 5-3 illustrates the above concept. Notice how the total reactance (X_T) decreases up to the frequency where X_M is the same as X_S. At this point there is no reactance as the difference between X_M and X_S equals zero. The only opposition to sound energy at this frequency is due to any resistance that may be present. (And resistance will stay the constant across all frequencies.) At frequencies above this point, reactance again increases. Any given medium will have a particular frequency that it passes with the least amount of opposition. This occurs when $X_M = X_S$, and is said to be the **resonant frequency** of the medium. Remember that reactance, whether in its negative form (X_S) or its positive form (X_M), is an opposition to energy flow. Thus, the X_T in Figure 5-3 is the difference between X_S and

RESONANCE OF SYSTEMS

Resonance is a complex phenomena related to the mass and stiffness of not only the medium within which the sound energy is traveling, but also the mass and stiffness of the objects and structures that are vibrating. The mass and stiffness of the material making the boundaries of the sound field are also important. We discuss briefly those factors most relevant to audiologists.

The resonance of a medium (for example, air) is determined by the stiffness and mass of that medium. We already know that reactance due to stiffness (X_S) provides opposition to the flow of energy and that the

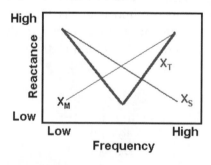

Figure 5–3. The relationship between frequency, reactance due to stiffness (X_S), reactance due to mass (X_M), and total reactance (X_T). Total reactance is the *difference* between X_M and X_S. The frequency where total reactance is lowest is the resonant frequency.

X_M and is the amount of reactance present irrespective of sign.

STANDING WAVES AND RESONANCE OF TUBES

Next we explore more about what happens when a sound wave reaches a barrier, such as a wall. The degree to which the mass and stiffness of the walls differ from the mass and stiffness of the air that fills the space (the impedance mismatch) will determine how much of the sound energy is reflected from the boundaries. When sound is reflected from a surface, the reflected energy combines with the original sound (also called the incident sound wave). If the reflected sound is **in phase** with the original sound, the original sound is increased. This was illustrated in Figure 4–8 from the previous chapter. In Figure 4–8C, waves 1 and 2 are in phase and sum to produce wave 3. In Figure 4–8D, waves 1 and 2 are 180 degrees out of phase and cancel. Whether the reflected wave is in phase or out of phase depends, in part, on the frequency of the original wave

and the distance from the reflecting surface. This phenomenon of **standing waves** is responsible for "live" and "dead" spots in certain auditoriums and music halls.

Resonance in tubes (such as pipe organ tubes, or your throat, mouth, or ear canal) also has to do with the reflected sound energy summating to create an enhancement of the sound energy. Resonances of tubes are related to the size and shape of a cavity or space into which a sound is introduced. The next section describes this phenomenon further.

Standing Waves

Let's examine some properties of vibrating strings before examining standing acoustic waves in a room. If you pluck a guitar string, it may vibrate for a while with a visible pattern of waves on it (Figure 5–4). When you see these areas where the waves cancel out and/or areas where they appear to be enhanced, you are seeing **standing waves.** The areas of enhancement of vibration are the antinodes; the areas where the string has diminished vibration are the

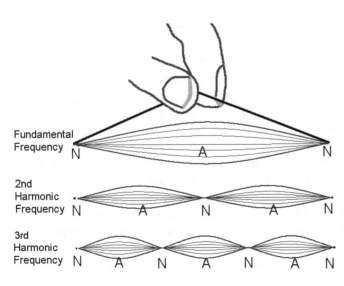

Figure 5–4. Illustration of standing waves on a string. *N* represents node of vibrations, *A* stands for antinode. The string will create standing wave vibration patterns at its fundamental frequency, at twice the fundamental frequency, and at three times the fundamental frequency. For a plucked string, the length of the string corresponds to the wavelength of the second harmonic frequency. Note what looks something like a sine wave at this frequency. The fundamental frequency's wavelength is twice as long as the string length.

Fundamental Frequency N   A   N

2nd Harmonic Frequency N   A   N   A   N

3rd Harmonic Frequency N   A   N   A   N   A   N

nodes. Depending on the characteristics of the string, it may vibrate only at its fundamental frequency (also called first harmonic), or it may additionally vibrate at higher order harmonics. If it vibrates at more than one harmonic frequency, the vibration seen is not each one in isolation, but a blur of the combined harmonic frequency vibrations.

Standing waves occur in reflective sound fields as well. If the reflected wave is out of phase (Figure 5-5A), there is **destructive interference**: the sound wave cancels. If the reflection is in phase, the energy is enhanced (Figure 5-5B).

In a room with a speaker producing pure tones, there can be some areas where there is destructive interference, and therefore a "dead spot," and other areas where there is sound wave summation enhancing the energy. To avoid this, sound rooms used for hearing testing attempt to absorb the sound energy rather than reflecting it. Also, the typical stimulus is not a pure tone, but either a tone that changes frequency slightly over time (a **frequency-modulated tone**) or a band of noise with energy in one concentrated frequency region (band-pass noise).

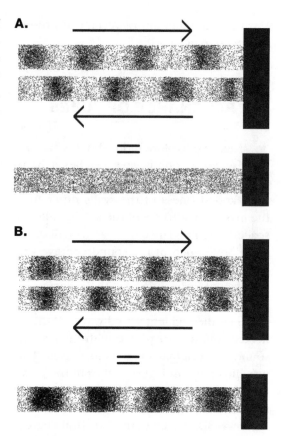

Figure 5–5. Illustration of destructive interference (**A**) when a sound wave reflects back out of phase, and constructive interference (**B**) when the sound wave reflects in phase.

Resonance of a Tube Closed at One End

Of particular interest is the resonance produced by a closed tube or cavity; that is, a tube opened on one end so that a sound can enter, but closed on the other end. (Closed tubes are things such as the ear canal, which ends at the eardrum, and the vocal tract, which is closed at the vibrating vocal folds and open at the mouth.) If we introduce a sound into a closed tube, we are setting the column of air that fills the tube into vibration. The frequency that best sets the column of air in a closed tube into vibration (the resonant frequency) is one whose wavelength is four times as long as the tube. (Said another way, the tube length is one-quarter the resonant frequency sound's wavelength.) Another equally good frequency is the second harmonic, which is the frequency that has a wavelength three-quarters the size of the tube. Let's examine why.

At the closed end of the tube, the sound cannot continue to propagate the vibration; it has to be reflected back. When the sound reflects, it does so 180 degrees out of phase. As shown in Figure 5-6, when the barrier is at this precise location, three-quarter wavelengths through the incident wave, something interesting happens to the sum of the

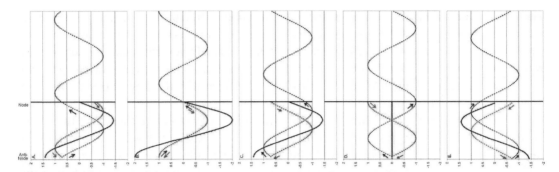

Figure 5-6. This figure shows how a sound travels and is reflected in a closed-at-one end tube. The phase of the waves are shown on the horizontal axis and the sound wave's amplitude of displacement is on the vertical axis. The vertical line represents a barrier, like the closed end of a tube. The longest sine wave shows the original, or incident signal, as if it were passing through the barrier. If the sound does not pass through the barrier, it is reflected back 180 degrees out of phase, as shown by the direction of the arrow next to the reflected wave. The sum of the two is shown with the thicker line. The combined incident and reflected wave alternates between building to double its amplitude and canceling out. (**A**) through (**E**) show the wave going through various phases of vibration. Note that the sum of the reflected and incident wave is always zero at the location of the barrier. That is a vibration node. The summed wave is varying most at the far left. That is a vibration antinode.

reflected and incident wave. This summed wave does not vary in amplitude at the end of the tube: it is always at zero amplitude, it is cancelled out at that point. Just as the string in Figure 5-4 has a node of vibration, so does the sine wave in the ear canal. The greatest amount of vibration of the summed wave is at the far left side of the figure. In the case of the ear canal, the barrier is the eardrum, and the far left side of the figure represents the location of the ear canal opening.

Let's look at Figure 5-6 in more detail. Part (D) is the easiest figure to see that the reflected wave is 180 degrees out of phase from the incoming (incident) wave. Look at (A). The incident sound wave entering the "ear canal" is at 135 degrees of phase. (Note that it has passed the 90 degree phase mark and the sine wave is "coming down.") The length of the ear canal is three-quarters of the sound wavelength, so the sine wave hits the barrier (the eardrum) 270 degrees later (270 is three-quarters of 360). Adding 270 to the starting phase of 135 equals 405 de-

grees, which is 45 degrees into the next sine wave cycle. The sine of 45 degrees is 0.707. That's the amplitude of the sine wave when it "hits" the barrier. The reflected wave is 180 degrees out of phase, so it is at 225 degrees. The sine of 225 degrees is –0.707. The summed wave at that reflection point is zero. There is cancellation at the eardrum, which is a node of vibration. At the opening of the ear canal, the summed wave is 1.414.

In Figure 5-6B, the incident wave starts at 90 degrees. At the eardrum it is at 360 degrees. The reflected wave is at 180 degrees. Of course, the sine of both 180 degrees and 360 degrees is zero. The reflected wave is in phase, and the sine wave of the combined incident and reflected wave is double that of the original. As you scan through the different sections of the figure, notice that the largest amplitude is always at the opening of the ear canal.

The sum of the reflected and incident waveforms from each of Figure 5-6 segments (A) through (E) are combined and shown in

Figure 5-7. The overlapping of the waves at these different moments in time show that the summed wave always cancels out at the reflecting, closed end, at the node of vibration. The summed incident/reflected wave is always greatest in amplitude at the opening. The standing wave created looks similar to the vibrating string. Had more phases been illustrated, the resemblance would be even greater. You would see the same standing wave pattern if you have a frequency with a wavelength that is one-quarter the size of

the tube. (Though the illustrations are easier to understand using the three-quarter wavelength.) The lowest resonant frequency is the one with the one-quarter wavelength. We would term that the first harmonic frequency. The second harmonic frequency is the one that has the wavelength that is 4/3 the size of the tube. Said another way, three-quarters of the wavelength of that second harmonic frequency is the tube length. Figure 5-8 shows these two frequencies. There are more as well. The third harmonic frequency would have a wavelength 5/4 the size of the tube. Now, let's examine what would happen if we keep the sound wave frequency the same, and make the tube length shorter. That is, let's move the location of the barrier, as shown in Figure 5-9. There is still summation and cancellation of the sound, but the barrier is not a node of vibration. This is also seen in Figure

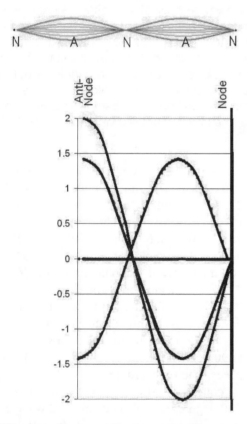

Figure 5–7. The vibration pattern of a standing wave on a string is again illustrated at the top. The sum of the reflected waves shown in Figure 5-6 is superimposed. Note the node of vibration at the reflected barrier, the eardrum, and the antinode to the left, representing the location of the ear canal entrance. Resonance occurs when you have this standing wave vibration pattern.

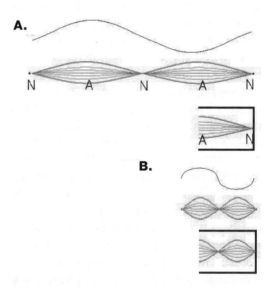

Figure 5–8. A. The first harmonic frequency has a wavelength that is four times the size of the tube. The antinode of vibration is at the opening of the tube. **B.** A sound with a wavelength 4/3 the size of the tube also resonates. That is the second harmonic frequency.

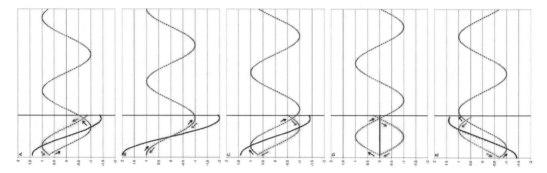

Figure 5–9. The sine wave frequency, and thus wavelength, remains the same as illustrated in Figure 5–6, but the location of the barrier has changed. As the barrier is not at one-quarter or three-quarters of the sound wavelength, a standing wave is not created. Note that there is no node of vibration at the barrier.

5-10, where the summed waves from Figure 5-9 are illustrated on top of each other.

Let us look at an example of calculating the first resonant frequency of a tube closed at one end.

Suppose we have a tube whose length is 1.5 inches (about the size of the ear canal). The column of air in that tube will resonate to a sound frequency that has a wavelength of 4 × 1.5, or 6.0 inches (one-half foot). (We are looking for the frequency that has 1/4 of the wavelength equal to the tube size, which is 1.5 inches, so we multiply the tube length by four.) Recall that wavelength is equal to the speed of sound divided by the frequency. Thus, in this example, the resonant frequency is the number that, when divided into 1100 (the speed of sound is 1100 ft/sec), will equal 6 inches (0.5 ft). (Six inches is four times the distance of the tube.)

$$0.5 = 1100/f$$
$$0.5f = 1100$$
$$f = 2200 \text{ Hz.}$$

Thus, a 1.5-inch column of air will vibrate best to a sound that has the frequency of 2200 Hz. The resonant frequency of a 1.5-inch closed tube is 2200 Hz.

Resonance of a Tube Closed at Both Ends

The resonance of a tube closed at both ends (such as an ear canal closed because of an inserted hearing aid) is different (Figure 5-11). The resonance occurs when the node is at each of the two ends. This situation occurs when we have the zero and 180 degrees of phase points at the tube ends. This can occur either when the tube size corresponds to one-half the resonating sound's wavelength or the full wavelength (or 1.5 wavelengths, etc.). The resonant harmonic frequencies of a closed tube occur at even multiples of the fundamental.

Let's look at another example. Assume there is one-half inch between the end of the hearing aid and the eardrum. What is the lowest frequency that will resonate? One that has a wavelength of 1 inch, which is 0.0833 feet. What frequency is this? Using the formula frequency = speed of sound / wavelength

$$\text{Resonant frequency}$$
$$= 1100 \text{ ft/sec} / 0.0833 \text{ feet}$$
$$= 13,205 \text{ Hz}$$

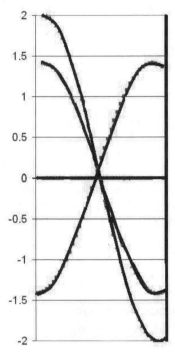

Figure 5–10. The summed reflected and incident waveforms from Figure 5–9 are combined to illustrate that when the tube length is not one-quarter or three-quarters the wavelength, we don't create a node of vibration at the tube end, nor an antinode at the opening. This is not the resonant frequency.

The resonant frequency has been shifted up dramatically from the 2200 Hz resonant frequency of the open ear canal calculated earlier. The original resonant frequency has been destroyed by inserting the hearing aid

SUMMARY

This chapter has discussed impedance. Impedance comes partially from the frictional component, which remains the same for a given medium, regardless of frequency. The mass reactance of the system limits high-frequency sound transmission, and conversely

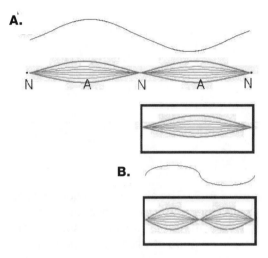

Figure 5–11. Tubes closed at both ends resonate when the node is located at each barrier. As shown in (**A**), this can occur when the sound has a wavelength that is twice as long as the barrier. (**B**) Resonance can also occur when the barrier length equals the wavelength, as this also creates the situation where the node of vibration is at the barriers.

stiffness reactance prevents low-frequency sound transmission. The frequency at which the total reactance is at its minimum is the resonant frequency. At that frequency the mass and stiffness reactance values balance out, and transmission is limited by the frictional component so the total impedance is lowest at that frequency.

We have also seen that, for columns of air, the length of the column of air affects the resonant frequency. The longer the tube, the lower the resonant frequency. Closing the tube at just one end, the lowest resonant frequency is the frequency with wavelength four times the size of the tube. If the tube is closed at both ends, look for the frequency with wavelength twice that of the tube length.

Sound travels between two media best when each has equal impedance. The greater the difference in the impedance of the two media, the less sound is transmitted (the more is reflected away). This has significance in hearing science as airborne sound needs to be conducted into the fluids of the inner ear; this impedance mismatch creates a 30 dB loss in signal power.

6

Electricity and Analog Systems

Physiologic processes that occur in the inner ear, auditory nerve, and the brain are electrochemical in nature. For this reason it is necessary to comprehend some basic concepts related to electricity if one is to understand how the auditory system works. However, for purposes of this text, it is not necessary to go beyond the simple relationship of voltage, current, and resistance.

The information in this chapter also forms the basis for understanding the electronic equipment used by audiologists. Hearing aids and audiometers use electricity and have analog systems.

ELECTRON FLOW

You may recall from basic chemistry that neutrally charged atoms have an equal number of positively charged protons and negatively charged electrons. Different elements have different numbers of protons and electrons. For example, the simplest atom (hydrogen) has only one proton and one electron, whereas gold has 79 protons and 79 electrons. Depending on the arrangement of electrons (in motion around the nucleus), some atoms may rather easily "lose" electrons to other atoms, or "pick up" electrons that are loose. The positively charged

protons are located in the nucleus of the atom and cannot be readily separated from it. Therefore, whether an atom is **positively charged** or **negatively charged** depends on whether it has the proper number of electrons.

The notion of **electrical charge** is related directly to electrons. If there is an excess of electrons (more electrons than protons in an atom), the atom is negatively charged. If there is a deficit of electrons (fewer electrons than protons in an atom), the atom is positively charged. The magnitude of the charge depends on two things: how many electrons each atom has lost or gained, and how many of those charged atoms are present in a given space.

As nature always seeks a balance, there is a tendency for these "out-of-balance" atoms to seek a rebalanced or equilibrium state. Therefore, atoms with a deficit of electrons will attract electrons, and atoms with an excess of electrons will freely give them up. The greater the charge, that is, the greater the disparity of electrons, the greater the potential for electrons to move in seeking equilibrium. Thus, the magnitude of the charge can be expressed as the **potential** for electron movement or flow. The magnitude of this potential is expressed in units called volts (V). The volt, then, is a statement of potential electron flow. The potential can be stated in positive or negative units depending on whether the atoms in question have a deficit or an excess of electrons. If there is a deficit of electrons, there are more positively charged protons than negatively charged electrons, and a positive charge exists. If there is an excess of electrons, a negative charge exists. Whether the point in question (object being measured) is positive or negative is a relative matter. For example, in Figure 6-1, point A is 10 volts negative relative to point B, point C is 10 volts positive relative to point B, point C is 20 volts positive relative to point A, point B is 10 volts negative relative to point C, point B is 10 volts positive relative to point A, and point A is 20 volts negative relative to point C.

As already mentioned, nature (if unimpeded) always seeks equilibrium, and an unbalanced condition will result in electron flow from the negative (where there is an excess of electrons) to the positive (where there is a deficit of electrons) until the atoms are again in a balanced state. The greater the electron excess or deficit, the greater will be the force to equalize. Again, the measurement of this force represents the magnitude of the potential in volts.

The electron flow that results from this potential is called **current**, and the **ampere** (or **amp**) is the unit of measure of the *rate* of current or electron flow. Obviously, the larger the potential, the higher the rate of flow, if all other things are equal.

OHM'S LAW

In order to maintain a voltage of any significant magnitude, one must provide an opposition to electron flow. Otherwise, electrons will move freely and rapidly from negative to positive until equalization occurs. The rate of flow, then, is determined by (a) the magnitude of the potential and (b) the amount of opposition to electron flow, called resistance. The unit of measurement of resistance is the **ohm**, sometimes noted as Ω, the Greek symbol for omega. In simple situations the entire opposition is made up of resistance. The relationship between potential, current and resistance is expressed by Ohm's law, which states that the rate of electron flow (current) is equal to the potential (voltage) divided by the opposition (resistance), or:

$$\text{Current (I, in amps)} = \frac{\text{Potential (E, in volts)}}{\text{Resistance (R, in ohms)}}.$$

Consider the following examples:
Example 1: What is the current when 120 volts are applied to 60 ohms?

$$I = E/R = 120 \text{ volts}/60 \text{ ohms} = 2 \text{ amps}$$

Example 2: What is the current when 120 volts are applied to 120 ohms?

$$I = E/R = 120 \text{ volts}/120 \text{ ohms} = 1 \text{ amp}$$

Example 3: What is the current when 120 volts are applied to 240 ohms?

$$I = E/R = 120 \text{ volts}/240 \text{ ohms} = 0.5 \text{ amps}$$

At a constant voltage, current decreases as resistance increase, and increases as resistance decreases; thus it is possible to regulate the current by varying the resistance.

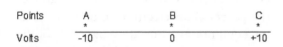

Points	A	B	C
	*	*	*
Volts	-10	0	+10

Figure 6–1. Illustration of the relative voltage difference between points. For example, point B is 10 volts more positive than point A.

A high-power hearing aid might use 0.9 mA (milliamps) of current. A lower power hearing aid might only use 0.3 mA. The same size battery (a source of electrons) would last only one-third the time in the high-power hearing aid.

ELECTRICAL CIRCUITS

When a potential is present, when there is a path through which electrons can flow, and when there is some opposition to electron flow in that path, one is said to have an **electrical circuit**. We can schematically represent a simple circuit as shown in Figure 6–2A. The symbol between (*a*) and (*f*) is standard for a battery. Electrons leaving the negative pole of the battery (*a*) must travel through the wire (*b*). The symbol between (*c*) and (*d*) is for a resistor. The electrons flow through this resistor and then through the wire (*e*) in order to return to the positive pole of the battery (*f*).

Figure 6–2B includes the actual values of the battery and resistor, and illustrates a switch in the circuit. When the switch is open (off), the path (circuit) is broken and there is no electron flow. When the switch is closed (on), the circuit is complete and electrons flow at the rate of 2 amps ($I = E/R = 12/6 = 2$). The current that flows when the switch is toggled on twice is illustrated in Figure 6–3A.

Now suppose we substitute a **variable resistor** (such as the volume knob on a radio) for the fixed value of resistance in this circuit (Figure 6–2C). We can then continuously vary the amount of opposition with a resulting fluctuation in current. If the resistor is continuously varied back and forth between 6 and 24 ohms, the current would vary back and forth between 0.5 and 2.0 amps as shown in Figure 6–3B. What we have here is a direct current (in the sense that electron flow is always in the same direction) but one which is alternating in the rate of flow. The rate of flow is increasing and decreasing. If we draw a line (light horizontal line in Figure 6–3B) at the center of the fluctuation, it is obvious that the rate of flow is varying around some midpoint, that is, 1.25 amps in the example. In electrophysiologic studies, this type of variation is sometimes described as **alternating current (AC)** even though the electron flow never actually reverses direction. (In AC electrical circuits, the electron flow direction does alternate. The power company is pushing and pulling electrons through the electronic device.)

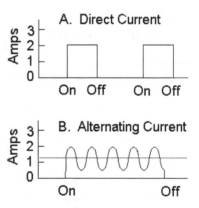

Figure 6–3. Illustration of current in (**A**) a direct current circuit, and (**B**) in a circuit where an alternation is superimposed on a direct current.

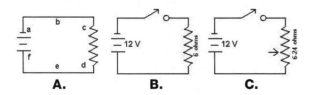

Figure 6–2. Schematic diagram of three simple DC (battery operated) circuits.

ION FLOW

Knowledge of current and potential helps in understanding cochlear physiology, because there are biological chemical potentials in the inner ear. In physiology, ion flow rather than electron flow may occur. An ion is a particle that is electrically unbalanced. If it is a positive ion, it has fewer electrons than protons; if a negative ion, it has more electrons than protons. Although protons are not free to leave the atom (as electrons may be), positive ion flow can result from the movement of positive ions in which the entire atom moves. That is, positively charged or negatively charged ions can move across a resistive membrane or barrier. The laws governing ion flow are similar to those governing electron flow. For example, there will be less ion flow if the membrane has greater resistance.

COMMON ANALOG COMPONENTS

Analog electronic acoustic systems create an electrical signal that mimics the sound waveform. For example, if the sound is a 1000-Hz pure tone, then within the circuit, electrons will be moving back and forth 1000 times per second, and the variation in the current flow will look just like the sine wave. The word analog comes from analogous—the movement of electrons in the circuit is directly analogous to the sound wave motion.

An acoustic system typically consists of a microphone to convert the sound to an electrical signal, an amplifier to make it a stronger signal, and a speaker of some form to convert it back into sound. The system may also filter the signal, that is, change its spectrum by reducing energy at some frequency components. We will discuss these various components, starting with an overview of the function of the amplifier. (Chapter 8 provides more information on hearing science equipment.)

The electronic device used to make sound louder is called an **amplifier**. However, the sound must first be converted into electricity. The electricity can then be fed into an amplifier, increased by some decibel level in the amplifier, and sent to a device, which converts it back to sound. The resultant **gain** in sound energy is the decibel difference between the level of the sound leaving the amplifier and the level entering the amplifier. Output minus input equals gain. In physics, it is not possible to get something for nothing and the "gain" in energy has to come from somewhere. It comes from the battery if the system is battery operated, or from an electrical outlet if operated by ordinary house current.

A good quality (high fidelity) amplifier increases the intensity of a sound without changing it in any other way; that is, it does not change the frequencies nor otherwise distort the sound.

Microphones

The first step, the conversion of sound energy to electrical energy, is the function of the microphone. As this can be done in several ways, there are several different types of microphones (see Chapter 8). The one thing they all have in common is that they depend on sound energy to move the diaphragm of the microphone. The diaphragm is a thin, light sheet that moves in response to the changes in air pressure from the sound wave. Movement of the diaphragm in the microphone produces a current that mimics the sound wave. If the sound at the microphone diaphragm is a 2000-Hz pure tone, then the electrons in the wire will be flowing back and forth 2000 times per second. The amount of flow will change gradually over time in proportion to the amplitude of the sine wave. This merits a little further thought. Chapter 4 described the trigonometry behind the sine wave. The sine of a 30 degree angle is .5; the sine of 45 degrees is .707. Let's assume for a moment that the 2000-Hz sine wave was large enough to produce a change in voltage that ranged from +1 volt (at 90 degrees of phase) down to –1 volt (at 270 degrees of phase). When the sine wave in front of the diaphragm is at 30 degrees phase, the voltage will be 0.5 volts (the sine of the angle times the maximum voltage). When the sine wave reaches 45 degrees of phase, the voltage will be 0.707 volts.

Amplifiers

Most amplification is achieved by using electronic devices called **transistors**. Transistors are made of a **semiconductor** material, which allows electrons to pass, but which provides a high resistance to their passage. A transistor used as an amplifier consists of three components: an **emitter**, a **collector**, and a **base** (Figure 6-4). Am-

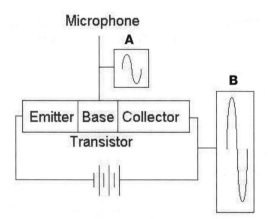

Figure 6–4. The use of a transistor as an amplifier. The small alternating current from the microphone (**A**) causes a large alternating current in the transistor circuit (**B**).

plification is accomplished by using a small voltage to control a larger voltage. This is possible because unlike charges attract and like charges repel. Electrons (which are negative) are in excess at the negative pole of the battery and are attracted to the positive pole of the battery. However, in order to get there, they must pass through the transistor. The polarity of the transistor base influences the rate at which electrons pass through the transistor on their way from the negative to the positive pole of the battery. These electrons will continue through the base of the collector and on to the positive pole of the battery. If the base is made negative, it will reduce electron flow by repelling electrons trying to move from the negative pole through the transistor (like charges repel). This reduces the number of electrons reaching the positive pole of the battery.

The electrical power (P) in a circuit is equal to the voltage (E) times the current (I); that is, P = EI. Furthermore, Ohm's law tells us that E= IR; that voltage is equal to the current times the resistance (R). If E=IR, then P = EI can also be written as P = IRI, or P = I^2R. As noted above, transistors are semiconductors and have a high resistance. As power equals the current squared times the resistance, the power output of a transistor can be high when only a small voltage is applied. In Figure 6-4 note that the small alternating current (A) from the microphone applied to the base of the transistor results in a large alternating current (B) through the transistor.

There is a limit to how much amplification a single transistor can produce. If one tries to obtain too much gain, the transistor is overdriven which causes distortion. When high levels of amplification are needed, the output from one transistor is fed into the input of the next for as many stages of amplification as are needed to achieve the desired gain.

Filters

Because hearing-impaired people often have worse hearing for some frequencies than others, hearing aids need to amplify some frequencies more than others. Analog filters reduce the amplitude of the sound energy that is at a frequency where high gain is not desired, so that the sound frequencies that we do want amplified are increased in intensity. Diagrams of filters show the reduction in the sound energy that the filtering will create. As shown in Figure 6-5, this filter does not reduce energy that has a frequency above 1000 Hz. It reduces energy at 500 Hz by 15 dB, and energy at 250 Hz by

30 dB. Note that the decrease in the energy that can pass through the filter between the octave of 250 and 500 Hz is 15 dB. This filter would be said to have a **rejection slope** of 15 dB per octave. This filter is called a **high-pass filter**, which is synonymous with **low-cut filter**.

Figure 6-6 illustrates a 24-dB/octave **low-pass** or **high-cut filter** with a "cutoff" frequency of 1000 Hz. Two other filter types are common: band-pass and band-reject. Figure 6-7 shows **band-pass filters.** Only a limited range of frequencies is transmitted. Conversely the band-reject filter (Figure 6-8) allows all frequencies to pass except those in a certain range. **Band-reject** or **notch filters** aren't used very often in audiology applications. One exception is the 60-Hz band-reject filter. AC power supplies run on 60-Hz

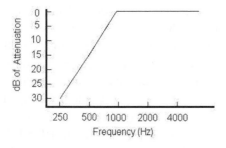

Figure 6–5. Illustration of a high-pass filter with a cutoff at 1000 Hz and 15-dB/octave rejection slope. Frequencies above 1000 Hz are passed at full amplitude. Below 1000 Hz, amplitudes are reduced at a rate of 15 dB per octave.

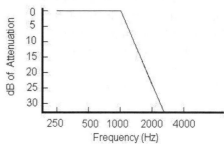

Figure 6–6. Ilustration of a low-pass filter with a cutoff at 1000 Hz and 24-dB/octave rejection slope.

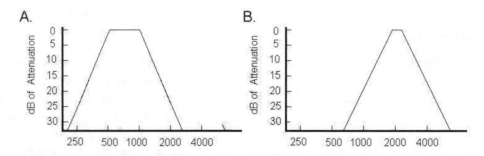

Figure 6–7. A. Illustration of a band-pass filter with cutoffs at 500 and 1000 Hz and 24-dB/octave rejection slopes. **B.** This is a one-third octave band-pass filter centered at 2000 Hz.

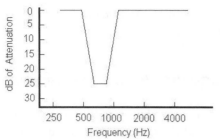

Figure 6–8. Illustration of a band-reject or notch filter centered at 707 Hz (one-half octave above 500 Hz).

electron flow (in North America). If this signal crosses into the audio signal, one may hear a buzzing sound that comes from the 60-Hz sound, and its harmonics. A 60-Hz notch filter reduces that distortion.

Band-pass or band-reject filters may be described by their center frequency and width, rather than the upper and lower cutoff frequencies. For example, a filter that is centered at 1000 Hz and is two octaves wide ranges from 500 Hz to 2000 Hz. A one-octave wide filter would range from 707 Hz to 1414 Hz

Calculating Filter Cutoff Frequencies

If a filter is one-octave wide, centered at 1000 Hz, then it extends from one-half octave below 1000 Hz to one-half octave above. The formula for octave calculations is:

$$F_c = Fo \times 2^{\text{octaves up or down}}$$

where Fc is the cutoff frequency, Fo is the original frequency (e.g., the center frequency of the one-octave wide filter) and that is multiplied by 2 raised to the power of the number of octaves up or down that is desired. Example 1. One-half octave below 1000 Hz is:

$$F_c = 1000 \text{ Hz} \times 2^{-.5}$$
$$= 1000 \text{ Hz} \times .707$$
$$= 707 \text{ Hz}$$

Example 2. One-half octave above 1000 Hz is:

$$F_c = 1000 \text{ Hz} \times 2^{.5}$$
$$= 1000 \text{ Hz} \times 1.414$$
$$= 1414 \text{ Hz}$$

Cutoff Frequencies Defined at 3-dB Down Points

The figures above show idealized (theoretical) filters. In reality, the pass-band of an analog filter is not perfectly flat, nor are the corner points either perfectly angled or perfectly rounded. Because of these two realities, the cutoff points of a real filter refer to frequencies where the signal is attenuated by 3 dB—that is, the frequencies at which the energy is 3 dB less than in the pass band (Figure 6–9). Recall that 3 dB loss of power is equal to one-half the power of the signal, so the filter cutoff frequency shows you the frequency where the power is reduced by that amount.

Speakers

The speaker is the device for converting the amplified electrical energy back to sound. Like microphones, speakers come in a variety of types. However, the most common type is based on using the electrical output from the amplifier to vary a magnetic field causing a **cone** (or diaphragm) to move. The cone has magnets in it, so it moves when the magnetic field changes. Movement of the cone sets particles of air in front of the cone into motion, producing sound. Speakers come in all shapes and sizes. Small ones mounted in headbands for wearing over the ears are called **earphones**. Miniaturized speakers developed for hearing aids are called **receivers.**

Large speakers with large cones (**woofers**) are more effective at producing low-fre-

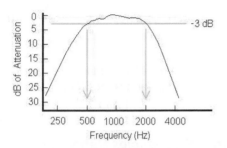

Figure 6–9. Actual filters typically have some irregularity in the pass-band. The nominal cutoff frequency for the filter is where the energy is 3 dB below peak. This bandpass filter is two octaves wide, with the 3 dB down cutoff points at 500 and 2000 Hz.

quency sounds whereas small speakers with small cones (**tweeters**) are more effective at producing high frequencies. Good quality stereo sound systems often use a number of different sized speakers, including a **midrange** speaker.

Transducers

Transducers change one form of energy to another form of energy. A microphone is a transducer, and a speaker is also a transducer. The microphone changes sound energy into electrical energy; the speaker changes electrical energy to sound energy.

Volume Controls

Most volume controls are special forms of variable resistors They usually consist of a rotary knob that increases resistance when turned one way and decreases resistance when turned the other. Recall that, according to Ohm's law, current decreases as resistance increases and vice versa. Thus, decreasing or increasing the resistance of the circuit can vary the output from the amplifi-

er. This results in more or less sound energy at the speaker.

Frequency Response Controls

Controls that vary the filtering of a circuit, and thus change the amount of sound energy at the different frequencies, alter the system's frequency response and are referred to as **tone** controls or **frequency response controls** They work by splitting the signal into frequency regions and then adding resistance to one or another of these frequency regions. For example, a circuit that emphasizes high frequencies does so by attenuating (adding resistance to) low frequencies, and a circuit that emphasizes low frequencies does so by attenuating (adding resistance to) the high frequencies. In effect, tone controls emphasize some frequencies by de-emphasizing the rest.

Figure 6–10 puts the above components into the simplified circuit of a hearing aid. Sound energy is picked up by the microphone (*1*, with a built-in preamplifier), which converts it to electricity. This electricity is applied to the base of the transistor, which regulates the current flow through the amplifier (*2*, the symbol for a transistor). The amplified electrical current output of the amplifier is increased or decreased by the volume control (*3*, a variable resistor). From the volume control the signal passes through the filter (*4*) that enhances the high or low pitches. (This is not a standard symbol for a filter but shows that an analog filter is made up of a resistor and a capacitor, shown by the symbol below the number *4*. A **capacitor** is an electronic component that blocks (resists) the flow of direct current.) The signal then arrives at the speaker (*5*, which would be called a receiver in a hearing aid) where it is converted back to sound. The battery (*6*) provides the power source for the energy gain.

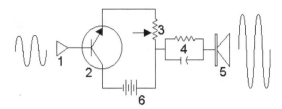

Figure 6–10. A simplified schematic of an analog hearing aid. See the text for a description of components and functions.

SUMMARY

Analog circuits, such as hearing aids and audiometers, have two transducers: a microphone and a speaker. They contain an amplifier to increase the signal voltage.

Hearing aids filter out the amplification at frequencies where the added gain is not desired.

Analog circuits keep the signal in electric form. Within the circuit, electrons are alternating back and forth, just as the sound waveform causes the microphone diaphragm to move back and forth.

Some electronics principles of electron flow are similar to the rules for ionic flow. Negatively charged chemical particles will be attracted to positively charged ones, just as a source of free electrons is drawn to the positive pole of the battery. Resistors control the rate of flow of electrons in a circuit. Within the body, membranes function to resist the flow of ions.

7

Digital Systems and Digital Signal Processing

Chapter 6 highlighted the features of analog systems. The outer ear, middle ear, and inner ear are analog systems. The cochlea in the inner ear has a form of a microphone; it operates on ionic potentials and has a form of a variable resistor. When the cochlea has done its job, neurons fire. The neuron's firing is "all or nothing"—either a neural potential is created and a signal is sent to the next neuron in the chain, or else the signal is not large enough and the nerve doesn't fire. Thus, in this one sense, the auditory neural system is analogous to a digital system. Digital systems operate by transmitting signals that are coded by 1 and 0 signals, where 1 represents "on" and 0, "off."

The equipment used by audiologists is increasingly digital, but will always have analog components. By changing electrical energy into digital signals, computers and computer chips can readily process the sound waves. This allows different forms of sound conditioning than available with analog systems, and allows us to more precisely control things that analog systems also do, such as filtering.

BITS AND SAMPLING RATES

Whereas analog systems have electrons moving back and forth within the circuit, digital systems transmit numbers. This section describes how digital systems use groupings of 1's and 0's (**binary numbers**) to represent signal frequency and intensity. We will examine the process of **digitization**, the representing of an analog signal, such as the output of a microphone, with numbers.

How Big Is That?

The digital number describing the amplitude of a voltage is composed of a series (a combination) of zeros and ones. By combining series of these zeros and ones together, the digital system can represent sizes other than just 0 and 1. The number of **bits** tells you how many series of zeros and ones are used to describe amplitude. The number of bits is the exponent in 2^n. The number of zeroes/ones is the answer to 2^n. For example, if two bits are used (2^2), then the amplitude of the signal could be described as being one of four size steps: 00, 01, 10, or 11. That would be like measuring something with a ruler that only allows four measurements, without your being able to interpolate the size. If our "ruler" is three bits, we can have eight steps ($2^3 = 8$). The possible amplitudes are digital numbers 000, 001, 010, 011,100, 101, 110, and 111.

Figure 7-1 (A and C) illustrate 5-bit quantization; whereas (B) and (D) show 3-bit resolution. In the early days of digital systems, the accurate representation of amplitude was more of a problem than it is today. Technology advances now allow us to use very accurate amplitude resolution (e.g., 16-bits, with 65,536 different amplitude measurements), even in devices powered with hearing aid batteries. A 16-bit system will **sample**, that is, measure, the amplitude to create a **word** that is made up of these 16 0's or 1's.

How Often Should Amplitude Be Measured?

Another issue in the accuracy of the digitizing (measuring) system is how often the amplitude is sampled (measured). The time waveform shown in Figures 7-1C and 7-1D is measured only 12 times during the duration of this signal; each measurement is presumed to be correct until the next measure is taken. The characteristics of the sound wave are not being well represented. When the sine waveform is sampled more often, as shown in Figures 7-1A and 7-1B, the shape of the underlying sound wave becomes more evident, though it is still somewhat misrepresented. An even faster sampling rate would yield better results.

Figure 7–1. A. The waveform (*smoothed line*) is digitized with a 5-bit quantizer, giving 2^5 or 32 possible amplitude steps. It has a relatively high sampling rate, giving many samples in the timeframe shown. **B.** The signal is sampled at the same rate, but with a 3-bit quantizer, creating greater digitization error. **C.** A 5-bit quantizer with a slow sampling rate also creates digitization error. **D.** With a slow rate and 3-bit quantization, even more error is introduced.

Digitization rate is the number of samples taken in one second of time. Said another way, digitization rate is the frequency at

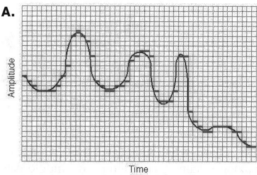

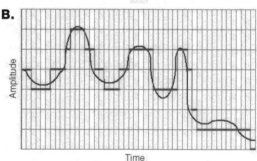

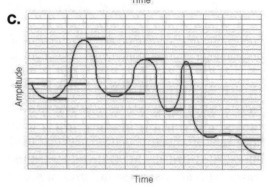

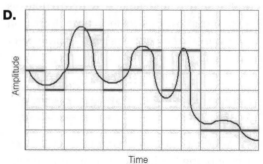

which the samples are measured as a sound wave is converted into digital format (as it is **digitized**). If a sound wave amplitude is measured 16,000 times per second, then the digitization rate is 16,000 Hz. Audio CDs use a sampling rate of 44,100 samples per second. At this writing, 32,000 Hz is a common sampling rate for hearing aids, as is 20,000 Hz.

Building an Analogy to Use Later

The nervous system conveys information in a digital-like format. Either a neural impulse is sent, or it is not sent. After a neuron fires, there is a recovery time before the neuron can fire again. It is as if the neuron that will code for the presence of sound has a slow sampling rate.

As the neuron either fires or it doesn't, each neuron acting individually sends a one-bit signal. However, there are many different neurons within the auditory system. If we examine the firing of three neurons, either one, two, or three neurons may have fired. Although it is tempting to extend the analogy further, to say that there are eight combinations of firings of the neurons, it is not helpful. There is no evidence that the auditory system uses information about which neuron is firing in quite that specific a manner. However, there are classes of neurons, some of which are harder to stimulate. That feature of auditory neural coding will be explored in Chapters 21 and 22. For now, just remember that a neuron has only a 1-bit choice: it fires or it doesn't.

ADDITIONAL DIGITIZATION CONCEPTS

Analog to Digital Converters

The component that measures (samples) the analog signal and turns it into a digital number is the **analog to digital converter (ADC)** (also called **A to D converter**). As discussed above, ADCs vary in their sampling rate and their bit size.

Early ADCs made sequential (step-by-step) judgments about the signal intensity. For example, let's say the voltage that the ADC can measure ranges from +5 volts to –5 volts and the ADC has 2-bit resolution. Remember that means there are only four (2^2) 0/1 digits to represent the signal amplitude at each moment in time. Let's assume that the measurement to be digitized is 3.1 volts. The first decision the older style ADC would make is whether the signal is above or below 0 volts, the midpoint of the +/–5 volt range. In this case, the 3.1 volt signal is above 0. That would be coded by the first value being a 1 rather than a 0. The next digit would be used to record whether the signal is at the upper or lower half of the remaining range: is it above or below +2.5 volts? Here the 3.1-volt signal is above the +2.5 volt dividing point, so the second digital amplitude value is also a 1. The remaining range is 2.5 volts to 5.0 volts, and the halfway point is 3.75 volts. The 3.1-volt signal is lower than 3.75 volts, so the third value is a 0. Lastly, we compare whether the voltage falls from 2.5 to 3.125 volts or from 3.125 volts to 3.75 volts. As it is in the upper range, the last digital value is 1. This signal's digital representation is thus "1 1 0 1."

Engineers found that this was an inefficient way to measure, or **quantize** the amplitude of the signal. For example, a 16-bit ADC has to make 16 decisions for each sample, always starting with asking if the signal is above or below zero volts. In the real world, the next sample is going to be close in amplitude to that of the one before it. That is particularly true with the high-speed sampling typically used today. Therefore, a better way is to examine the most recent data point, and see if the amplitude is now above or below that level. It's a more efficient, more exact, way of coding amplitude. A high sampling rate is used, and the system is determining whether the signal measured has increased or decreased since the last measurement. The type of ADC that uses this logic is called a **sigma delta ADC**, which has the Greek symbols ΣΔ. This is now the industry standard for A to D conversion.

Nyquist Frequency

The sampling rate not only affects the accuracy of the representation of the signal, it also limits the highest signal frequency that can be recorded. For example, if the ADC measured the signal amplitude 1000 times per second, and a 1000-Hz signal were present, only one data point would be recorded for each cycle. That's clearly not enough to tell about the signal frequency (Figure 7–2).

To be able to conduct a spectral analysis of a signal, at least two samples must be taken for every cycle of the wave. This principle leads us to the concept of the **Nyquist frequency**. One-half the sampling rate used in digitizing the sound wave is the Nyquist

frequency, and the Nyquist frequency is the highest frequency signal that can be analyzed. For example, if the sampling rate is 44,100 Hz (the rate for compact disk (CD) sampling), then the Nyquist frequency is 22,050 Hz, and frequencies higher than this cannot be accurately represented.

Aliasing

If a signal that is higher than the Nyquist frequency is digitized, a problem occurs. The digitization creates **aliasing**, the false recording of a low-frequency signal rather than the true high-frequency signal. Figure 7–3 illustrates this.

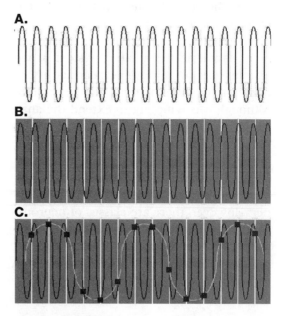

Figure 7–3. A. A high-frequency waveform is shown. **B.** Only 14 of the points on the black waveform are measured, illustrated here as if the waveform is only seen in the brief periods shown by the vertical white bars. **C.** The result is that it appears that a different frequency pure tone is present—here the lower frequency wave shown in white. An "alias" (false identity) of the original signal is digitized.

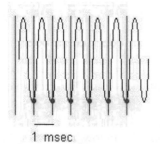

1 msec

Figure 7–2. This 1000-Hz signal (with its 1-msec period) is sampled with a 1000-Hz sampling rate. A sample is measured (*dots*) each millisecond (*vertical lines*). The presence of the signal is not detected, instead the ADC would instead record that a large negative DC signal is present.

Antialiasing Filtering

To prevent aliasing, before the waveform is digitized, the frequencies above the Nyquist need to be filtered out using an analog filter, so those high frequencies can't become misrepresented. Most of the time this filter is built into the ADC. For audiology applications, the microphone may act as the anti-aliasing filter. If the microphone doesn't respond to high-frequency sounds (above the Nyquist), then they cannot be digitized.

DIGITAL TO ANALOG CONVERTERS

Eventually, the signal must return to analog form if it is to be heard. The **digital to analog converter (DAC)** performs this task. DACs, like ADCs, have a bit rate and a sampling rate.

Imaging

When the digitized signal is reconverted into an audio signal, it has some irregularities in it (Figure 7–4A (stair-step lines). These stair-steps are rapid changes, and a signal that changes rapidly is a high-frequency signal. A signal with this irregularity has a high pitched sound superimposed—it sounds artificial and tinny.

Anti-imaging Filters

In order to smooth out the waveform to prevent imaging, the signal is sent through an analog low-pass (high-cut) filter (Figure 7–4B). This is called the **anti-imaging** filter. It may be a part of the DAC itself. In hearing aid applications, if the hearing aid speaker (receiver) doesn't transmit high frequencies well, it will serve the same purpose as the anti-imaging filter.

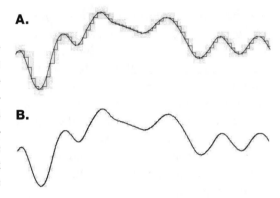

Figure 7–4. A. The original waveform (smoother line) was digitized (stair-step lines), but contains rapid transitions in amplitude that introduce a high-frequency distortion to the signal. **B.** An anti-aliasing filter removes the highest frequencies, smoothing out the waveform.

OVERVIEW OF WHAT A DIGITAL SYSTEM CAN DO

Most hearing aids sold today are digital. The difference between fitting a digital hearing aid, rather than an analog hearing aid, can be compared to the difference between typing with an electric typewriter and computer word processor. You can type a letter on a typewriter, but it's easier to correct errors on a word processor. You can select an analog hearing aid that the patient may do well with, but if you are not satisfied with how the hearing aid works for the patient, it's harder to make adjustments.

Digital hearing aids can allow more flexibility in adjusting the amount of amplification per frequency region than analog hearing aids. Digital aids allow the audiologist to customize the fit of the hearing aid to the patient's hearing loss more precisely. Most digital hearing aids are automatic and don't require the user to adjust the volume at all. If the sound levels increase, the volume is decreased so that the patient never hears amplified sound present that is too loud. Digital hearing aids use more sophisticated methods of decreasing the hearing aid volume as the sounds at the microphone increase.

Because the digital hearing aid uses numbers to code the signal, some types of signal processing that are not possible in an analog hearing aid can occur in the digital device. The hearing aid can sense when certain types of noise are present and alter the hearing aid characteristics to minimize the noise interference.

Another improvement with digital hearing aids is they may be less prone to having feedback. **Feedback** occurs when the signal, amplified by the hearing aid, escapes the ear and is picked up at the hearing aid microphone. The hearing aid amplifies that escaping signal, which again escapes, and is reamplified. You have probably heard the same phenomenon in an auditorium when the speaker's microphone is turned up too high—a squealing sound occurs, which is called feedback. That same problem can occur with hearing aids. Digital hearing aids typically have ways to detect the feedback and stop it from occurring.

Currently, one disadvantage to digital hearing aids is higher cost. The component costs for the hearing aid itself are rapidly decreasing; however, the manufacturers cite research and development costs as the reason for the expense of digital devices. Just as the next generation of home computer has more features, but costs about the same as the obsolete PC, new features are added to new generations of digital hearing aids.

FAST FOURIER TRANSFORM ANALYSIS OF AUDITORY SIGNALS

One of the advantages to digitizing a signal is that the frequency content of the signal can be analyzed using a **Fast Fourier Transform** (FFT). (As mentioned in Chapter 4, Fourier is pronounced "fŏor-e-a". In International Phonetic Symbol, that would be /fur' i e'/). FFT analysis mathematically determines what frequency components are in a waveform. Figure 7–5 illustrates. The analysis also determines the phase of the wave components. Fourier analysis is a standard method of conducting a spectral analysis, and it is used in several audiology applications.

Windowing

FFT analysis "looks at" different segments of the digitized time waveform, analyzing each segment separately, as illustrated in Figure 7–6A. Here, three windows are illustrated. The FFT would analyze each of these windows separately. When talking about how many samples are analyzed in one window, any of a number of terms may be used. You may hear it called the **FFT frame size, FFT size, window size,** or **window length.** (Sorry, the field of audiology didn't create these synonyms; engineers did.) These terms are all referring to the same thing—how many data points are being analyzed in each segment of data—each "window."

This is a bit confusing. The amplitude of the signal digitization is described in bits. So is window size. The window size is also referred to in "power of two" numbers, where the bits are the exponents in 2^n. A 2-bit FFT examines 4 samples ($2^2 = 4$); a 6-bit FFT, 64 samples ($2^6 = 64$); an 11-bit FFT uses $2048 (2^{11} = 2048)$. Again, remember, when talking about digitizing a waveform, the amplitude resolution is described in bits. Here, when talking about bit size of the FFT frame, we are referring to the number of samples.

During the analysis, the FFT mathematics makes the assumption that the waveform being analyzed is continuous. That is, you

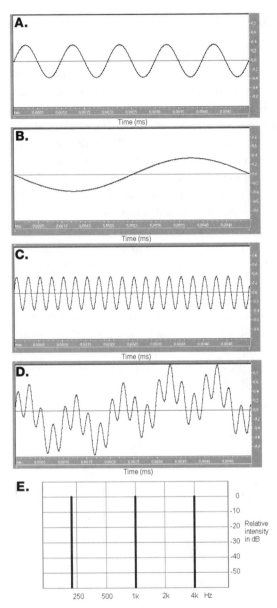

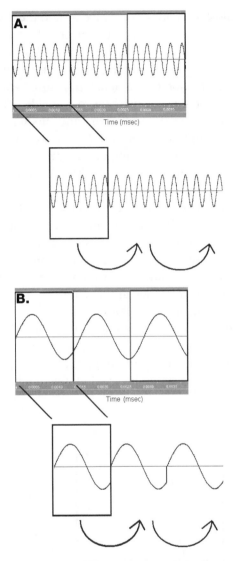

Figure 7–5. Three tones, 1000 Hz starting at 0 degrees of phase (**A**), 200 Hz beginning at 180 degrees of phase (**B**), and 4000 Hz starting at 30 degrees (**C**) phase are added. The result is a complex wave (**D**). FFT analysis will give information on the frequencies within the complex wave, as shown in (**E**), and can provide the phase of the signal components.

Figure 7–6. FFT analysis occurs in segments, called windows. When one window is mathematically manipulated during FFT spectral analysis, there is the assumption that you can take a copy of the waveform and add it to the end of the windowed segment. If the window coincides with the period of the signal, as in (**A**), this is not problematic. However, in most cases, it will create an abrupt shift in the signal, which changes the waveform, as shown in (**B**) This creates the false presence of a high-frequency, rapidly changing signal. This problem needs to be overcome.

could add a copy of the waveform to the end to make it a longer signal. (You could "wrap" the signal on itself.) The FFT analysis assumes that this wrapping won't cause a misrepresentation of the signal. In Figure 7–6A, the frame size just happens to coincide with five cycles of the waveform, and this wrapping doesn't cause a problem. However, in most cases this is going to be a problem, as illustrated in Figure 7–6B. The beginning and end of the waves don't match up, and as a result, there is an error in the waveform appearance. If this were analyzed, it would not show that the signal was a pure tone.

There's a way to get around this problem, called "windowing" the data. Figure 7–6 illustrated "rectangular" windowing. A rectangular segment (a block) of the waveform is analyzed. The amplitude of the signal is not changed at all. Rectangular windowing is not a good thing to do. Instead, most FFT analysis uses a nonlinear windowing, where

the amplitude of the signal at the beginning and end of the window is reduced. (There are different types of windowing "functions" [mathematical ways to decrease the amplitude of the signal at the beginning and end]. Blackmann, Hamming, and Hanning windows are all good choices. They have slightly different ways of gradually reducing the energy at the start and end of each window.) As shown in Figure 7–7, windowing reduces the irregularities that occur when the signal is looped (wrapped) onto itself.

The same problem occurs with speech waveforms, and the same solution, windowing, is used (Figure 7–8). This waveform is the word "digital," recorded at a sampling rate of about 41,000 Hz. Each 50-msec "**window**" contains 2048 samples. (In the mood to be picky? As there are 2048 data points sampled each 50 msec, there are 40,960 samples per second, so that is the actual digitization rate.)

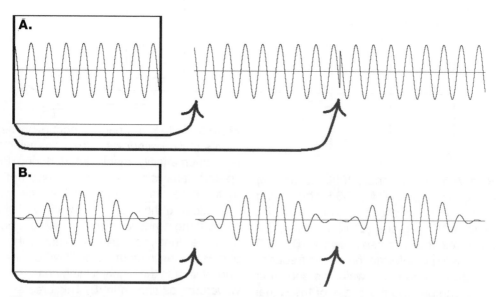

Figure 7–7. A. Rectangularly windowed waveforms when wrapped on themselves have irregularities in them, which will cause an error in the frequency analysis. **B.** Reducing the amplitude at the beginning and end of the window (superimposing a nonlinear envelope) eliminates this problem.

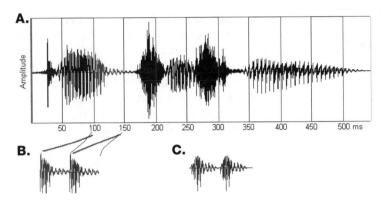

A.

Amplitude

50   100   150   200   250   300   350   400   450   500 ms

B.

C.

Figure 7–8. A. The word "digital" is recorded digitally and the time waveform is shown. This FFT will be analyzed in 2048 point segments, which correspond to 50-msec segments or "windows." If the segment from 100 to 150 msec is wrapped on itself without windowing, as shown in (**B**), the ends do not meet up and the frequency analysis will be in error. Windowing (**C**) is used to prevent the inaccurate frequency analysis.

Overlapping Windows

Windowing solves one problem (the ends of one segment will now meet up with the start of the next copy of the segment), but it creates another problem. Figure 7-9 illustrates that windowing might eliminate portions of the speech waveform. When the signal is rapidly changing in frequency, that loss of information causes misinterpretation. The solution is for the FFT analysis to use windows that *overlap*. When properly done, there is no loss of information, and the distortion that comes from wrapping windowed segments on each other is still avoided. The FFT then gives accurate information. Figure 7-10 shows how that would work.

Goal of FFT Analysis

The purpose of conducting an FFT is to be able to measure the amount of energy in a certain frequency analysis region. Analog filtering could allow you to find this information as well. For example, you could analyze a recorded speech signal over and over using different band-pass filters. That would

tell you how much energy is in each band-pass region. Analog band-pass filters typically come in either one octave or one-third octave widths. That means that while you could measure the total energy in a band (e.g., between 707 and 1414 Hz if using one-octave analysis or between 794 Hz and 1260 Hz if using a 1000-Hz, one-third octave wide filter), you cannot measure the signal with any more precision. (You don't know if that total energy in the band came from a single 1100-Hz pure tone, or a wider band signal that spanned from 800 Hz to 1100 Hz.) FFT analysis has the potential to be much more accurate. In theory, it could even tell you exactly how much energy is at each single frequency. In practice, that may not happen, but the FFT can analyze fairly precise or "narrow" frequency regions. The degree of accuracy depends on two things: how big the window is (number of samples) and how fast the waveform is sampled.

FFT Resolution

Generally speaking, we would like to obtain a precise measurement of the frequencies within the signal. Let's use the parlance

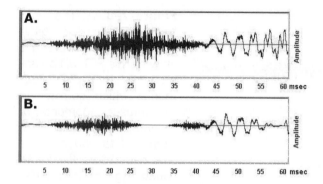

Figure 7–9. A. Original waveform. **B**. Waveform after windowing. Windowing speech signals creates a loss of segments of the waveform. When the spectral qualities of the signal change rapidly, this means that certain segments aren't analyzed and the frequency analysis will be in error.

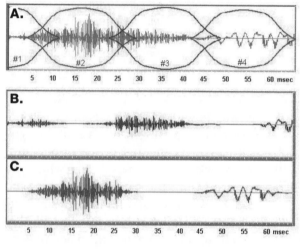

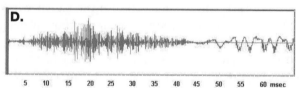

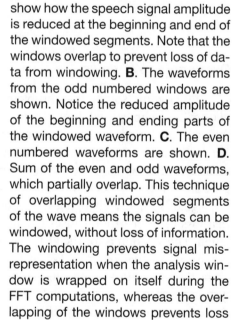

Figure 7–10. The original speech waveform is shown in (**A**). Superimposed are the window functions that show how the speech signal amplitude is reduced at the beginning and end of the windowed segments. Note that the windows overlap to prevent loss of data from windowing. **B**. The waveforms from the odd numbered windows are shown. Notice the reduced amplitude of the beginning and ending parts of the windowed waveform. **C**. The even numbered waveforms are shown. **D**. Sum of the even and odd waveforms, which partially overlap. This technique of overlapping windowed segments of the wave means the signals can be windowed, without loss of information. The windowing prevents signal misrepresentation when the analysis window is wrapped on itself during the FFT computations, whereas the overlapping of the windows prevents loss of information.

of FFT. (*Parlez vous Français?* "Parlance" comes from the French word, and means manner of speaking.) In FFT lingo, we would say that we want a narrow **bin width.** The bin width is the range of frequencies that the FFT distinguishes between. For example, if the bin width is 100 Hz, then the FFT is reporting how much energy is in each 100-Hz-wide section of the spectrum.

You calculate bin width by taking the sampling rate and dividing by the frame size, measured in samples rather than milliseconds. For example, if analyzing something recorded at the rate for a music CD (44.1 kHz) using 2048 sample frame sizes, then the results of the FFT will be reported in 21.5-Hz (44,100/2048) segments. (The bin width is 21.5 Hz.) If you were still able to analyze 2048-Hz segments, but you dropped the sampling rate to 10,000 samples per second, the analysis is more precise: you would have the results in 4.9-Hz-wide bins

(10,000/2048). Recall that dropping the sampling rate limits the highest frequency that can be recorded; so in this example, you would have good frequency analysis precision, but you could not analyze the frequency content above 5000 Hz, the Nyquist frequency for a 10000-Hz sampling rate.

Reducing the frame size widens the bin width. If the CD sound were analyzed with a 256 sample (8-bit) analysis window, it has 172-Hz bin widths. (44,100 Hz / 256 = 172 Hz.) That means that if you were analyzing a pure tone signal, you could not determine if the signal was 1000 Hz or 1170 Hz. You would only know the total energy in each 170-Hz-wide frequency region.

Example FFT Results

Figure 7–11 shows the FFT analysis of the word "digital." On the top part of the figure, the scale is linear (2000 Hz per grid). The bottom part of the figure shows the frequency scale in octave intervals. Obviously, if you want to see the higher frequencies with precision, use the linear scale; the log scale (octave scale) is better for seeing the low frequencies.

The amplitude scale in Figure 7–11 requires special consideration. The FFT measured the voltage of the incoming signal. It doesn't know if the talker was speaking into the microphone from a distance of 3 inches or 3 feet away. In each case, the speaker's overall voice level would be the same, but when the microphone is only 3 inches away, the level picked up at the microphone and digitized would be greater. Rather than referencing the levels in dB SPL, the computer records the data in terms of how much softer it was than the maximum amplitude it could possibly record. To interpret this frequency analysis, you have to compare relative amplitudes. For example, you can say that the level at 6000 Hz (which reads as 48 dB less than the largest amplitude the system could

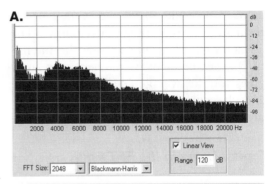

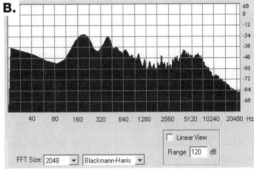

Figure 7–11. The results of an FFT of the word "digital." Frequency is along the x-axis. **A.** Each grid represents a 2000-Hz change in frequency. **B.** The scale is in octave increments: every other grid represents that frequency has doubled. The amplitude scale lets the viewer determine the relative intensity of different frequencies. You can determine how much higher or lower the intensity is at one frequency or another. The scale is in negative dB, meaning that as you move down the y-axis, the signal is less intense. The most intense signal would be 0 dB, and would correspond to a signal that takes up the full amplitude range of the analog-to-digital converter.

measure) is 6 dB less intense than the energy at 4000 Hz (where it reads about -42 dB, which is higher up on the *y*-axis.) The actual values of –42 and –48 dB are meaningless unless you know what SPL would cause you to read a 0 dB reading in this analysis.

Typically, you can choose whether you want to see your FFT results separately for each different FFT analysis frame, or whether you would like to see the average of the results across the measured windows. The former would let you see how the intensity changes moment by moment; the latter gives you the average energy for the entire speech segment, and is what is shown in Figure 7–11.

Digital Noise in the FFT Analysis

Digitization is not error free; that is, the process creates "noise." The digitization error causes some misrepresentation of all signals, at all frequencies, and this error is random. Anything digitized has this digital noise added to it. If you could see just the added noise, you would find that it has approximately equal energy at each frequency (Figure 7–12 A). The white noise is more accurately described as random noise, and because it is random, the noise levels at each frequency will not be *exactly* equal, but approximately so, and will vary a bit across time.

The FFT analysis of the digitized noise alone would show how intense the noise is in each bin. The per-bin noise reading depends on the size of the analysis band (the bin width). If analyzed in small bin widths, the total noise is not as large as if analyzed in wider bands (Figures 7-12B and 7-12C). That is because the FFT tells us the *total* energy in each frequency band, which is the sum of the energy at each single frequency. When you have a narrower analysis band, there

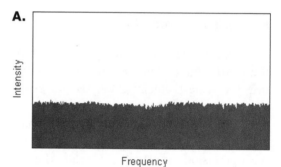

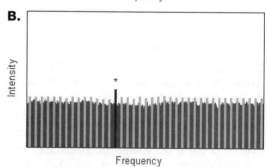

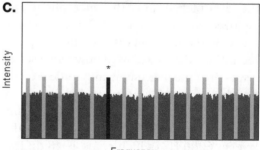

Figure 7–12. A. Illustration of digitization noise, if it could be viewed at each single frequency. The noise is generally equal in intensity at all frequencies, but because of the random nature of the noise, there is slight variation from frequency to frequency occurring just by chance. **B.** If the FFT measures the energy in a narrow band, the energy of the noise in the band is summed together and that overall intensity per band is analyzed and reported. That is shown with the vertical bars. The black vertical bar with the asterisk above it represents the signal plus noise bin. The signal can be detected because the level in that bin is greater than the noise level in adjacent frequency bins. **C.** If the analysis uses wider bins, then the summed noise is of greater intensity. Note that the bars are wider, which represents the inclusion of more frequencies, and the bars are taller, as they contain greater intensity per bin. The low-intensity signal is not significantly greater than the energy in the neighboring bins. Because of the wide bin widths, the signal is not distinguished from the background noise.

are fewer cycles of energy to sum. We hope Figure 7-12 and a little more discussion will help you grasp this concept.

Sometimes we are measuring very low-amplitude signals. (Otoacoustic emissions [Chapters 18 and 19] are a case in point.) With otoacoustic emissions, and in other audiology applications, we often know which frequency bin should have the response that we seek to detect. But, if the digitization noise in the frequency bin that should have the signal is greater than the signal level, the signal cannot be observed—the signal is no larger than the background noise. In that case, small bin widths are needed to detect the signal.

Not only can digitization noise be a potential problem, but ambient noise can obscure recording of a low-amplitude signal. Again, if the analysis is in a narrow bin, then the background noise in that bin is also lower. (Just as with digitization noise, the total background noise in a bin is the sum of the energy at each single frequency, so the smaller the bin, the less the summed noise.) If the bin is narrow, it is easier to detect a low-intensity signal as having greater energy than seen just from background noise.

If we know which bin should have the response, we can see if that bin has significantly higher amplitude than neighboring bins. FFT analysis of signals embedded in noise often compares the total energy level in a bin (coming from the noise plus the signal) to the energy level in surrounding bins (coming just from noise). If the energy is significantly larger in the response bin than in the bins a bit lower and a bit higher in frequency, then we can be confident that a signal is present.

Calculating Noise Per Bin and dB of Bandwidth Per Bin

In Chapter 2, it was shown that doubling power increases the signal level by 3 dB. The formula is 10 log 2/1. If energy were present at two separate frequencies, for example, 1000 Hz and 1001 Hz, and each were separately 20 dB SPL, the two frequencies together would give 23 dB SPL of sound. If there were four frequencies instead of two, you double again the number of frequencies, and you are now 3 dB higher still: 26 dB SPL. Go from four single frequencies combined to eight, and you now have 29 dB SPL. There is a general formula that lets you know how much more intense the total signal level is when different equal-intensity signals are combined. It is:

$$\text{dB increase} = 10 \log (\text{number of cycles})$$

For example, $10 \times \log 8 = 9$ dB. If each single frequency were 20 dB SPL, the level of eight simultaneously presented 20 dB SPL signals is 29 dB SPL.

We are going to use this same concept to add noise components at different frequencies. It is customary to call the intensity of the noise at a single frequency the **level per cycle (LPC)**. Generally, the frequencies that are "added together" are right next to each other, and form a band of frequencies. Typically, we will describe the band of frequencies by their **bandwidth (BW)**. For example, if examining the increase in intensity for pure tones with frequencies from 1000 Hz to 1187 Hz, or for noise components at frequencies 1000 Hz to 1187 Hz, there is a range of 187 Hz between the low end and the high end. The bandwidth is 187 Hz. The total level of the sound, which is the sum of the level per cycle at each single frequency (the level that results from combining all the sounds in the bandwidth), is called the **overall (OA) level.** The formal formula for calculating the overall level is:

$$\text{OA} = \text{LPC} + \text{BW in dB}$$

Note that this formula says bandwidth in dB. To obtain that, take $10 \times \log$ BW, where BW

Clinical Correlate: Bins in Audiology

The method of analyzing the signal level within one bin, compared to the "noise" level in neighboring bins, is used in clinical audiology. Otoacoustic emissions (OAEs) occur at known frequencies. The energy in the band at that frequency is contrasted to the energy at neighboring frequency regions to see if the signal is present. The results are described as a signal-to-noise ratio. The signal level is the amplitude in the bin that should have the OAE. The noise level is the average level in nearby frequency bins.

Auditory steady-state evoked response testing also uses this same technique. The special warbling signal creates a brain wave response that should occur at a given frequency. The computer system again determines whether there is energy in the frequency range of interest (the warbling frequency), and contrasts it to the brain wave energy at nearby bins. The energy in the nearby bins is not related to hearing the warbling signal—it is "just noise."

is the number of cycles in the frequency region within that band. For example, if the BW = 187, the BW in dB is 19.4.

Returning to the concept of FFT analysis, let's apply this principle. Recall that digitization creates noise that is spread out across the frequency range. Let's see how increasing the FFT analysis size reduces the noise level in each bin. A CD-quality recording (44.1 kHz sampling rate) is analyzed with a 6-bit FFT size (64 samples per frame) and then again with an 11-bit FFT size (2048 samples). How much more intense is the noise in the bigger bin than the noise level at one single frequency? First, find the bin size. The 44,100 sampling rate/64 samples per frame = 689 bin width. This contrasts to 44,100/2048, which is 21.5-Hz bin width. Now, put each bin width in dB: 10 x log 689 = 28.4 dB. Whatever the digital noise level per cycle is at each frequency, the overall level is now 28 dB higher. If the 2048 frame size is used, with its tiny 21.5-Hz wide analysis

bin width, the increase from the level per cycle is only 13.3 dB (10 × log 21.5 = 13.3 dB). The noise level per bin is about 15 dB higher in the wider bin. Again, using a wider bin means that you not only have limited ability to analyze the small frequency-by-frequency changes, it also means that the difference between background noise and the signal might be very small. You might not be able to detect a low-amplitude signal embedded in the background noise (see Figure 7–12).

TIME-DOMAIN SIGNAL AVERAGING

Among the advantages of using a digital system is the ease with which **time-domain signal averaging (TDSA)** can be conducted. This is a powerful tool for reducing background noise, which, as you know, can limit our ability to detect low-amplitude signals. TDSA involves measuring the same phenomenon repeatedly. For this technique to work, we want to "evoke" a response, that is, to purposefully cause the response (if present) to occur. The more often we evoke it, the easier it is to detect the response, which always occurs at the same time after each evoking stimulus.

One of the types of responses we may evoke is an **auditory brainstem response**, which occurs when nerves in the lower brainstem fire in response to sound stimulation. In order to make the example more straight-forward, let's assume that 5 msec after the presentation of sound a group of auditory nerves all simultaneously fire. Their firing creates an electrochemical change. Charged particles (ions) are going into and out of the nerve cells. These polarity changes radiate out, including outward to the skull. Electrodes placed on the surface of the skull are capable of detecting this type of chemical change deep within the brain. The difficulty is that other neurons are also active, as the person is breathing, the central nervous system is regulating the heartbeat, and the person is thinking. The firing of those neurons that are not related to hearing also causes chemical changes that the

Clinical Correlate: Digital Hearing Aids

Digital hearing aids also filter signals within bands. The specifications for a Phonak Claro digital hearing aid (one of Phonak's older digital hearing aids) say they use 128-point FFT processors with a 20-kHz sampling rate. If we take the sampling rate, and divide by the 128-point FFT size, we find that their filter band width (bin width) is 156 Hz. You can theoretically adjust the hearing aid gain in each 156-Hz-wide band, which means across the frequency range the hearing aid can handle (from 1 Hz to the Nyquist frequency of 10 kHz), gain can be manipulated in 64 individual bands. (10,000 Hz/156 Hz = 64 bands.) The audiologist may not want to have that level of control; it could be difficult to work with that software. However, the fact that there are that many bands available allows the hearing aid to have some processing advantages. For instance, if the hearing aid were to sense **feedback** in one frequency band (when the hearing aid "whistles" because amplified sound escapes and is picked up by the microphone), the amplification (gain) in just that one band could be reduced. That would (potentially) only affect one 156-Hz-wide range, it would not cause the loss of acoustic information in other frequency regions.

Digital hearing aids also have noise reduction strategies, but description of those **algorithms**, or methods for computer software to operate, is beyond the scope of this book. Many of the algorithms will work better if the hearing aid has small analysis bands.

surface electrodes will record. The audiologist is trying to find a 3-µV change from the nerves of hearing firing while the polarity of the overall brain could well be fluctuating between +20 and –20 µV.

TDSA is going to involve adding signals, so let's first review this concept. As was shown in Table 4–2 and Figure 4–10, if you have two time waveforms, and you combine them, you simply sum the amplitude. The amplitude is not in dB format, so it is OK to simply add.

The next major concept is that if you were to add together random noise segments, the summed level would become less and less. Observe Table 7–1. Numbers were generated pseudorandomly to represent the amplitude (voltage) of noise at 8 moments in time (amplitude at each of 8 samples). This was done five times, just as we might evoke and then measure the brain activity of the patient five separate times. Table 7–1 shows the sum of those amplitudes after five trials. Note that the sum has lower amplitude than the individual trials. Summing reduced the amplitude of the random signal.

In time-domain signal averaging you can either sum the waveform, or sum it and then divide by the number of samples tak-

en, depending on your needs. The latter way of taking an average gave rise to the name time-domain signal *averaging.*

For those who like the visual image, Figure 7–13 shows the first time the signal was measured, and the sum.

Now, let's discuss what would happen if, each time the measurement were taken, there was an event at one of those moments in time, and it was always evoked at the

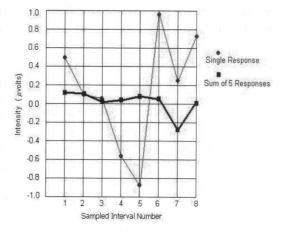

Figure 7–13. The single "sweep" (measurement) has higher amplitude than the sum of five trials. The measurements are taken from Table 7–1.

Table 7–1. Example of What Might Occur if Eight Sequential Voltage Measurements (samples at 8 time intervals) Are Obtained in Five Separate Trials

Repetition	Time Interval (Sample)							
#1	0.51	0.11	0.08	–0.57	–0.87	0.98	0.25	0.73
#2	–0.23	0.21	0.51	0.25	0.35	–0.25	0.36	–0.54
#3	0.36	–0.6	0.32	0.37	0.47	–0.74	0.08	–0.21
#4	–0.29	0.19	–0.61	–0.24	0.11	–0.22	–0.64	0.62
#5	–0.23	0.2	–0.27	0.25	0.02	0.3	–0.29	–0.59
Sum	**0.12**	**0.11**	**0.03**	**0.06**	**0.08**	**0.07**	**–0.24**	**0.01**

Values are amplitudes µV. The sum of those values is less than the individual values. In this illustration, the signal being measured comes from noise alone. Because the samples are in essence random, sometimes positive, sometimes negative, the sum is smaller than the individual trials.

same time relative to the start of our measurement. Table 7–2 shows these same numbers, but a value of 0.1μV has been added to the 5th sampling interval. As shown in Figure 7-14, the sum of the samples clearly shows the response. The minor change is not noticeable in the single sweep.

In audiology, there are times when we will average multiple trials. In auditory brainstem response testing, the signal is so minute that the average is of thousands of sweeps! Measurement of otoacoustic emissions uses dozens to hundreds of averages. Digitization of each sweep makes it easy for the engineers to calculate and display the ongoing, averaged waveform.

SUMMARY

When a signal is digitized, the precision of the measurement of the analog wave is determined by the bit size (number of amplitude steps that can be measured) and the sampling rate. The sampling rate determines the Nyquist frequency; signals higher than half the sampling rate cannot be included.

One of the major advantages of working with digitized signals is that the frequencies can be analyzed using a Fast Fourier Transform (FFT). The FFT measures the signal level present within narrow frequency ranges, called the bin widths. The bin width increases as the sampling rate increases. It decreases as the size of the FFT (the num-

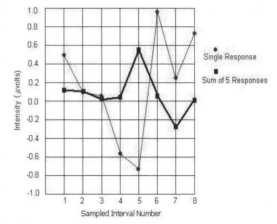

Figure 7–14. When the sum of the values is plotted, the addition of 0.1 to each of the five trials at sample number 5 (see Table 7–2) is clearly evident.

Table 7–2. The Fifth Measurement in Each Sample Was Increased by 0.1 to Illustrate What Would Happen if a .1-μV Response Occurred at the Same Time in Each of the Five Trials

Repetition	Time Interval (Sample)							
#1	0.51	0.11	0.08	−0.57	**−0.77**	0.98	0.25	0.73
#2	−0.23	0.21	0.51	0.25	**0.45**	−0.25	0.36	−0.54
#3	0.36	−0.6	0.32	0.37	**0.57**	−0.74	0.08	−0.21
#4	−0.29	0.19	−0.61	−0.24	**0.21**	−0.22	−0.64	0.62
#5	−0.23	0.2	−0.27	0.25	**0.12**	0.3	−0.29	−0.59
Sum	**0.12**	**0.11**	**0.03**	**0.06**	**0.58**	**0.07**	**−0.24**	**0.01**
Average	0.024	0.022	0.006	0.012	**0.116**	0.014	−0.048	0.002

The sum shows that the average value is noticeably larger than the amplitude at other sampled points. This illustrates that when a response is evoked at the same time, relative to the start of the measurement, the sum is noticeably larger: the average of the values is also larger in the fifth sample in this illustration.

ber of points analyzed in each FFT sampling frame) increases. Generally, small bin widths are desired. For example, in a hearing aid, if you can filter and then amplify the signal in each separate band, you can have extremely precise customization of the patient's amplification needs if the FFT analysis was in small bins.

There are a number of digital algorithms used in both hearing aids and audiologic equipment. Time-domain signal averaging was described (which is used in some audiologic evaluation equipment, but not in hearing aids). In this technique a response is evoked numerous times. The waveform is sampled each time, after the evoking stimulus is presented. The sum of the numerous trials (often called "sweeps") is averaged. This is an effective technique for reducing background noise and enhancing the part of the response that is time-locked to the start of the recording of the separate trials.

8

Some Equipment Used in Audiology and Hearing Science

The audiologist's job is to determine how much hearing loss is present, and what part of the ear is causing the loss. As later chapters will discuss, the parts of the ear are the outer ear (the part you can see and the ear canal), the eardrum, the middle ear (a space behind the eardrum that sound passes through), and the inner ear (where sound becomes a nerve signal). After that, the nerve signal has to be sent to the brain for interpretation. At this point, you only need to accept that there are different parts of the ear, and that the audiologist determines what part (or parts) of the ear create(s) the hearing problem. This chapter discusses the equipment the audiologist uses to determine which part of the ear is causing the loss and to determine how severe the loss is. We will examine how the equipment functions, but not how it is used to diagnose the hearing problem.

Audiologists also provide hearing aids when the hearing loss cannot be medically treated. This chapter examines the equipment that is used to determine if the hearing aid is working properly and introduces equipment used to fit hearing aids.

This chapter's section on microphones applies not only to measuring sound, but also applies to hearing aids. This chapter also overviews the equipment used in a hearing science laboratory, used to conduct research experiments.

AUDIOMETERS

The most fundamental piece of audiologic equipment is the audiometer (Figure 8–1). It produces pure tones at octave frequencies from 125 Hz to 8000 Hz (and some interoctave frequencies) at calibrated intensities. Octaves are doublings of frequency, so the audiologist can test hearing at 125 Hz, 250 Hz, 500 Hz, and so forth, but not 300 Hz. Interoctave frequencies are also available above 500 Hz, so hearing at 750, 1500, 3000, and 6000 Hz can also be tested. Typically, an audiometer has two sound generators and two "channels" to control the presentation of sound to the two ears. The audiometer allows the audiologist to adjust intensity, and has a button that the audiologist presses to present the signal to the patient. The patient presses a button (or raises his or her hand) to signal that the tone has been heard. If the response button is used, pressing it illuminates a light on the audiom-

A.

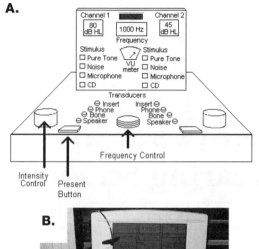

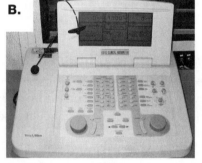

B.

Figure 8–1. A. Schematic illustration of the parts of an audiometer. **B.** Photograph of a Grason-Stadler 61 audiometer, showing that the actual device has more options than those highlighted in this chapter.

eter. The audiologist will increase and decrease the intensity of the tone to find the hearing **threshold**, the lowest intensity that can be heard at least half the time. As described in Chapter 3, the decibel used in hearing testing is dB HL—decibels hearing level—where 0 dB HL is the lowest intensity the average normal hearer can detect.

Pure tones are not the only signal that can be presented using an audiometer. Noise signals are available. The noise stimuli are typically routed to the ear that is not being tested (the nontest ear) to prevent that ear from hearing the test signal. That noise is called **masking noise**.

The audiologist is able to talk to the patient who is seated inside a sound room and

to test the patient using speech stimuli. The audiometer has a button on it that activates the **talk-forward** system, allowing the audiologist to speak to the patient, for example, to give instructions. The audiologist typically wears a microphone on a headset, and another microphone mounted in the sound room allows the audiologist to hear the patient. That is called the **talk back** system.

Tests of speech understanding, administered by the audiologist using his or her own voice, are termed **live-voice testing**. The audiologist conducting live-voice testing has to adjust the loudness of the sound coming from the microphone into the audiometer in order for the level to be calibrated. If the audiologist speaks quietly, then a little more amplification of his or her voice is needed. If the audiologist is speaking loudly, the signal needs to be turned down. The voice level is shown on a **VU meter**. VU stands for volume unit, and the meter scale shown in decibels. If the audiologist's voice is at +3 dB, then what is heard by the patient would be 3 dB louder than the calibrated level. The goal is to adjust the VU meter, which amplifies or attenuates the signal, until the audiologist's voice is peaking at 0 dB—that is, the loudest syllables are at 0, and syllables that are naturally a bit quieter are, of course, lower than 0. If sound is too loud, if it peaks in the range much higher than 0 dB, then the voice is likely to be distorted and garbled, in addition to being out of calibration.

Most assessment of how well the patient understands speech is conducted using recorded materials, so the audiometer typically has, or has a connection to, a CD or DVD player. The recorded material also has to be calibrated, and the same VU meter is used. Rather than holding down the present button for the total time of the testing of speech understanding, the audiologist toggles on the **reverse button**, which makes the present button act in the opposite (reverse) of its usual function. Pressing the presentation button would interrupt the signal (it would go silent). The reverse button is sometimes called the **interrupt button**.

The audiometer has several options for how to present the signal to the patient, that is, which **audiometric transducer** to use. The most common transducer is an **insert earphone**, shown schematically in Figure 8–2A. A foam tip is inserted into the ear canal. The foam tip is rolled up to compress it, and then it is inserted into the ear canal and it expands to seal the ear. The sound speaker is in a small box that can be clipped to a shirt collar. A thin plastic tube connects the foam tip to the speaker box. **Supra-aural headphones** are also an option (Figure 8–2B). Alternatively, the sound can be routed to **sound-field speakers**. These three types of transducers are all **air-conduction transducers**: they create vibrations of the air, which enter the outer ear. A final transducer used is the bone vibrator, or **bone oscillator** (Figure 8–2E). This device creates a mechanical vibration. The bone oscillator is placed on the bone behind the ear and cre-

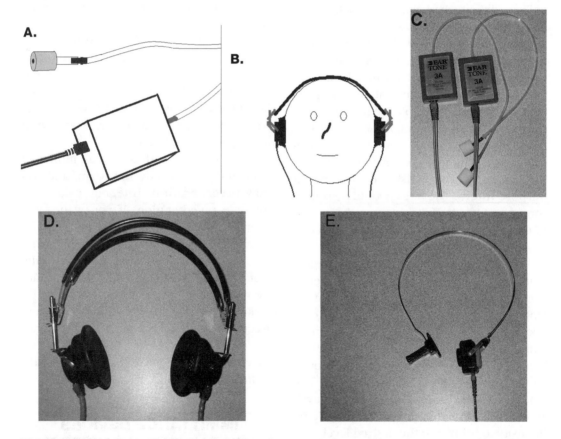

Figure 8–2. Schematic illustration of an insert earphone (**A**) and supra-aural earphones (**B**). Actual insert earphones (**C**), supra-aural earphones (**D**), and (**E**) bone oscillator. The insert earphone has a foam tip that is compressed and inserted into the ear. A sound speaker is worn clipped to the lapel, and the sound travels up a flexible tube to the ear. Supra-aural earphones are worn on top of the ears. The bone oscillator, or bone vibrator, is worn on the mastoid bone behind the ear.

ates a vibration of the skull. Chapter 14 will introduce how bone conduction testing creates a signal that is sent to the inner ear and how this allows the audiologist to deduce what part or parts of the ear is/are creating the hearing loss.

SIGNAL GENERATORS

The audiometer is the signal generator used for hearing testing; however, researchers may use more basic equipment. Whereas an audiometer costs about $6000, a signal generator can cost as little as a few hundred dollars (though they can cost much, much more). **Signal generators** typically produce not just pure tones, but also square waves, triangular waves, and sawtooth waves at a variety of frequencies. They may be able to produce noise as well. Dedicated **noise generators** also are available, which typically produce white noise, pink noise, and brown noise (noise that has greater high-frequency energy). If filtered noise is required, then the laboratory also is likely to use special purpose **filters**. The noise would be routed through a filter, such as an octave band-pass filter, to create a narrow-band noise that can be sent to earphones.

Increasingly computers are used to generate the signals needed for experiments. Computers can create any signal that an analog generator can produce. They may connect to an amplifier, which may be under computer control. Rather than the amplifier being adjusted, however, most laboratories would use an adjustable **attenuator.** The amplifier turns the signal to its full on level, and then the attenuator reduces the signal intensity to bring it to the desired level.

SOUND BOOTHS

The typical **sound booth** or **sound room** used for audiometric testing is a free-

standing metal room. The booth is called double-walled if it has interior and exterior walls separated with an isolation space. Single-walled booths are available but provide less sound isolation. The interior paneling of either a single- or double-walled both is made of metal sheets that have many small holes. Sound from inside the room (e.g., from the sound-field speaker) will be **absorbed** rather than reflected because the interior has a high **coefficient of absorption**, that is, it absorbs a large percentage of the sound wave that strikes the wall. The solid exterior wall helps reflect sound away from the booth, limiting the amount of sound that is transmitted into the sound booth. Or, using the terminology of Chapter 3, we say the booth has high **transmission loss**.

The patient is seated in the sound room. Typically there is a window for the patient to see out, and this window is double-paned glass. One window pane is flush with the interior wall, one with the exterior wall, with an air space in between.

The sound booth seeks to minimize sound reflection inside the room, and has a low **reverberation time**, but it does not eliminate reverberation. If you want even better sound absorption, you would need an **anechoic chamber**, which, as the name implies, doesn't echo. The interior has wedges of foam on all surfaces to absorb sound. The wedges are positioned in alternating directions to help catch reflections from any direction. The floor is a metal grid that can be walked on, and below the grid is an air space, and then below are the sound-absorbing foam wedges.

IMMITTANCE DEVICES (MIDDLE EAR ANALYZERS)

Tympanometers

Audiometers test hearing. Immittance devices measure how well sound is transmitted through the tympanic membrane (eardrum) and the air-filled space behind it, the middle ear. These devices are also called **middle ear analyzers.** "**Immittance**" is a word that means it relates to either **impedance**, which was discussed in Chapter 5, or the opposite of impedance, **admittance**. Admittance is a measure of how easily sound is transmitted, whereas impedance is a measure of how difficult it is for sound to be transmitted. The two terms are the inverse of each other. Immittance testing is used to determine if the sound transmission systems of the eardrum and middle ear are, or are not, normal. This text will not describe how the information is used clinically, as this is a text in hearing science, not audiology, but we will review the principles of how the equipment works—the science behind the equipment.

The aspect of immittance testing that relates to the hearing sciences is that the device can tell us about the impedance/admittance and resonant frequency of the sound-conducting system, which in this case is the human ear. This section briefly overviews this technology, and discusses the principles behind the operation of the device.

First, some general concepts have to be understood. Imagine taking a portable radio into a gymnasium. While holding it at your side, you adjust the volume to be comfortable in loudness. Now, you walk into a small empty broom closet adjacent to the auditorium. Your perception is that the sound is louder because the sound is now reflected off the closet walls that are, at most, a few feet away. The concept here is that the size of the enclosed space affects the overall intensity of the sound.

An immittance device will deliver a 226-Hz **probe tone** into the ear canal. The immittance probe is seated in the ear canal and creates an airtight or **hermetic seal** using a soft plastic dome (Figure 8–3). The intensity of the probe tone is measured. If the tympanic membrane and middle ear are nor-

mal, then sound level in the ear canal will be less than if the eardrum had a pathology that

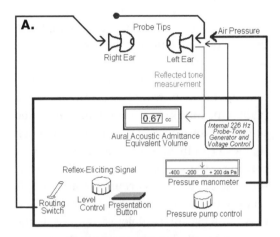

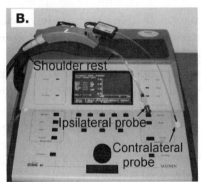

Figure 8–3. A. Schematic of an immittance measurement device. The audiologist is able to control the pressure delivered the ear, shown as the left ear in this figure. A 226-Hz tone is delivered. The sound level of the reflected 226-Hz tone is converted into an equivalent volume reading (see text). The signal to trigger the acoustic reflex can be adjusted in frequency and intensity and presented. The signal can be routed ipsilaterally or contralaterally. **B.** Photo of a Madsen Zodiac 901 middle ear analyzer. The portion containing the probe tone generator and sound measuring microphone is shown on the shoulder rest. The ipsilateral probe connects to this portion of the device. The reflex-eliciting sound can be routed through the ipsilateral probe, or directed to the contralateral probe.

keeps sound from vibrating the eardrum. If pathology limits eardrum vibration, then the sound would reflect off the eardrum instead of passing through it. This brings us to the second concept to understand. How loud the probe tone is in the ear canal tells us something about how well sound enters the middle ear.

Let's examine how this immittance system operates. It would be simpler to explain if the immittance system measured the sound pressure level of the probe tone when the device delivers sound at a given voltage. However, the device actually will increase the voltage until a certain sound level is reached (such as 85 dB SPL). The voltage level is not what the audiologist records as the measurement, though. Instead, the device makes a calculation of **equivalent volume**. If a machine could think out loud, it would be saying, "I increased the voltage to X volts in order to make the 226-Hz sound reach 85 dB SPL. If I take the probe out of the ear and put the probe into different size cavities and keep the voltage at X volts, it would read 85 dB SPL only if the cavity is of this size." (Keep the first concept in mind—how loud the sound is depends on the size of the enclosed space.) The immittance system reports the size of the cavity, called the equivalent volume. If a high voltage is required to produce the 85 dB SPL level, then the probe will read 85 dB SPL only when it is put into a large cavity. If only a small voltage is needed, then this is equivalent to measuring the sound with the probe in a small cavity.

Now, let's link this back to the impedance of the ear. If the ear has low impedance/high admittance (it transmits sound very easily), then most of the sound goes through the eardrum, not much is reflected back, and the reading is of a large equivalent volume. An eardrum that doesn't transmit sound well has high impedance, low admittance, and it only takes a low voltage for the 226-Hz probe tone to reach 85 dB SPL. This relates to a low equivalent volume reading.

The astute student may see a fundamental problem with this measurement. Let's consider what happens if an adult with a large ear canal and a baby have the same impedance of their sound-conducting middle ear systems. When the probe is put in the adult ear, the equivalent volume is going to be higher because the ear canal is larger. We really want to know about how well sound goes through the eardrum, not the size of the ear canal. There is a solution to this problem. Make a measurement of the size of the ear canal alone, and subtract that equivalent volume from the total. That will tell you about the immittance of the eardrum and middle ear alone.

Time for a second take on this topic; it's a tough one at first read. The probe is put in the ear, and the sound level is measured. If the ear has high admittance (sound goes through well), then the equivalent volume is large. But that reading is also partly affected by the size of the ear canal itself. So, our desired solution is to make a measurement of the total measure (sound transmission plus ear canal effects), then make a second measure of just the ear canal size. Subtract the ear canal size, and we have a measure of how well the sound goes through the eardrum.

To do this, we need to create a situation where sound doesn't transmit through the eardrum very well at all. We can do this by creating an **impedance mismatch** between the ear canal and the middle ear space. We now spend a few paragraphs on how this works.

In Chapter 5, impedance mismatches were introduced. It was said that if sound goes from one medium to another, it does this best when the two media have equal impedances. One example in Chapter 5 was that sound does not transmit well between air and seawater; it bounces off the seawater back into the air.

With that thought in the back of your mind, it's time for some mental imagery. Envision two adjacent airtight rooms with a large circular window connecting them. Imagine that window as taking up nearly the entire wall between those rooms, and that the two rooms are the same size. The window is covered with an airtight flexible plastic membrane. Envision a sound speaker in the room to the left, and a sound level meter in each room. Now, pressurize the room on the left. Specifically, let's pump in a lot of positive air pressure into that airtight room. The window membrane between the two rooms now bulges toward the room on the right. The pressure keeps the membrane from vibrating well in response to the sound, and so less sound is transmitted through the window, as can be measured by the sound level meter in the room on the right. Meanwhile, the sound level meter in the room on the left reads a higher level because there is now more reflected sound in that room. When the two rooms were at equal pressure, sound went through easily, and the sound level meters in the two rooms read just about the same level. If an equivalent volume reading were made at this point (equal pressure in the two rooms), we would see that the sound level in the room on the left is low, meaning that the equivalent volume is the volume of the two rooms combined. If we do a good job of creating a big pressure difference between the rooms, creating a large difference in impedance between the air in the two rooms, then very little sound will go through the membrane-covered window. The sound level in the left room will increase considerably, and the equivalent volume measurement would be about half what it was before.

Now let's see how this works with measures of the ear. The immittance device probe is sealed to the ear canal. To make the measurement of the equivalent volume of the ear canal, the ear canal is pressurized to about +200 daPa. (That's enough pressure that the patient definitely feels fullness in the ear, but it's not painful. It's similar to the pressure feeling you might have when flying, which is another time you have an impedance mismatch that decreases sound transmission through the eardrum.) While the ear canal is pressurized to +200 daPa, the equivalent volume measurement is made, and this is considered the **ear canal volume**. Next, the pressure is gradually eased, and measurements of the equivalent volume are made as the pressure goes to ambient (0) and then continues to decrease toward –200, or even –400 daPa. The purpose of gradually changing the pressure is to determine the pressure where the equivalent volume is the highest, meaning sound is transmitted best at this pressure. This portion of the test is called **tympanometry**. You would expect the best sound transmission (largest equivalent volume) at normal ambient atmospheric pressure; however, one type of ear pathology creates a partial vacuum behind the eardrum. If you have felt stuffiness in your ears with a cold, you have had this phenomenon. Tympanometry will provide a measure of how severe the pressure problem is, as well as giving the reading of **aural acoustic admittance**, the ease with which the tympanic membrane and middle ear accepts energy. This is also called the ear's **static admittance value**.

A brief note on pressure measurement is warranted. Today, the **manometer** (pressure measuring device) in tympanometers measures pressure in daPa. In prior years a different unit of pressure was used: **mm H$_2$O**. If you filled a tall cylinder of water, and connected the pressure pump to bottom, if the pressure lifted the water 100 mm, then that was a pressure of 100 mm H$_2$O. Fortunately, 1 daPa is very close to 1 mm H$_2$O.

As old habits die hard, audiologists may still report tympanometry pressure readings in mm H_2O even though the actual measurements were made in daPa.

The standard tympanometers produces a 226-Hz probe tone to make the aural acoustic admittance measures. In general, low-frequency sounds do not transmit well through a stiff system, whereas high-frequency sounds aren't affected by the stiffness of a system. (High-frequency transmission is impeded by mass.) Some tympanometers produce additional higher frequency probe tones as well as having the 226-Hz probe tone, and this can give the audiologist indirect information about the mass and stiffness of the ear.

A few models of tympanometers are even capable of measuring the sound conducting mechanism's resonant frequency. As was discussed in Chapter 5, although resistance is the same at each frequency, reactance varies frequency to frequency because it has two components: mass reactance and stiffness reactance. Mass reactance is minimal when the sound frequency is low—massive objects vibrate well at low frequencies. However, if the sound frequency increases, the mass reactance becomes greater. It's hard to vibrate a massive system at a high frequency. Stiffness reactance works in the opposite direction. Stiffness reactance is a major impeding force for low frequencies, but not for high frequencies. The total reactance is the mass reactance (X_m) minus the stiffness reactance (X_s). Any system with mass and stiffness will have one frequency where sound is transmitted most efficiently—the mass and stiffness reactance values balance each other out, and the sound transmission is affected only by the frictional resistance of the system. That is the system's resonant frequency. A few tympanometers are capable of measuring the **resonant frequency of the middle ear** and tympanic membrane.

Acoustic Stapedial Reflex Measurement

The diagnostic-quality middle ear analyzer will have an additional capability: measurement of whether there has been contraction of the acoustic reflex muscle. There is a muscle within each middle ear that contracts (stiffens) when the listener perceives a loud sound. That muscle contraction reduces the sound transmission through the middle ear. To measure whether the acoustic reflex has occurred, both the 226-Hz probe tone and a reflex-eliciting tone are presented. The probe tone is always on, and the level of the probe tone that is reflected back into the ear canal is always being measured. Loud, brief pure tones or noise bursts are presented. If the reflex has been triggered, and the muscle stiffens, sound doesn't transmit as well through the middle ear. More sound is reflected back into the ear canal, and the equivalent volume reading momentarily decreases. The audiologist can adjust the level of the reflex-eliciting sound to find the **acoustic reflex threshold**, the lowest intensity of sound that triggers the reflex, and compare that threshold to normal values. In some cases, the reflex cannot be triggered: it is said to be absent.

If an acoustic reflex occurs, it is normal for the reflex to occur in each ear, that is, to be bilateral. This is true even if the loud sound is heard only in one ear. During reflex testing, the reflex-eliciting signal can be routed either to the same ear as received the tympanometric testing (**ipsilateral** routing), or to the opposite ear (**contralateral** routing).

There is also diagnostic value to knowing whether the reflex can be sustained for several seconds. If the reflex occurs at first, then rapidly dies down, that is called **reflex decay**. The immittance device measures the drop in equivalent volume that occurs initially, and then over the next 10 seconds. If the reflex abates, then sound is transmitted through the ear more readily and the equivalent volume reading gets larger: reflex decay has occurred.

OTOACOUSTIC EMISSIONS DEVICES

As the chapters on physiology later in this text will describe, the healthy ear actually produces sound, sometimes in response to being stimulated, and sometimes without any stimulus present. This sound is not a ringing of the ears (it is not tinnitus). It is called an **otoacoustic emission (OAE)**. The discovery of otoacoustic emissions was monumental and is discussed beginning in Chapter 18. This chapter describes the equipment used to make those measurements.

Spontaneous otoacoustic emissions occur without a sound being presented. **Evoked otoacoustic emissions** are triggered by a sound presented to the ear. The **transient**, also called **click-evoked otoacoustic emissions**, are triggered by a click, whereas **distortion product otoacoustic emissions** are elicited using pairs of tones.

Spontaneous Otoacoustic Emission Measurement

A spontaneous otoacoustic emission is a sound, produced by the inner ear, that travels to out of the ear into the ear canal. These are very low-intensity signals; they are just a few decibels SPL. To measure a spontaneous otoacoustic emission, the ear canal is sealed. The seal helps keep sound from the environment out of the ear canal, but it is best to do this testing in the quietest possible environment. The probe that is inserted into the ear canal is connected to a microphone that picks up the emitted sound, and the system displays the spectrum of that sound. Typi-

cally, an otoacoustic emission is composed of several different tonal signals.

Transient-Evoked Otoacoustic Emissions Measurement

Chapter 4 defined the click, or transient signal, as a brief pulse of sound. The spectrum of the sound is said to be "white"—it contains energy at all frequencies in equal amounts. In click-evoked, or **transient-evoked otoacoustic emissions testing** (TEOAE testing), the ear canal is sealed. A click is produced and sent to the sealed ear canal. This sound travels through the different parts of the ear, and if the ear is normal, produces something similar to an echo in responses. The OAE system records the response, and shows what frequencies are in the spectrum of that response. As the click has wide-band energy, the response should have energy across the spectrum, too. However, the middle ear has some characteristics of a filter: Some sounds are transmitted through the ear better than other sounds. The OAE spectrum is shaped by the middle ear filter. For example, the middle ear doesn't transmit very low- and very high-frequency sound well, so those frequencies are not expected in the emission. The inner ear doesn't produce emissions equally at all frequencies, and this too is shown in the clinical results.

Distortion-Product Otoacoustic Emissions Measurement

Chapter 4 introduced one common type of signal distortion: harmonic distortion. A nonlinear (distorting) transducer produces this type of distortion that occurs at octave increments above the signal frequency. The ear is a signal transducer that does not send the sound through with perfect fidelity—it is a nonlinear transducer and it creates harmonic distortion and other types of distortions as well. Although distortion is typically thought of as something unwanted, it is normal for the ear to produce some forms of distortion, and in fact, it is a signal of a healthy ear. In **distortion-product otoacoustic emission testing** (DPOAE testing), the testing seeks to see if one of these normally occurring distortions is present. The distortion of interest is called the **cubic difference tone**. When two single pure tones are sent into the ear, a third frequency distortion is created. The equation for the third distortion frequency, the cubic difference tone, is $2f1 - f2$, where $f1$ is the lower frequency pure tone, and $f2$ is the higher of the two frequencies. For example, if 1000 Hz and 1212 Hz are both put in the ear simultaneously, the expected cubic difference tone distortion product will be at 788 Hz ($2 \times 1000 - 1212$). The otoacoustic emission system will determine whether it can detect this 788-Hz component as being present. There is always some background noise in the measurement, so the instrument seeks to determine if the energy the microphone reads at the cubic difference tone frequency is larger than the background noise at neighboring frequencies (e.g., 768 Hz and 808 Hz).

Different pairs of tones are used in DPOAE testing. The complete test might determine if the cubic difference tone is present for each of five to twelve tone pairs. There is no magic number for the number of test tone pairs used, that is up to the audiologist. If a patient has normal hearing in the low frequencies, and inner ear hearing loss for the higher frequencies, then we would expect to see DPOAEs only for the low-frequency tone pairs.

DPOAE testing systems will use two internal speakers, one producing each of the two tones. This is required because the speaker itself can produce a cubic differ-ence tone, and if that happened, you could not tell if the tone was present as part of the stimulus, or as the response. Each of the two speakers is causing air wave compression and rarefaction cycles, but at different frequencies: Each speaker is separately pushing and pulling the air molecules. The two forces are combined, and the vibration pattern of the air molecules is the same as it would be if the sine waves had been added together electronically by a single speaker (e.g., as shown in Figure 4–10A, part 3). By using two speakers, any cubic difference tone distortions are created by the ear.

An otoacoustic emission system is shown in Figure 8–4. The probe that is sealed to the ear is shown resting on the laptop. For this device, the signal generators are inside the hardware case.

Signal Processing Used in Analysis of All Types of OAE Measurements

OAE systems use digital technology to record and analyze the responses. For

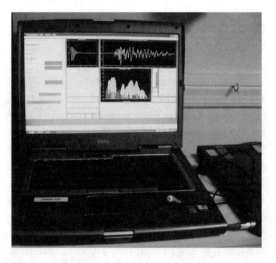

Figure 8–4. An Otodynamics otoacoustic emission system.

evoked emissions, the signal is presented, and then multiple samples of the ear's response are acquired. With spontaneous otoacoustic emissions, again multiple samples are taken—the samples are not linked to any triggering stimulus.

Each of the samples of the OAE measurement is digitized. The principles covered in Chapter 7 apply. If a response is at a frequency above the **Nyquist frequency**, it won't be included in the response. We trust that the manufacturer has used proper antialiasing filtering to prevent any erroneous recordings from occurring.

The multiple samples are stored, and **time-domain signal averaging** is used to reduce the background noise, which varies in amplitude and frequency from recording to recording (sweep to sweep) during the averaging. The clinician often is allowed to change how many sweeps, or samples, are taken during the measurement. The more samples used, the better the audiologist's ability to find weak responses; however, this increases the testing time. OAE measurement is often used as a screening tool for hearing of infants and young children, so rapid test completion is important. The audiologist has to balance the time and accuracy tradeoff.

The OAE system uses digital FFT analysis. Some OAE systems allow the user to modify the FFT analysis parameters. Recall that the FFT system provides the spectral analysis results. Different FFT parameters determine whether the **FFT bin width** is narrow or large—that is, whether the FFT shows the amplitude in large frequency segments or very narrow frequency increments. The smallest possible bin width is desired, as was described in Chapter 7. That chapter also discussed that widening the **frame size** (the number of points digitized in each sample segment) creates narrower analysis bins and better frequency resolution accuracy. The frame size may also be called by any of the following names: FFT frame size, FFT size, window size, or window length. The bin width is calculated as the sampling rate divided by the frame size. To achieve the desired narrow frame size, either lower the sampling rate, or increase the frame size. As mentioned above, lowering the sampling rate lowers the Nyquist frequency which limits the highest frequency that can be analyzed, so the sampling rate can only be lowered to a certain degree. Increasing the bin width improves accuracy, but the disadvantage there is that it requires longer samples per window, which takes longer to acquire. As with increasing the number of samples, increasing the sample frame size improves results, but at the cost of longer test time.

The internal analysis system is using **windowing** to define segments of the sample to analyze. Except perhaps for some research systems, the user will not be able to alter the windowing characteristics (things like percentage of overlap or the shape of the windowing function). Typically those attributes are preset by the manufacturer.

As mentioned in Chapter 7, the goal is to provide narrow frequency bins for precise signal analysis. The otoacoustic emission will be low intensity. It will be possible to differentiate the response from the background noise provided that (a) the background noise is not too loud, and (b) the analysis bins are narrow enough so that the sum of all noise within the bin is still lower than the response.

AUDITORY EVOKED RESPONSE MEASUREMENT SYSTEMS

Evoked otoacoustic emissions are responses evoked from the inner ear by producing either clicks (TEOAEs) or pairs of tones (DPOAEs). In contrast, auditory evoked responses originate from the auditory nervous system, rather than the inner ear. Electrochemical changes in the nerve cells occur when the nerves fire. These minute electrical charges are time-locked to the signal that generates them: they always occur at the same time after stimulation. Many different stimulations are made, one after the other, and time-domain signal averaging is used to obtain the response. This is discussed in more detail below. Some common types of evoked responses are the **auditory brainstem response,** the **auditory steady-state response**, and the **middle-** and **late-latency responses.** This text will not cover the clinical use of these tests, but will describe how the equipment that records them operates.

Common Mode Rejection

Electrodes are placed on the surface of the head to pick up the electroencephalographic (EEG) waves—brain waves. A common setup is shown in Figure 8–5. One

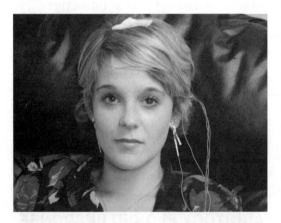

Figure 8–5. Surface electrodes, filled with electrode paste and placed on the head, are used to measure auditory evoked responses. The electrodes can be taped in place, or for the earlobes, attached with clips. Those placed within the hairline are usually held in place only with the paste, and then covered with a gauze pad.

electrode, termed the positive or **active electrode** or noninverting electrode, is placed on the vertex (top) of the head. Two negative or **reference electrodes** (also called inverting electrodes) are clipped to the earlobes, or alternatively, taped to the mastoid bone area behind the ear. (For this discussion, we'll just focus on one of those reference electrodes, though the evoked potential system typically has one for each ear.) A final electrode is the neutral or **ground electrode**, shown here taped to the forehead. The signal that each electrode detects is compared to the signal at the ground. Stated another way, the electrode is actually recording how much more positive or negative the voltage is relative to what the ground electrode detects. For example, at one moment if the active electrode detected +20 μV, and the ground detected +5 μV, then the active electrode will send a signal of +15 μV to the amplifier. If one of the reference electrodes records –17 μV, this voltage is –22 μV compared to the +5 μV detected by the ground electrode (Figure 8–6A). The reference electrode signal is sent to the inverting or negative input of the **differential amplifier**. The active electrode is connected to the positive input. The differential amplifier inverts the signal at the negative input (changes it from negative to positive or from positive to negative voltage). The two inputs are then added together. Figure 8–6 provides a schematic.

The differential amplifier controls the comparison to the voltage at the ground electrode within the amplifier itself. A more common schematic therefore shows the ground as a separate input to the amplifier (see Figures 8-6B through 8-6D).

The differential amplifier performs what is called **common mode rejection**. Inputs that are the same at the reference and inverting electrode are canceled (see Figure 8-6B). This feature is critical when measuring evoked potentials because the signal of

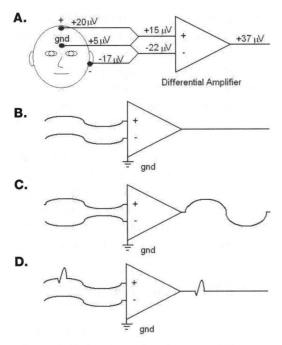

Figure 8–6. A. The positive, or active, electrode voltage is compared to ground and sent to the positive or noninverting input of the differential amplifier. The reference electrode voltage is also compared to ground and then sent to the negative or inverting input of the amplifier, which then changes the signal polarity. The differential amplifier then adds the two inputs together. **B.** If the same signal is present at both inputs, the output is no signal. **C.** If the two inputs were the same amplitude, but 180 degrees out of phase, the signal out of the amplifier would be double in amplitude. **D.** Any difference between the signals is amplified.

interest, the electrical activity from the auditory system, is embedded in the background of the EEG activity, which comes from thinking and controlling all of the autonomic nervous functions, like breathing and heart rate control. The size of much of this EEG activity will be similar at the two electrodes, and will (partially) cancel out.

If the voltage measured over time were exactly the opposite at the two electrodes,

then the differential amplifier would show the signal as double in amplitude (see Figure 8–6C)—as the name implies, the amplifier amplifies what is different at the two electrodes. This would happen during evoked potentials measurement if the generating signal were halfway between the two electrodes, traveling up the brain. The vertex electrode would "see" that as a voltage that increases over time. The electrode on the earlobe would "see" it as a voltage that decreases over time. Adding the two together in the differential amplifier would cause the signal to be read as twice the voltage. If a signal is detected in by just one of the electrodes (see Figure 8–6D), that difference is also amplified.

Time-Domain Signal Averaging and Artifact Rejection

During evoked potentials testing, earphones are inserted into the patient's ears, and the stimulus, often a click, is produced. A recording of the EEG is made and stored. Another click is produced, and that response is stored. The evoked response testing uses **time-domain signal averaging**, summing many sweeps. In auditory brainstem response testing, 1500 to 2000 sweeps will be averaged. As described in Chapter 7, the portion of the response that is similar in each sweep is increased; the part that changes sweep to sweep (e.g., thought-related activity or the heartbeat) is decreased in amplitude.

The patient is asked to recline and relax during evoked response testing, and refrain from moving. Even the most cooperative patient will have to swallow, and may occasionally cough or sneeze. If the patient is an infant, even less cooperation is expected. The sleeping baby may momentarily wake, or turn his or her head. Whenever muscle groups contract, very large potentials are generated. If these "contaminated" sweeps are averaged in, these sweeps, with their large voltages, bias the average. The principle behind **artifact rejection** is that if a sweep contains any voltage readings that are large, then that sweep will be assumed to contain a muscle artifact, and the sweep will not be entered into the average: it is rejected. Most evoked response systems allow the user to adjust the threshold for rejection. If very clean recordings are desired, the trigger for rejection can be lowered so that even minor muscle contamination is eliminated. This increases the recording time, however.

Filtering the Evoked Response

We are used to thinking about filtering auditory signals. For example, we might take white noise and send it through a low-pass (high-cut) filter to create pink noise. But auditory signals are not the only kinds of waveforms that can be filtered. Any signal in electrical form can be filtered. The electrical wave doesn't have to have come from a microphone or sound generator. The electrical signal that is filtered can be the EEG waveforms coming from the differential amplifier.

Chapter 6 introduced **band-pass filters**. Recall that a band-pass filter allows energy within a range of frequencies to pass through, but attenuates energy that is lower than the low-frequency cutoff and higher than the high-frequency cutoff. Chapter 6 described octave-wide and one-third octave-wide pass bands, but the pass band can be of any width. In evoked-potentials testing, we might set the high pass to 100 Hz and the low pass to 3000 Hz, creating a 2900 Hz-wide pass band.

Why filter the evoked response? To better visualize the evoked response! For example, if we expect to see a waveform with peaks every millisecond, then we expect a waveform with 1000-Hz information in it (1 peak per 1 msec is equivalent to 1000 waves

per 1 second: 1000 Hz). If that were the only information of interest, we would filter out all the energy except 1000 Hz to best see the response. However, evoked potential waves don't have just one sine-wavelike response in them, so we don't use a narrow band-pass filter. But by filtering out those frequencies we don't need, not only do we improve the image we see and analyze, we reduce **myogenic artifact**, that is, muscle activity contamination. Myogenic artifacts are large, slowly changing voltages. If we filter out the low-frequency energy in the EEG, the myogenic artifacts contained in the EEG are reduced.

HEARING AID ANALYZERS

Hearing aids have the goal of making soft sounds audible, making sounds that are comfortably loud to normal hearers comfortable in loudness to the hearing aid wearer, while ensuring that loud sounds are not uncomfortably loud. The hearing aid should do this without creating much distortion, or producing excessive amplifier hum.

Hearing aid analyzers are used to determine if a hearing aid is amplifying as intended by the manufacturer. This testing gives some information about whether the product is suited to a given patient, but hearing aids are customized with the aid of real-ear measurement systems, described below. The hearing aid analyzer is helpful as a quality control tool.

The hearing aid analyzer components are shown in Figure 8–7. The analyzer produces pure tones at calibrated intensities. The amplified signals are then picked up by a microphone and analyzed. One of the fundamental measurements is the **frequency response curve**. To make this measurement, 50 dB SPL pure tones are input one at a time, and the amount measured at the microphone is displayed frequency by frequency (Figure 8–8A).

A.

B.

C.

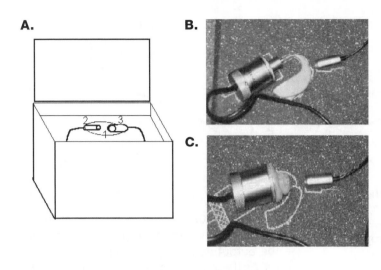

Figure 8–7. A. A hearing aid analyzer has a sound attenuating box, into which the hearing aid is placed. There is a speaker under the fabric floor of the box (*1*) a reference microphone monitors the sound and ensures that it is presented at a calibrated level (*2*). A coupler (*3*) has another microphone inside. **B**. The coupler for a behind-the-ear hearing aid is shown. **C**. The in-the-ear hearing aid is held into the coupler with putty. The amplified signal is channeled into a coupler, and then sent to a microphone. The results are displayed or printed. Figure/photos © Nova Southeastern University and reprinted with permission.

As later chapters will discuss, the most common type of hearing loss (cochlear loss, from inner ear damage) has an unusual characteristic. Soft sounds can't be heard, but loud sounds are still perceived as loud (a phenomenon called **recruitment**). Therefore, we need to ensure that the hearing aid does not create sound that is too loud. The output sound pressure level 90 (OSPL90) curve shows how much sound is produced by the hearing aid when 90 dB SPL is at the hearing aid microphone. Again, pure tones are input one frequency at a time, and the output graph is shown (Figure 8–8B).

The hearing aid analyzer can also show the amount of amplification, or **gain** of the hearing aid. Figure 8–9 shows that there is less gain when the signal input level is high. The hearing aid doesn't increase loud sounds as much as it increases softer sounds.

The hearing aid will adjust the amount of gain on a moment to moment basis, de-

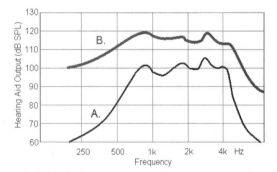

Figure 8–8. Frequency response curve (**A**) and output sound pressure level-90 (OSPL90) curves for a hearing aid (**B**). The frequency response curve shows the hearing aid output when 50 dB SPL is present at the hearing aid microphone. The OSPL90 curve shows the hearing aid output in response to 90 dB SPL.

pending on how much sound is present at the microphone (or, depending on the hearing aid design, how much is present at the

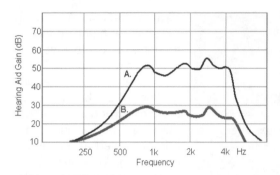

Figure 8–9. Gain curve for the same hearing aid illustrated in Figure 8-7. The amount of amplification (gain) is shown when the hearing aid input is 50 dB SPL (**A**) and 90 dB SPL (**B**).

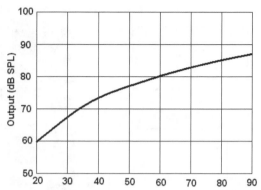

Figure 8–10. Input-output curve showing how a hearing aid might gradually increase the output as the signal input level increases. As the input changes from 20 dB to 90 dB SPL, the output increases only by 28 dB.

output of the hearing aid, but that's too picky a point to delve into in this text). An **input-output curve** shows how the hearing aid reacts as sound levels increase (Figure 8-10).

If the sound at the microphone suddenly changes from low intensity to high intensity, the hearing aid will decrease the gain; however, the electronic circuitry takes some amount of time to reduce that gain. That is called the hearing aid's **attack time**. Similarly, the **automatic gain control** hearing aid takes some time to return to providing full gain if the signal level goes from loud to quiet. That is the hearing aid's **release time**. Attack and release may sound like odd terms, but it makes sense if you think of the automatic gain control attacking the problem of having too much amplification of loud sounds, and releasing that control mechanism when it is no longer needed.

One more term: **compression.** This time it has nothing to do with the phase of air molecule vibration, but it is related to squeezing. The total range of hearing aid sound output is compressed relative to the range that comes into the hearing aid. In Figure 8-9, the input varied from 20 to 90 dB—a 70 dB range. The output only ranges

60 to about 88 dB SPL—only a 28 dB range. The hearing aid has compressed the output range by a factor of 70 to 28, which is a 2.5:1 **compression ratio**. (In an effort to avoid confusing the reader should he or she be on the track for the Au.D. degree, you will learn in your courses on amplification that the compression ratio is typically described over a more limited range of intensities, not the entire 70 dB input range.)

Hearing aid analyzers measure how much **harmonic distortion** is produced. They also measure something called **equivalent input noise**. Any amplifier produces some hum of its own, although the less the better. Equivalent input noise measurements provide an idea of how "noisy" the hearing aid amplifier is.

Hearing aids are battery powered, and different hearing aids drain the battery at different rates. A simulated battery can be inserted into the hearing aid, and this **battery pill** can detect the amount of current the hearing aid uses. The current is measured in mA, that is, milliamperes, thousandths of an amp. High current drain results in shortened battery life. Internal damage to the hearing aid sometimes causes excessive current drain, so if a patient complains of short battery life, the hearing aid analyzer provides a way of determining if the fault lies with the hearing aid, or if not, then one presumes the problem is with the brand of the batteries.

REAL-EAR MEASUREMENT SYSTEMS

Real-ear measurement systems do what hearing aid analyzers do not do. They measure how the hearing aid performs in the patient's ear and can be used while the audiologist adjusts the hearing aid as needed for the patient. Real-ear systems allow the audiologist to determine if quiet sounds are audible, whether conversational/comfortable level sounds are present in the ear at the prescribed level that should be comfortable to the listener. Additionally, real-ear systems allow verification that loud sounds are not uncomfortably loud. We first review the more modern speech mapping real ear measurement systems, then describe how the original technology worked, which is the basis for some of the measurements made in analyzing the resonances of the outer ear.

Speech Mapping Technology

A speech mapping system creates speech signals, or noise signals that have the same spectrum (frequency content) as speech and additionally have similar fluctuation of amplitude over time. The signal is delivered via sound-field speakers at different calibrated intensities.

This technology uses a **probe microphone**. This is a small microphone that is located near the ear. A flexible hollow plastic tube (the probe tube) connects to the microphone housing. This tube will be inserted into the ear to measure the sound in the ear

canal. (Figure 8-11 shows the equipment.) The hearing aid is then inserted in the ear. The microphone probe tube that is inserted the ear is not so soft that it will collapse when the hearing aid is inserted in the ear, so the amplified sound in the actual ear canal is measured.

To decide how much amplification is needed at each frequency, the audiologist

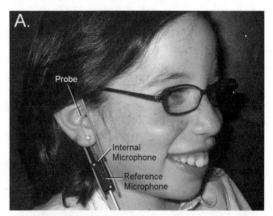

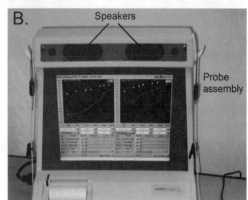

Figure 8–11. Speech mapping system. **A.** A flexible probe is inserted into the ear canal. The sound measured in the ear canal is measured by the microphone inside the probe system and compared to the level at the reference microphone. The hearing aid would then be inserted into the ear while the probe is still in the same location. **B.** The AudioScan real-ear system is shown. The unit has a probe assembly for each ear and speakers to produce the speech signal.

uses a prescription formula that is derived from the amount of hearing loss. Depending on the hearing loss, different amounts of amplification will be needed to restore sounds to audibility at each frequency. The printout shown in Figure 8-12 is from the **AudioScan** speech mapping system. As shown in Figure 8-12, the hearing test results have been entered, and a formula computes the desired amount of amplification, labeled as "target" in this figure. The AudioScan system produces speech, and shows the intensity of the speech in the ear canal, after being amplified by the hearing aid. The audiologist adjusts the hearing aid until the amplified speech signal is at the proper level. Figure 8-12 shows the range of speech intensity produced. Digital hearing aids can be computer adjusted to increase or decrease the amount of amplification across the frequency range. They can also separately amplify soft, medium, and loud intensity sounds, so that the prescription targets can be met.

The AudioScan speech mapping system uses digital technology. A number of different prerecorded digital wave files can be presented. For example, there is a child's voice, a male voice, and a female voice, so the response of the hearing aid to different types of voices can be analyzed. The system can also show the amount of amplification of any sound in the environment. This is useful if the patient reports not being able to hear a desired sound, such as the ring of a cell phone. The probe microphone system can display the amplified sound when the cell phone rings. The audiologist can note the frequencies in the sound and adjust the hearing aid to increase the amplification in the desired frequency range.

Hearing aids process speech (with its energy spread across the frequencies) differently than they do other sounds, such as music or pure tones. To ensure that tonal sounds, such as musical notes from a flute, with energy concentrated in one frequency

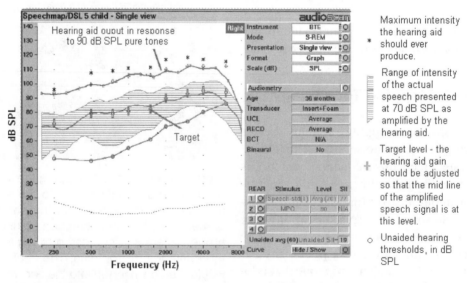

Figure 8–12. Speech mapping results, modified from http://www.audioscan.com/resources/usersguides/Currentverifitguide.pdf Reproduced and modified with permission courtesy of AudioScan® division of Etymonic Design Inc., Dorchester, Ontario, Canada.

region, aren't excessively loud, the speech mapping system can produce tonal signals. A common test produces 85 or 90 dB SPL pure tones at various frequencies and measures the output in the patient's ear. While the test is in progress, the audiologist can note whether the patient finds any of the tones uncomfortably loud—a reflexive grimace will occur!

These types of measurements are also called **real-ear aided responses**. The intensities of signals present with the aid in the ear are measured. There are other measurements that can be made using the same equipment setup, the traditional real-ear tests, which are described next.

Traditional Real-Ear Testing

Chapter 13 and 15 will explain that the outer ear, without a hearing aid inserted, is essentially a tube that is open at one end and closed at the other (at the eardrum). Chapter 5 described how this sort of acoustical chamber has certain frequencies that will resonate. If the resonances of the outer ear are of interest, this can be measured. Note that this is described as resonances—plural. The ear is not a simple tube and there are different frequency regions that will be amplified because of the size and shape of the tube, and because of the resonances of the pinna (the part of the ear on which eyeglasses rest). When measuring the **real-ear unaided response**, the audiologist will determine how much amplification of sound occurred because of these resonances. This can be thought of as the "before" measurement. (How does the size/shape of this patient's ear enhance the amplification of different sound frequencies?) The **real-ear aided response** is the "after"—the amount of sound present after the hearing aid is in place. As long as the same signal is used to make both of these measurements, then

the two responses can be compared. The amount (in dB) that the aided response is above the unaided response is the **gain** that the hearing aid provided. When these results are plotted frequency by frequency, the curve that shows the results is the **real-ear insertion response**. (When the word "gain" is used, it refers to testing at one frequency. "Response" refers to the gain shown graphed across frequencies.) If you read Chapter 15, you will learn more about real-ear testing and see how it is used to measure the response of the ear.

POWER SUPPLIES FOR HEARING INSTRUMENTS AND TESTING EQUIPMENT: SAFELY CONCERNS AND ELECTRONIC NOISE

Relative Safety of AC and DC Power Supplies

Sound measurement equipment and hearing testing equipment can be powered in one of two ways: with a battery, or with connection to an electrical power outlet. **Batteries** produce **direct current** (DC)—the electrons flow from the positive pole of the battery to the negative side. In contrast, the power from a wall outlet is AC—**alternating current**. There are several advantages to using batteries.

The voltage batteries provide is limited, which means there is a limit to the amount of current that can be produced. Remember that:

Current (I, in amperes) = Potential (E, in volts) ÷ Resistance (R, in ohms).

If the maximum potential for electrons to flow is 9 volts, even if you connected the negative and positive poles of the battery together with a very low impedance conductor (like a wet dog nose, a trick known to boys world wide), not much current can flow. Let's assume the dog's nose has 100 ohms of resistance. That would produce a current of just less than 0.1 amp. That's enough to make the dog jump back, but not enough to cause any harm. If you place your dry finger over both the positive and negative pole of that same battery, because your finger has high resistance to electricity flow (about 50,000 ohms), the current is so low (.000018 amps) that you can't even detect it.

The AC voltage from the power company is 110 volts. Connecting the negative and positive AC power terminals together with a "load" of only 10 ohms would allow current to flow at 11 amps. You would not want your body or your dog's nose to be subjected to that current flow!

Although the advantage to batteries is increased safety because of the low voltage, that is exactly what limits their utility. You cannot run equipment such as a power amplifier with batteries.

What Is AC Electricity?

Let's expand on the material introduced in Chapter 6 on electricity and analog systems and consider first, just what is electricity? We go back to the atom. From chemistry

and Chapter 6 you know that the atom has a positively charged center, and electrons that orbit in rings. **Conductors** have weakly held electrons in their outer (valence) ring. It's relatively easy to have the electron leave that outer ring and move over to a neighboring atom. Figure 8–13A illustrates the electrons in the copper atom. As shown, there is just one electron in the outermost ring, so it is easy to displace. Similarly, there are many empty "places" for extra electrons to attach. An **insulator** by comparison is a material that does not readily give up or accept electrons.

In North America, the atoms move back and forth in the electrical wire 60 times per second. The electric company is "pushing" and "pulling" the electrons back and forth. This energy is what causes the light bulb to glow, or what powers an amplifier. (The loose electron in the outer ring of the molecule is hopping from one molecule in the wire to the next, down the chain, then back, 60 times per second. See Figure 8–13B.) What then is a sound wave in a circuit? Let's take the example of a 2000 Hz sine wave in electrical form. The electrons in the wire are moving back and forth 2000 times per second. After passing through an amplifier, the amount of back and forth motion of those electrons is going to increase, but the rate of the vibration stays the same.

A.

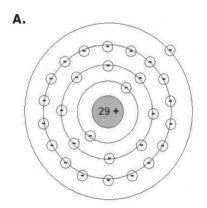

Figure 8–13. A. Orbit of electrons in the copper atom, which has 29 protons and 29 electrons. Each electron shell can only hold so many atoms, so for copper, the 29th atom is alone in its valence (outermost) shell, and it is easily dislodged. **B.** A conductor readily gives up and accepts electrons. Electricity is the movement of electrons from atom to atom.

B.

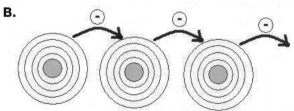

Ground Noise

If connecting audiology equipment to an AC power supply, there can be a problem: introduction of noise from the power supply. The power company is pushing and pulling electrons in the wire back and forth 60 times per second. Sometimes the electrical signal contaminates the audio signal. In the example begun above, the equipment would not only have a pushing/pulling of electrons back and forth 2000 times per second, but also, if we aren't set up just right, the electrons have a movement at 60 Hz as well. When this happens, it's not just the 60 cycles that is introduced, but all the harmonics as well. You may have heard that sort of buzz from your stereo system if it is not connected properly. This "ground hum" is not inevitable, but it requires careful equipment setup in a hearing science laboratory, where the researcher assembles the systems him or herself. This is one reason clinical audiology equipment is expensive. It has been engineered to keep the signal and power noise separate. An advantage to using battery-powered equipment is that you don't have to worry about this source of noise.

Grounding Equipment, Fuses, and Circuit Protectors

Next we introduce the idea of equipment grounding, which is a way to improve the safety of electronic equipment, and a way to lessen the chance that your equipment will pick up the humming sound from the power supply. That requires more introduction to the nature of electricity.

When the electric company is moving electrons back and forth through the power system, the electric company needs a source of extra electrons. All electrons are created equal, so just because the wire is copper, it does not mean that the electrons have to come from copper. The earth, the ground outside, is a good place to get electrons, and a good place to receive any extra ones. The power company is connected to a "ground," and the building you are in also has a connection from the "ground" electrical wire to the ground outside the building. (That might be a connection to a metal rod stuck into the ground, or it might be a connection to the building's metal plumbing pipes that run underground.)

Most appliances that are plugged into AC wall outlets have three prongs. The two longer, narrow prongs are the ones that push and pull the electrons through the appliance—the "positive" and "negative" wires coming from the power company connect here. The round third connector is a "redundant ground." That third prong is connected to your house ground as well as the power company's ground. Anything metal that the user could touch is connected to that ground wire.

If the "hot" positive wire pushing and pulling electrons were to break inside a piece of equipment, but not touch anything else, then the equipment would just stop working. But instead, if the "hot" wire connected directly to the negative wire (without the resistance of the electrical components in between), then current would flow very, very rapidly. One hopes this excess current is detected, and either a **fuse** "blows" or a **circuit breaker** "trips." A fuse is a wire filament through which the electrons flow (Figure 8–14). Fuses are designed to burn up if too much current flows, which stops the current flow. Fuses are designed to either burn out quickly or slowly, and are rated by the number of amps that can pass through before burning the fuse. If you have a piece of equipment that "blows a fuse" then either the fuse is just old and worn out, or you may have a defect in the internal components. You can open the equipment and inspect and replace the fuse yourself. Sometimes a

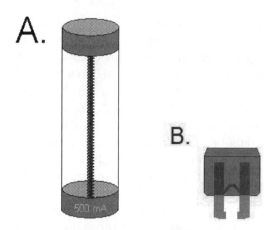

Figure 8–14. Illustration of fuses. **A.** The most common type of fuse in electronic equipment. Fuses generally have silver colored metal tops and bottoms, with a glass base that allows you to see the filament inside. **B.** This type of fuse is common in automotive applications, but occasionally seen in electronics. Replace fuses with ones with the exact same specifications.

spare fuse is stored inside the instrument. If not, fuses can be purchased as stores like Radio Shack, Home Depot, or Lowes. Bring the original and purchase an exact replacement. You should not just change the fuse to one that allows more current, as the reason the fuse is blowing may be because of a defect. Using a fuse with a higher amperage rating may keep the equipment working without blowing fuses, but it doesn't provide the same safety from too much current flowing inside the equipment.

Circuit breakers are similar—they too are designed to stop current flow. Rather than being inside a piece of equipment, they are a part of the building's electrical system, and detect excessive current from one or more of several outlets. Circuit breakers are able to be reset by flipping a switch, which is why we say that circuit breakers are "tripped" rather than "blown." The switch on the circuit breaker physically moves to the off position if too much current is flow-

ing. Putting too many pieces of heavy-duty amp-pulling equipment on the same circuit can blow the fuse. In a household application, you might find that if your refrigerator, toaster, microwave oven, and hair blow dryer are on the same circuit, the circuit may trip if too many of these appliances are on at the same time. The solution is to move one or more appliances to a different circuit. Excessive AC current flow in the wires can cause overheating and an electrical fire.

Now let's return to the purpose of the redundant third ground. Circuit breakers and fuses are good protection, and one hopes they prevent electric shock from occurring and fires from starting because of the excess current flow. However, the third ground wire can also prevent electric shock. Recall that the extra ground wire is connected to anything metal that a user could possibly touch, and then this is connected to the earth itself. If the positive wire touches the case of the equipment or appliance, then that current is routed to the outside ground wire for the time before the circuit breaker trips. If there isn't a grounding wire connected to the case, and just the positive wire touches the case, there may not be any current flow. However, if that metal case is touched by a person (or dog nose), suddenly there is a pathway for the current to reach the supply of electrons beneath one's feet (or paws). Electric shock results.

There are adapters that allow one to plug a three-prong device into a two-prong outlet. If the screw in the center of the outlet is connected to the building's grounding wire, and if you take the time to screw in the adapter, you might take that route at home. However, that should never be used in a clinic, as it is not approved for use with equipment used for medical testing or research.

Ground fault circuit interrupters (GFCI) are another safety device. They detect even a momentary fault in the grounding of equipment and trip. These are sometimes built into the power plug of appliances used near water (e.g., hair dryers) and therefore aren't common on audiologic equipment. GFCIs can also be built into electrical outlets, and are common in kitchens and bathrooms. You may find them on the power outlets, including ones in clinical facilities. Often, they are recognized by a black "test" and red "reset" buttons on the power outlet. (Sometimes the test and reset buttons are not colored differently from the outlet itself.)

Grounding is an important safety issue, but it also influences signal quality. Incomplete or improper grounding, or an improper mix between the audio signal ground and the power supply ground, can create the previously mentioned audible hum. Ensuring that equipment doesn't produce this noise requires considerable engineering care. Many an hour has been spent in hearing science labs trying to find the source of the electrical hum!

Floor Noise

Hearing science equipment's working components are designed to do their job without introducing additional noise; however, no piece of equipment is perfect. Even with no signal coming in, the internal components will produce some signal of their own. This is called the **floor noise** of the equipment. Audio equipment also has a highest intensity it is capable of producing (a ceiling of sorts), but it also has this lower "floor" that limits your ability to measure or accurately present signals that are lower in intensity than the floor noise, or for your patient or research subject to hear these weak signals. (They are lost in the floor noise.)

MICROPHONES

The microphone is one of the most basic components in the hearing sciences.

Without a microphone, you cannot measure sound or record or amplify it. Microphones were introduced in Chapter 6, where you learned that the purpose of the microphone is to create an electrical voltage that mimics the sound wave. The main component inside a microphone is a thin metal sheet, called the diaphragm that is light enough to vibrate to sound rarefaction and compression cycles (Figure 8–15). The circular diaphragm is held firmly to the sides of the microphone case (the "housing"), but the center can move easily. The microphone diaphragm is moved back and forth by the pressure wave in front of it. When the air molecules are in compression, the diaphragm moves inward; when in rarefaction, the diaphragm is sucked outward.

Types of Microphones

The most common microphone types are the condenser microphone and the dynamic microphone. One type of **condenser microphone** is the **electret microphone**, used in hearing aids. This type of microphone has a charged metal plate (or "back plate") right behind the diaphragm. The back plate's charge will change de-

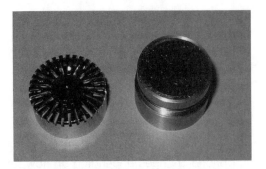

Figure 8–15. A microphone, seen with its protective grill (*on left side of photo*) removed to show the diaphragm. Dust has collected on the surface of the microphone diaphragm.

pending on how close the diaphragm is to the back plate. In Figure 8–16A, there is no sound present, and the microphone produces a steady neutral voltage. If the diaphragm moves inward (Figure 8–16B), the voltage increases; the voltage decreases as the diaphragm moves away (Figure 8–16C). Figure 8–16 suggests that the diaphragm is moved to one position and holds there. Of course, sound waves have cycling compression and rarefaction, so the output of a microphone usually doesn't stay steady very long. If the sound were a 1000-Hz sine wave, then the microphone output would cycle positive and negative 1000 times per second. The microphone produces an electrical output that is the analog of the sine wave—it directly mimics the sound wave. If the signal were a triangular wave (Figure 4–13A), then the microphone output would be an electrical triangular waveform.

The condenser microphone design is not the only way to create electron flow in response to sound. A **dynamic microphone** has a wire coil that can move inside a magnetic field. The movement creates the electrical current.

There are a few less common microphone types. **Crystal microphones** change the diaphragm movement to electricity by changing the shape of certain types of crystals, but this microphone type does not have a very flat frequency response and they are not suitable for professional applications. **Carbon microphones** have carbon crystals between the front and back plate, and the electrical current passes through the carbon. Again, this is not a type widely used today.

Microphones can also be classified by their use. **Lavaliere microphones** are the type clipped onto a lapel or worn hanging from the neck. They are usually attached to a wire, and then connect to a transmitter box to send a wireless radio or light signal to a receiver box that picks up the signal and amplifies it. **Headset microphones** are also common. They are meant to be worn right at the corner of the mouth, typically about 1 inch away. You should not wear a headset microphone right in front of your mouth. Some speech sounds (like "p") create a burst of air. If the headset microphone is 1" away, right ahead, the air burst creates a sudden noise. Moving the microphone to the side corner of the mouth prevents this problem. There are also **tabletop microphones** designed to sit on a conference table and record lectures.

One final classification merits introduction. **Field microphones** are meant to be used to measure sounds "in a sound field," that is, in a room. **Pressure microphones** are used in some audiology calibration situations where the microphone is placed inside a metal cylinder (coupler). Hearing aid analyzers use a pressure microphone. Audiometer earphone calibration also requires a pressure microphone.

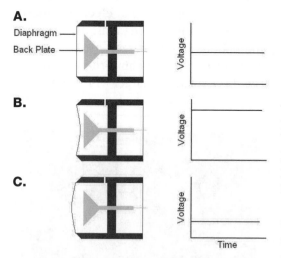

Figure 8–16. The voltage produced by a microphone changes depending on how far away the diaphragm is from the back plate, a metal plate that has an electrical charge applied to it. The voltage coming from the back plate varies depending on the position of the diaphragm.

Microphone Directionality

Another way to classify microphones is to see how well they pick up sound coming from different directions. An **omnidirectional microphone** picks up sound from all directions equally well. A **directional microphone** is designed to pick up sound from some directions better than for other directions.

Microphones can be tested to see how well they pick up sounds from different angles—from in front, to the sides, to the rear. The angle of the sound is referred to as the sound's **azimuth** (Figure 8–17). To test the directionality of the microphone, a sound source is kept a certain distance away from the microphone, for example, 3 feet away. The sound speaker is rotated around the microphone, and the microphone's output is recorded at each angle. The resulting trace of how well the microphone picks up the sound at different angles is called a **polar plot**. (The name polar plot brings to mind the poles of the earth, but any type of measurement referenced to an angle system is a polar measurement.)

A perfect omnidirectional microphone would pick up sound equally well from all angles. Its polar plot would show a circle. Let's assume that a microphone is tested with a 90 dB SPL signal. The signal output from the omnidirectional microphone would be 90 dB at all angles. As the idea is how much better or worse the microphone is at picking up signals at different angles, it doesn't really matter whether the test was done at 90 dB SPL or some other intensity. What matters is the relative change, if any, in the sound level as the source rotates around it. Therefore, the polar plot is usually labeled in dB of change across angle. In Figure 8–18, several common types of polar plots are illustrated. Notice that all of the types of directional

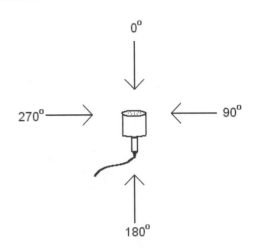

Figure 8–17. The directionality of a microphone is tested at different sound source azimuths. A sound source is kept a fixed distance from the microphone and is rotated around the microphone. The output of the microphone is recorded at each angle.

microphones attenuate sound that comes in from behind, that is from 180 degrees. The thicker lines show how much attenuation is provided. For example, the supercardiod microphone illustrated in Figure 8–18B attenuates sound from 100 degrees azimuth by 10 dB. The supercardioid and hypercardioid microphones have two directions where the signal is severely attenuated (illustrated as about 125 degrees and 235 degrees azimuth in Figure 8–18C) but sounds from a direction in between those angles are not as greatly attenuated.

The polar plots shown in Figure 8–18 would be typical of a microphone that is used in measuring in sound field. A microphone mounted in a hearing aid and worn at the ear would perform differently because the head would block some frequency sounds coming from the far side of the head. This is shown in Figure 8–19.

Polar plots are shown for only one frequency at a time. The microphone's response can vary substantially from frequency to fre-

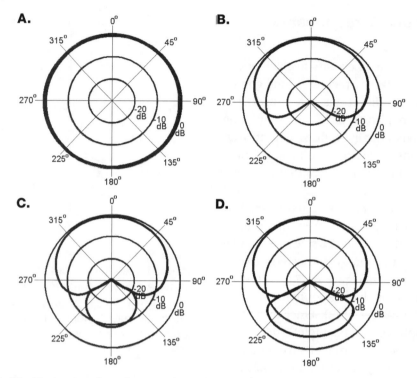

A. **B.** **C.** **D.**

Figure 8–18. Example microphone polar plots. **A.** Omnidirectional microphone plot shows equal sensitivity regardless of the direction of the signal. **B. Cardioid microphone** response showing least sensitivity for sounds coming from directly behind (180 degrees). **C.** This **supercardioid microphone** response has some sensitivity to sounds from behind, but this microphone attenuates signals from 180 degrees about 10 dB relative to those from straight ahead. **D. Hypercardioid microphone** response attenuates sound from behind less than does the supercardioid; as shown, sounds from behind are reduced 5 dB relative from those in front.

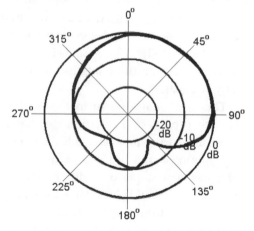

Figure 8–19. Illustration of potential hearing aid microphone response from a directional microphone worn in the right ear.

quency. That is particularly true with hearing aid microphones where the head and outer ear help to block sounds from certain directions. High-frequency sounds, with wavelengths shorter than the head, are blocked by the head—there is a **head shadow** effect. Lower frequency sounds are not attenuated. (See Chapter 3, section on diffraction and reflection, and Figure 3-3.)

Microphone Care

Good quality measuring microphones used for calibration of hearing testing equipment and for hearing research applications cost about $1000 each. They are designed to be highly accurate in measuring sounds of all frequencies. They are delicate and can be damaged by excessive vibration. For instance, even being dropped onto a surface from a height of just a few inches can change how the microphone responds to sound, and not for the better! The metal diaphragm inside the microphone is extremely fragile, so it is usually covered by a protective grill that is screwed in place (see Figure 8-15). This keeps anyone from accidentally touching the microphone.

Microphones of this quality are so sensitive that even a speck of dirt or condensation of moisture on the surface of the diaphragm can alter their performance. They are usually stored in a special case with dehumidifying desiccant crystals. Never blow on one of these microphones or allow anything to touch the diaphragm. If you see dust on them, the manufacturer who calibrates and services the microphones may be able to help.

SOUND LEVEL METERS

As the name implies, sound level meters are used to measure the intensity of sound. They have three types of use. They can be used to measure the intensity of sound in the environment, for example, to determine if the noise level is high enough to cause damage to hearing or whether it exceeds community noise annoyance standards. They may be used to measure the intensity of signals produced by audiometers or research equipment, which permits calibration (the adjustment of the equipment to produce the desired sound level). They can also be used change an acoustic signal into an electrical signal, so that the electrical signal can be analyzed or converted to a digital signal for analysis or manipulation.

The sound level meter microphone picks up the sound and converts it to an electrical signal, and then the sound level meter displays the decibel level. A high-quality sound level meter typically has a way for that electrical signal to be sent to another piece of equipment. For example, you could connect from the output of the sound level meter to the input of a digital tape recorder, or into a computer analog-to-digital converter. Figure 18–20A is a photograph of a sound level meter.

Calibration

The sound level meter will have a read out to allow you to determine the intensity of sound. For the measurement to be accurate, you must first calibrate the sound level meter/microphone, which is done by using a device called a **piston phone**. The piston phone is a rugged sound generator that produces one signal at a time (Figure 8-21). Often piston phones can produce a couple of different frequency sounds, sometimes each at two different intensities. The sound level meter has an adjustment on it. You can increase or decrease the sensitivity of the sound level meter until it reads the level that the piston phone is designed to put out. Once you have done this at one intensity, for one frequency, you can then check that all of the other piston phone tones are also measured correctly. (If not, then the sound level meter and microphone need to be factory serviced.)

The sound level meter, with its microphone(s) and piston phone should all be returned to the manufacturer or service center annually. The manufacturer's technician will check the devices and certify their calibration.

Types of Decibel Scales

Chapter 3 differentiated between dB SPL, and dB IL, and introduced the types

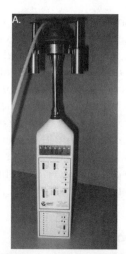

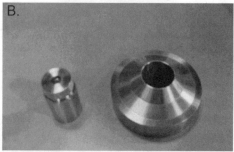

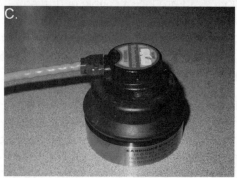

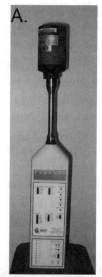

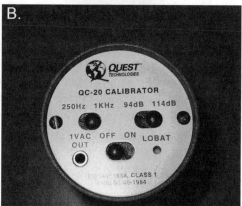

Figure 8-21. A. Calibration piston phone attached to the sound level meter. **B.** This piston phone allows presentation of two frequencies, at two different intensities.

Figure 8–20. A. Quest model 1800 sound level meter, shown here as set up for calibration of a supra-aural earphone. **B.** The couplers used for calibrating insert earphones (*left*) and supra-aural earphones (*right*). **C.** The earphone is placed on top of the coupler. The microphone fits inside the coupler, as can be seen in (**A**).

of decibels used in measuring hearing (dB HL and dB SL). There are four other types of decibels. These four types all refer to the in-

tensity of the sound after it has been passed through a type of filter.

One of the types of filters that might be available on a sound level meter is the **narrow band-pass filter** used to conduct spectral analysis. As you learned in Chapter 6, a band-pass filter has a region of frequencies that are not attenuated (passed through unchanged). The "corner frequencies" are the frequencies above and below the center of the pass band where sound is attenuated by 3 dB. Sounds with frequencies above the high-frequency cutoff point, or below the low-frequency cutoff point, are attenuated. The sound level meter may have a "bank" of these filters: you can select one filter at a time from a wide range of center frequency choices. The band-pass regions are typically either 1-octave wide or one-third octave wide. If you have octave-wide filters, you can conduct **octave band analysis** of the sound: You are able to measure how intense the sound is in each octave band. This gives you a general idea of the spectrum of the sound energy. **One-third octave band analysis** provides even more accurate frequency analysis. If the sound level meter has an output, another way to obtain a frequency analysis would be to take the output and send it to a computer that has software to conduct a fast-Fourier transform (FFT) analysis.

Figure 8–22 illustrates what the readings might be if five pure tones were present simultaneously. If a high-quality FFT analysis were made, it is theoretically possible to read just these five components, and determine that each is 50 dB SPL (Figure 8–22A). If measured with one-third octave band filters, the filter centered at 1000 Hz, with cutoff frequencies at 891 Hz and 1122 Hz, has two of the pure tones in that region. Recall from Chapter 2 that if two pure tones are summed (or detected in the same analysis band), the amplitude doubles. The 1000-Hz, one-third-octave band would read 53 dB SPL. Examine Figure 8–22B. Note that even though there are no pure tones within the 561 to 707-Hz cutoff frequencies, the one-third octave analysis would show energy in that frequency region. That is "spillover" from the 750-Hz tone. If a pure tone had been present at 707 Hz, that pure tone would be attenuated by 3 dB. (Remember by definition the signal is attenuate 3 dB at the cutoff frequencies.) 750 Hz is just 43 Hz away from the 707-Hz cutoff frequency, which is just 0.085 octaves above 707 Hz. The 750-Hz tone is only attenuated by about

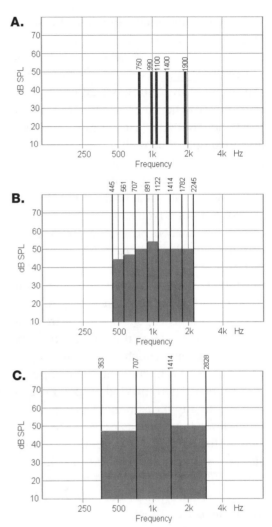

Figure 8–22. A. Five pure tone signals are present. **B.** If measured with one-third octave band filters, band-pass regions with more than one pure tone in that region show an elevated level because the energy of the different pure tones is summed together. Adjacent one-third octave band regions also show energy. The filter slopes of the one-third octave filters are not steep enough to completely attenuate frequencies not in the actual pass band. **C.** Octave band analysis provides less precise information about the frequency content of the original signal.

3 dB by the 561 to 707-Hz third-octave band-pass filter.

Even if the filters attenuate the signal by 48 dB per octave, the 750-Hz tone is only attenuated by 4 dB when reaching the 561 to 707-Hz pass band. For this same reason, some of the 750-Hz signal energy will be detected when measured in the 445 to 561 band. Similarly, just because there was no actual pure tone within the 1414 to 1782 band doesn't mean energy won't be read. That filter will pick up some of the 1400-Hz tone energy, and some of the 1900-Hz tone energy, both of which sum.

Octave analysis provides even less information about the spectrum. Note in Figure 8–22C that 56 dB of energy is measured in the 1000-Hz octave band. That comes from the sum of the four pure tones that are within that band. The 500-Hz center frequency band again detects the energy from the 750-Hz pure tone, which is attenuated somewhat because of the high-cut filter slope.

A limitation to any kind of spectral analysis and to any measurement made by the sound level meter relates back to the equipment's **floor noise.** You cannot accurately measure a signal that is at or is less intense than the floor noise level.

The other types of decibels are **dB A, dB B,** and **dB C.** These also are sound pressure level readings that are made after a signal is passed through a filter. The filter for reading dB C creates the least amount of change in the signal amplitude. As shown in Figure 8–23, it attenuates the energy of a 20-Hz pure tone, or the 20-Hz component of any complex sound, by about 8 dB. Signals with frequencies 50 Hz to about 5000 Hz are not changed at all. The B-weighted filter creates even greater attenuation of low-frequency sounds. The A filter attenuates them even more, but it also increases the reading of the mid-frequency sounds slightly. Chapter 28 will discuss the original rationale behind these filter curves; this chapter only briefly mentions the use of the A curve.

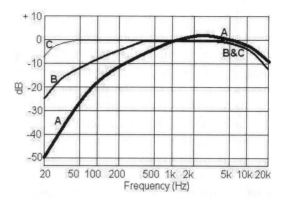

Figure 8–23. If the sound level meter is set to read dB A, dB B, or dB C, then the signal measured by the microphone is sent through one of the three filters before the intensity is measured. This figure shows how each of these filters attenuates sound and how the A filter adds a little to sounds with frequencies in the 2000 to 4000-Hz range. The amount of attenuation (or amplification) provided by the filters is shown. For example, the A filter would reduce the measurement of a 100-Hz sound by about 18 dB, whereas if read in dB B, the sound would be about 8 dB reduced from what it would read in dB C. The dB C reading and the "linear" or unfiltered reading would be the same for a 100-Hz sound.

The dB A curve is used to make noise hazard measurements. High-frequency sounds in the 1000- to 5000-Hz frequency range are more damaging to hearing than lower or higher frequency sounds, and in general, the lower the frequency, the less likely it is to damage hearing. The A filter reduces the measured intensity of these less damaging low-frequency sounds, matching the lowered risk when exposed to these frequency sounds, and slightly increases the readings for sounds with the greatest potential to harm hearing. The **Occupational Safety and Health Administration** (OSHA) has set workplace standards that limit an employee's exposure to sound, using the dB A scale. For example, if the person is exposed to 90 dB A or more sound for 8 hours, he or she must be provided with hearing protection and be enrolled in a hearing conservation program that monitors hearing status.

If you are not using either the narrow band filters or an A, B, or C filter, then you are using what is termed the "linear" scale. If so, when you read the sound level meter measurement, record the measurement as dB SPL. If using the dB A scale, and reading a measurement of 80 dB, it is reported as 80 dB A. If you selected the 1000-Hz band-pass filter, and it was a one-third-octave filter, you would note the reading as being however many "dB SPL in the 1000-Hz one-third-octave band-pass filter." It is important to always record the type of decibel, as the reading obtained depends on the filter selected.

Sound Level Meter Response Times

The sound level meter may also have settings that allow it to measure signals that vary over time in different ways. For example, the sound level meter may have a "peak hold" setting that records the highest sound level present. (The reading can be reset as desired.) The reading displayed may be the ongoing sound level instead, which would be more common. Even there, you have options on how the readings are obtained. The readings cannot truly be instantaneous— your eye could not register the readings if they changed every millisecond. The sound level meter time settings of "slow" and "fast" provide averages of the sound level readings, with that option changing how long the averaging takes, and thus how quickly the meter readings change.

Decibel Range Selection

The sound level meter can be set to more optimally read either very loud or very quiet sounds. High quality meters will have range selectors, for example, 20 to 60 dB / 30 to 70 dB / 40 to 80 dB, and so forth. The readings will be most accurate if you select the range that best describes the range of intensities you will be measuring.

Earphone Couplers

When the sound level meter is used to calibrate an earphone, the earphone needs to be connected to (coupled to) the microphone. There are standard couplers used for this purpose. The coupler is a metal cylinder designed to provide an easy and reliable way to connect the earphone to the coupler (see Figures 8-20B and 8-20C). In general theory, they are designed to imitate the ear. For example, the cylinder used to measure the insert earphone has a cavity size that is smaller than the coupler cavity used for supra-aural earphones, as the insert earphone has a smaller space between its end and the eardrum. However, these metal cavities are not accurate ear simulators. The decibel level read in the coupler is not exactly the level you would read at the eardrum of a human's ear. In contrast, the **Zwislocki coupler** does emulate the response of the average ear. It is not a simple cavity; it has a series of chambers. When the microphone is connected to a Zwislocki coupler, the sound pressure level read is what you would expect to measure at the eardrum of the average normal ear.

FREQUENCY COUNTERS

Sound level meters are one of the most fundamental pieces of equipment in a hearing research laboratory, and they are also indispensable to audiologists, as audiometers must be calibrated to ensure that it produces the proper intensity for hearing testing. In addition to calibration ensuring that the audiometer produces the proper intensity, calibration also verifies that the proper frequency is produced. Although the audiometer does not have to put out exactly the nominal frequency (e.g., it is OK to produce 1005 Hz instead of 1000 Hz), the signal frequency must be close. Diagnostic audiometers must produce frequencies that are no more than 1% off (1000 Hz may be 990 Hz to 1010 Hz). Frequency counters are used to determine the frequency produced. They may be attached to the output of the sound level meter, or they can measure the electrical signal itself, in which case the earphone is unplugged and the frequency counter is connected into that output.

AUDIOMETER CALIBRATORS

A frequency counter may be built into an **audiometer calibrator**. The calibrator is a device connected to the sound level meter output that can make other measurements to ensure that the audiometer is functioning properly. The system can measure the **harmonic distortion of the audiometer**. From Chapter 4 you know that harmonics occur at increments of the original signal. For example, 1000-Hz harmonic distortion would occur at 2000 Hz, 3000 Hz, 4000 Hz, and so forth. As the goal of hearing testing is to assess hearing at just one frequency, it's important to ensure that unwanted harmonics are not produced. If harmonics are present, and if the patient has better high-frequency hearing (more hearing loss in the low frequencies), he or she might detect the harmonic, rather than the frequency intended.

The calibrator can also measure the **rise time** and **fall time** of the pure tone: the time required for the tone to go from off to on, and from on to off. Too slow a time isn't desirable, but the real problem would be if the tone turns on or off too fast. If the earphone diaphragm is asked to move a far distance very quickly, as would happen if the pure tone turned on instantly, the earphone is not able to faithfully respond—it can't go from a dead stop to full-on amplitude that fast (and even if it did, the structures in the ear would not). The result is a popping sound. That pop sound has energy at more frequencies than just the pure tone frequency, so again, that would defeat the idea of testing hearing one frequency at a time.

Audiometer calibrators also can measure linearity of the audiometer. The audiometer intensity controls are "linear" if increasing 5 dB on the audiometer hearing control dial creates exactly 5 dB of increase in intensity. Measurement of the linearity of low-intensity sounds acoustically is limited by the equipment floor noise and the ambient noise in the room. The electrical signal linearity can be measured instead using the audiometer calibrator.

OSCILLOSCOPES

Sometimes "seeing is believing"—the hearing scientist may need to visualize the acoustic waveform. Once the sound is in electrical format, the waveform can be viewed on a device called an **oscilloscope** (Figure 8–24). One way to get the audio wave into electronic form is using the sound level meter. Most laboratory quality sound level meters will have an output that can be connected to the oscilloscope. Another option is to unplug the earphone and plug that signal output into the input of the oscilloscope. The oscilloscope displays the time waveform. Both the voltage (the vertical scale) and the time scale (horizontal) (Figure 8–25) can be changed. A storage oscilloscope will hold the waveform after a "sweep" is captured, or the ongoing signal can be viewed. If looking at the ongoing waveform, then the oscilloscope user

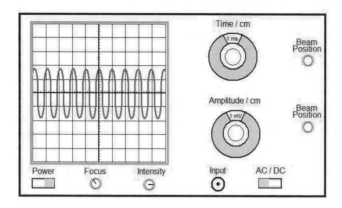

Figure 8–24. Illustration of an oscilloscope. The waveform is viewed on the screen to the left. The scale of the x-axis is adjusted using the "time/cm" scale, and the amplitude is also adjustable.

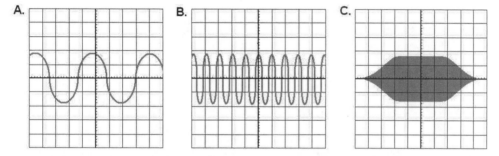

Figure 8–25. Example of adjustment of the time scale on an oscilloscope. The same signal is shown in (**A**) and (**B**), only the time scale has changed. In (**C**), the time per division is so long that the individual waveforms cannot be seen, but the envelope of the wave is evident. This can be useful when measuring the tone's rise and fall time.

will need to set the "trigger," which causes the oscilloscope to start displaying the signal once it reaches a certain amplitude. That allows an ongoing signal, like a pure tone, to appear stationary, as each sweep is started at the same voltage.

Computer software can also be used to allow the computer to function as an oscilloscope. An analog-to-digital converter is needed to digitize the signal, but once in the computer domain, the computer based signal analyzer has the advantage that it is easy to store waveforms and results. However, the computer may have higher internal noise, limiting the ability to make fine analyses.

SUMMARY

Audiologists use audiometers, middle ear analyzers (immittance devices), and real-ear measurement systems in daily practice. This equipment must be calibrated, which involves the use of measuring microphones, sound level meters, and dedicated audiometer calibration systems. Hearing scientists may use this same equipment, but may also create signals using dedicated signal generators or via computer software. Increasingly, experimental laboratories are using software-based systems to produce the signals, as well as to control experiments.

SECTION TWO

Introduction to Speech Acoustics

9

Classification of Speech Sounds

Phonetics is the study of how speech sounds are produced. Each unique speech sound or **phoneme** has been given an International Phonetic Alphabet (IPA) symbol. In this chapter, the reader is introduced to how phonemes are classified to show similarities and differences in how each is produced. Although the IPA symbols are used to help those who have had phonetics review this material, the reader need not know IPA or have had a course in phonetics. The purpose of this chapter is to introduce some of the major terms and ideas of phonetics, which will lead us to the next chapter on the acoustics of speech. Chapter 10 will discuss how the acoustic characteristics of speech depend on the shape and size of vocal tract—the throat, mouth, and nose. The goal of this chapter is to provide the overview needed to understand why different phonemes sound different—because they are produced differently.

CONSONANTS, VOWELS, AND DIPHTHONGS

Intuitively we know what consonants and vowels are, but from the acoustic phonetics standpoint, the classification might not be as obvious. **Vowels** are created with a relatively open vocal tract. **Consonants** are produced with a point of closure or constriction somewhere along the vocal tract. That point of constriction can occur at any point from the vibrating vocal folds (the glottis) to the lips.

Along with vowels and consonants is the class of speech sounds called **diphthongs**. Diphthongs are two vowels that transition one to the other to make a single sound. The vowel in the word "join" is an example. Although the dictionary may list the sound as the simple long "o" sound, in IPA it is written as /ɔɪ/ to show it is made by transitioning between the vowel /ɔ/, the "aw" in caught, to a second vowel /ɪ/, the short "i" sound, as in "it." Because diphthongs are a combination of two vowels, they won't be detailed in this chapter.

CONSONANTS ARE CATEGORIZED BY PLACE OF ARTICULATION, MANNER OF ARTICULATION, AND VOICING

The consonant sounds vary by where the tongue is placed to narrow or to close off the oral cavity, which is called **place of articulation**. The **manner of articulation** refers to how the sound is made. The manner of articulation refers to whether the sound is a stop, fricative, affricative, nasal, or glide. **Stop** consonants are made by creating a temporary blockage of the oral cavity. **Fricatives** are created when the breath stream passes a restricted, narrowed place. (Affricates will be defined later.) **Sonorants** are more melodious sounds created without much obstruction. Some of the sonorants are **nasal** sounds, made when the nasal cavity is open and sound escapes through the nose. A non-nasal sonorant is called a **glide**. Consonants also vary by whether the vocal cords are vibrating during the time the sound is made, which is called the feature of **voicing**. The concepts of place, manner of articulation, and voicing will be described again as we examine individual sounds.

Alveolar Sounds

Let's first describe the sounds made by placing the tongue in contact with the alveolar ridge, the bony part of the roof of the mouth that is right behind the front teeth. Figure 9–1 shows the tongue position for alveolar sounds "t" (/t/) and "d" (/d/). The "t" (/t/) sound is made without the vocal folds vibrating; a point easily understood if you rest your fingers on your voice box (larynx) and produce a few "t" (/t/) sounds in isolation. Now do the same while producing the "d" (/d/) sound and you will note the difference. Both "t" (/t/) and "d" (/d/) are brief sounds created when the tongue just momentarily blocks the oral cavity and some air pressure builds up behind and is then released. The "t" (/t/) and "d" (/d/) sounds are examples of **stop** consonants because the breath stream stops momentarily, then bursts forth. Try it yourself. Create an exaggerated "t" (/t/) sound and you will feel the pressure burst. Some texts call this class of sound a **plosive**, implying that a small explosion of air bursts forth. That term is losing favor, because you can actually create a

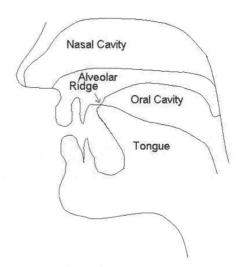

Figure 9–1. Representation of the manner of articulation for alveolar sounds. This sagittal cross-section of the head shows the outline of the oral and nasal cavities and the tongue. To create alveolar sounds, the tongue tip reaches up to the alveolar ridge, behind the front teeth. The non-nasal alveolar sounds are "t" /t/, "d" /d/, "l" /l/, "s" /s/, and "z" /z/.

"t" (/t/) sound without creating a true air burst. You can try that yourself also. Hold your breath and make a few "t" (/t/) sounds. Because you are holding your breath, there is no explosion of your breath when you release the tongue from the alveolar ridge, so the term stop consonant is preferred.

Other sounds are also made with the same tongue position—the sonorant sounds "n" (/n/) and "l" (/l/). **Sonorant** sounds are steady, even sounds that are created without a lot of friction from the breath stream. Feel what is happening as your prolong the sound "n" (/n/). You have closed off the oral cavity completely: the breath stream is going from the throat, via the velopharyngeal port (area at the back of the mouth that connects the oral and nasal cavities), into the nasal cavity (Figure 9–2). The "n" /n/ sound is called a **nasal** sound, for an obvious reason. Now produce "l" (/l/). The tongue is not fully occluding (blocking) the oral cavity and the ve-

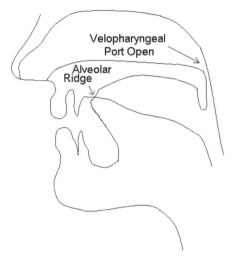

Figure 9–2. The "n" (/n/) sound is made with the same place of articulation as shown in Figure 9-1; however, the velopharyngeal port is open and the sound escapes through the nose.

lopharyngeal port between the oral and nasal cavity is closed. You can demonstrate the closure of your velopharyngeal port to yourself by sustaining the "l" (/l/) sound and pinching off your nose. There is no change in the sound, as none of the breath stream was exiting your nose. Try that while producing "n" (/n/) and you will not be able to create the sound. Sonorants will either be subcategorized as nasals or as **glides**, a name that nicely reminds us that the sound is made with a gradual onset and offset. The phoneme "n" /n/ is a nasal; "l" /l/ is a glide.

Two more sounds are produced at this alveolar ridge place, "s" (/s/) and "z" (/z/). Both are created with a hiss of air turbulence; they are considered **fricative** sounds. The "s" (/s/) is unvoiced; the "z" (/z/) is voiced.

Palatal Sounds

The sounds "r" (/r/), "zh" /ʒ/ as in the second consonant in the words "measure" and "beige," and "sh" /ʃ/ in "shoe" are made

with the tongue contacting a large area of the roof of the mouth, the palate. Figure 9–3 is not ideal in that it doesn't show that the tongue is somewhat rolled: the sides are in contact with the roof of the mouth, but there is a ridgelike depression down the center of the tongue that will allow the breath stream to flow past. There are no stop palatal sounds in English. There is one sonorant, the glide "r" (/r/). There is no palatal nasal sound. "Zh" /ʒ/ and "sh" /ʃ/ are the voiced and unvoiced fricatives for this place of articulation. There is also one glide, the "yuh" sound /j/, as in "**yes**."

There are a few more palatal sounds that are harder to classify. They are part stop and part fricative, and are called **affricatives**. The "tch" (/tʃ/) sound may be familiar to fans of the TV show *The Dog Whisperer* and its star Cesar Millan. To calm and get the attention of canines in his charge, he makes this voiceless sound in repeated series. It's the unvoiced sound of the "ch" in "ea**ch**." The other affricative is the voiced counterpart, which is the "j" sound in "**j**udge," or in the IPA it is /dʒ/.

Glottal Sound

The only English glottal sound, which has as its point of airflow constriction the glottis or space between the vocal folds, is "h" (/h/). It is unvoiced, and considered a fricative.

Velar Sounds

The roof of the mouth is composed of two parts: the anterior hard palate and the posterior soft palate. The latter is also called the velum and is the place for tongue contact for the velar stop sounds "k" (/k/) and its voiced counterpart "g" (/g/) (Figure 9-4). There is one sonorant sounds made at this place of articulation: "ng" (/ŋ/). The phoneme "ng" (/ŋ/) in "snori**ng**" is a nasal sound.

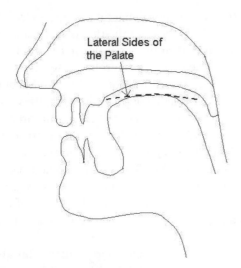

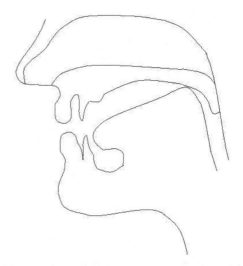

Figure 9–3. The place of articulation for the palatal sounds: the sonorant r (/r/) the fricatives zh /ʒ/ (as in mea**s**ure) and sh /ʃ/, the affricative sounds /dʒ/ as in **j**ustice and (/tʃ/) in **ch**est, and the glide "yuh" /j/ as in **y**es. The sides of the tongue come in contact with the palate.

Figure 9–4. The place of articulation for the velar sounds "k" /k/, "g" /g/. The back of the tongue touches the soft palate. The "ng" sound /ŋ/ is also made in this place, though with an open velopharyngeal port.

Linguadental sounds

There are two linguadental fricative sounds made with the tongue in contact with the front teeth: "th" (/θ/) and (/ð/) (Figure 9-5). Note that there are two IPA symbols and one English one. One is voiced (/ð/), the "th" as in "**th**is," one is unvoiced, the "th" (/θ/) in "**th**ank." Unsure of the difference? Try prolonging the "th" as you are saying "this," then add on the -"ank" from "thank" and you will more readily hear how it is a different sound. Again, you can feel your voice box to note that they are produced differently.

Bilabial Sounds

Next, let's discuss four sounds made with contact of the two lips (the labia) to restrict the breath stream (Figure 9-6). The sounds "p" (/p/) and "b" (/b/) are the unvoiced and voiced stop consonant pair for

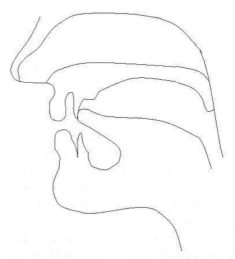

Figure 9–5. Place of articulation for the linguadental sounds, the voiced and unvoiced "th" (/θ/ and /ð/), in the words "**th**row" and "**th**ose." The tongue tip comes in contact with the back of the incisor teeth.

this place of articulation. If that closure is maintained, and the velopharyngeal port is opened, and the sound made longer in duration, then the sound is the nasal, sonorant

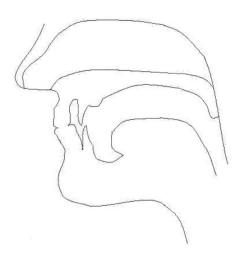

Figure 9–6. Place of articulation for the bilabial sounds "p" (/p/), "b" (/b/), "m" (/m/). The lips (labia) come together to produce each of these sounds. The "m" /m/ sound is nasal, so would be made with an open velopharyngeal port. The lips would be protruded for the sound "w" (/w/), which is also classified as a bilabial phoneme.

"m" (/m/). The "w" (/w/) sound is made at the same place, but with lip rounding. It is considered a sonorant sound, too, further categorized as a glide.

Labiodental Sounds

The lower lip contacts the upper incisors to produce the fricative labiodental sounds "f" (/f/) and "v" (/v/). The former is unvoiced, the latter voiced. Figure 9-7 shows the lip placement.

VOWELS DIFFER IN TONGUE HEIGHT, PLACEMENT, TENSION, AND LIP ROUNDING

The two primary ways that vowels differ are in where the tongue is placed front to back in the mouth, and how high the tongue is positioned during the production of that vowel. The vowels also differ in whether the lips are rounded or not, and in whether the tongue is tense or relaxed (lax).

Front Vowels

Five English vowels are made with the tongue tip located near the front of the mouth (Figure 9-8). The long "e" sound (/i/), as in "beet" or "heed," has high, front tongue placement with the tongue tensed. The approximate same position, with the tongue lax, is used to produce the short "i" sound (/ɪ /) in "bit" or "hid."

The long "a" sound (/e/) in "bait" or "hate," still has the tongue forward, but it is not as high in the mouth—this sound would be classified as being produced using mid tongue height. This vowel is produced with a tense tongue, where as the "eh" sound

---

Clinical Correlate: Limits of Lip Reading

People who aren't familiar with how speech is produced sometimes question why those with hearing impairment "don't just learn to lip read." Of course, the reason is that sounds made with the same place of articulation, but which vary in their manner of production, are not visibly different. Consonants made with a palatal, velar, or glottal place of articulation and vowel sounds are not easy to distinguish.

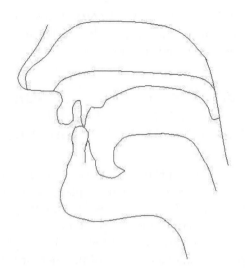

Figure 9–7. Place of articulation for labio-dental sounds f (/f/) and v (/v/). The lower lip is in contact with the incisors.

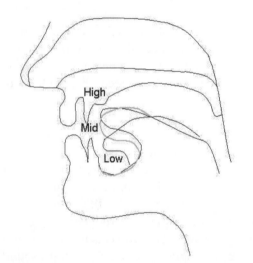

High

Mid

Low

Figure 9–8. Approximate tongue position for the front vowels. The long "e," /i/ in "*feet*," and the short "i," /ɪ/ in "*kit*" are made with high tongue height. The long "a" sound, /e/ in "*rate*" and the "eh" sound, /ɛ/ in "*end*", are made with mid tongue height, whereas the "ah" /æ/ in "*family*" is made with low tongue height.

(/ɛ/) in "b**e**t" or "h**ea**d," has the same approximate position, but a lax tongue.

Lower the tongue further, keeping it lax in tension, and the /æ/ in 'b**a**t" or "h**a**d" is produced.

Central Vowels

Among the most common vowels are the unstressed "uh" (/ə/) or schwa vowel in "**a**bout" or the same vowel when in an accented syllable, which is the stressed "uh" (/ʌ/) in "b**u**t" or "th**e**" (when pronounced "thuh" not "thee"). These vowels are produced with the tongue in a central position, mid way up in tongue height. A similar tongue position front to back is used to produce the "er" sounds: /ɚ/ and /ɝ/. (The former phonetic symbol is used if the "er" is produced in an unstressed syllable; the latter for stressed syllable "er" vowels.) It may seem odd to consider a "er" sound a vowel, as the consonant "r" is in it, but the sound of "er" (/ɚ/), as in "moth**er**" is made with a relatively open vocal tract, so it is classified as vocalic. If you produce "uh" (/ʌ/) in "moth-er," you can feel that your tongue has a similar position for both vowels, but different shape. The back of tongue is lower in the "uh" (/ʌ/) (Figure 9–9).

Back Vowels

The back vowels (Figure 9–10) leave more space in front of the tongue, and this feature is enhanced when the lips are rounded (protruded) for the vowels /u/, the "o͞o" in "**oo**ze" or "wh**o**'d" and the "o͝o", the /ʊ/ in "b**oo**k." The /u/ in "**oo**ze" is made with tongue tension, whereas /ʊ/ in "b**oo**k" has a lax tongue. The back vowels made with mid height are /o/ in "b**oa**t" and /ɔ/ in "c**au**ght" or "b**ou**ght." Lastly, /ɑ/ in "h**o**t" is made with the tongue low, lax, and back.

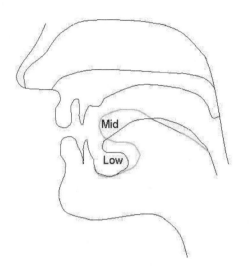

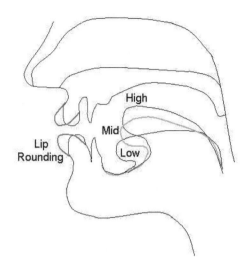

Figure 9–9. The vowels made with the tongue in the central position are (/ʌ/) "*of,*" the unstressed neutral schwa vowel /ə/ "*Lubbock*, Texas" and /ɚ/ and /ɝ/, which are the "*er*" sounds in unstressed and stressed syllables, respectively. The /ʌ/ is made with a lowered tongue position.

Figure 9–10. The high back vowels, /u/ in "*toot*" or /ʊ/ in "*took*" are made with *lip* rounding. The /o/ in "*token*" and /ɔ/ in "*caught*" have mid-tongue height, whereas the /ɑ/ in "*tot*" has low tongue height.

SUMMARY

The consonant sounds are made with some form of obstruction of the vocal tract—whether it is complete blockage for stop consonants or partial blockage for fricatives. Nasal sounds send the sound through the nasal cavity. Vowels are made with more open vocal tracts. Where the tongue is placed—how high/low and how far front or back—determines the vowel produced. Some are made with the tongue tense, some lax, and two are made with the lips rounded, which extends the length of the vocal tract further.

In the next chapter, we examine how tongue position affects the resonance characteristics of the vocal tract, and note how this affects the spectrum of the vowel sounds. We also briefly examine how different types of consonant place, manner, and voicing affect the spectrum of the sound.

10

Acoustics of Speech

Chapter 9 reviewed the ways in which speech sounds are produced. In this chapter, we examine how the shape and size and way in which the vocal tract is constricted change the acoustics and create the sounds we hear. Understanding the basics of speech acoustics is important for those studying the hearing sciences. Hearing loss is not like turning the radio volume down. Most often, the amount of hearing loss changes frequency by frequency. Knowing which frequencies are in which speech sounds gives you an idea of the frequencies that need to be heard for the sound to be identified. The basic information on speech acoustics lets you predict how different hearing losses will affect speech understanding. This knowledge helps one to understand the frequently heard complaint, "I can hear, but I can't understand."

We begin by reviewing the ways that the acoustic characteristics of speech can be visually presented. The chapter discusses how vowel sounds differ, and then examines some acoustic features of consonants. The chapter provides a general overview. There is much more to speech acoustics than what is highlighted here. An undergraduate audiology major with the option of electives and an interest in hearing science should consider taking a course in speech acoustics, as that knowledge is helpful in fully appreciat-ing how hearing loss affects speech understanding.

HOW SPEECH SOUND WAVEFORMS CAN BE VIEWED

Figure 4-10 showed two ways to give information about sound waves and is repeated and expanded here. In Figures 10-1A and 10-1B, the time waveform illustration shows the amplitude of the signal with time on the horizontal axis. In a spectral plot, (Figure 10-1A [right]) the horizontal axis is frequency in Hz, and amplitude remains the vertical axis. These plots are quite adequate when the signal is not changing over time, but if one wants to show how frequency varies at different times, a **spectrogram** is an appropriate plot. It shows time on the horizontal axis, with frequency on the vertical scale. Figure 10-1C shows this view.

These same three views (time waveform, spectrum, and spectrogram) are used with speech signals, as shown in Figure 10-2. This shows the vowel "ee" (/i/), produced here by an adult female, sustained for about a half-second. Figure 10-2A shows the time waveform, 10-2B shows the spectral energy, overall, averaged, for a middle segment of the sound. Unlike the spectrum of a pure

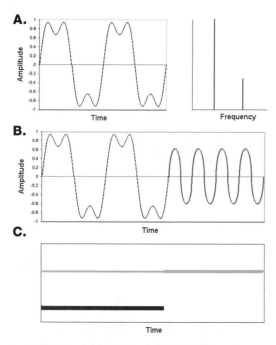

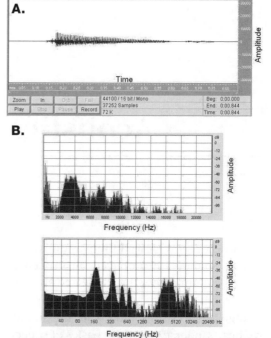

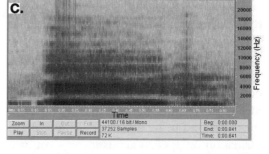

Figure 10–1. A. On the right, the time wave-form shows the amplitude (y-axis) of the sound wave with time on the *x*-axis. This is a complex wave that is composed of a low-frequency sound and a less intense high-frequency sound added together. The spectrum is shown on the right. **B**. The signal changes over time in this waveform view. The low-frequency component disappears, and the intensity of the high-frequency component increases. **C**. The spectrogram shows time on the *x*-axis. Frequency is shown on the *y*-axis. The intensity of the signals is shown with the shading used. Deeper colors mean greater intensity signals. That is, the darker color of the bar on the lower left of this figure is darkest because that is the most intense frequency component.

Figure 10–2. A. The time, or temporal wave-form, for the vowel "ee" (/i/) held for about 500 msec (.5 seconds). The *y*-axis is amplitude, the *x*-axis is time. **B**. Spectral analysis showing the average spectrum for approximately one-quarter second segment of the vowel. There is energy at most frequencies, though some areas show greater energy (peaks toward the top of the scale.) Two frequency scales are shown, as was done in Figure 7–11. **C**. The spectrogram view, which shows the same signal. Time is still shown on the *x*-axis. The different shades represent the intensity of the signal, whereas frequency is shown on the vertical axis. In this view, the frequency range shown is to over 20,000 Hz.

tone, the spectrum of speech sounds has energy over a variety of frequency regions. The spectrogram, Figure 10–2C, shows frequency regions of energy concentration by the colors. Note the darkest band for the lowest frequency region, indicating energy below about 1000 Hz. This corresponds to the greatest energy, as shown in Figure 10–2B. There is a less energy from 1000 to 2000 Hz as noted by the lighter color in that region. A wide band of energy is seen from about 2500 Hz to just above 4000 Hz, and the shading of the spectrogram is similar to that below 1000 Hz, showing that the intensity is similar.

FUNDAMENTAL FREQUENCY, HARMONICS, AND FORMANT FREQUENCIES

Next, let's examine a small segment of the time waveform of the same "ee" /i/ vowel (Figure 10–3). You can see that it is not a pure tone, but a complex signal that is repetitive. As shown in the center of the figure, 10 cycles of the complex wave occur in the 0.057 seconds. Having 10 cycles of the complex wave in 57 msec equates to 175 cycles in 1000 msec (one second). (Cross multiply and divide to solve the equation 10 cycles /57 msec = × cycles/1000 msec.) This is the **fundamental frequency** of the speaker's voice—the lowest frequency contained in the complex signal. The fundamental frequency is produced by the beating of the vocal folds, and will be essentially the same frequency for all vowels made by this speaker, although vocal tension changes will create some change from vowel to vowel, and even moment to moment. Also, some **jitter**, or minor cycle-to-cycle fluctuation in the fundamental frequency, is expected.

Look back at Figure 10–2C. Notice the *vertical* lines are strong then weak in alternating bands. The dark bands, representing louder signals, show that the signal is pulsing on and off with each beat of the vocal folds. These bands will not always be visible in the spectrograms shown in this book. Depending on the resolution of the graphics, they may not be readily distinguished.

As you know from Chapter 4, a signal will distort at its harmonics. The fundamental frequency, abbreviated F_0, is the same as H1, the first harmonic frequency. The second harmonic for this speaker would be 175 Hz × 2, or 350 Hz. The third harmonic is 525 Hz, and the next are 700, 875, 1050, 1225, 1400, 1575, 1750, 1925, 2100, 2275, 2450, 2625, 2800, 2975. . . and the series continues. However, even though all the harmonics are produced, that does not mean that each is equal in intensity. The shape of the vocal track will determine which of the harmonics resonate and which do not. Fre-

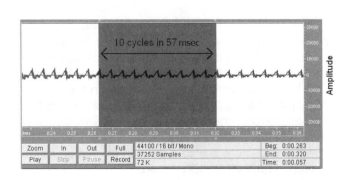

Figure 10–3. A small segment of the temporal waveform shown in Figure 10–2A, showing that the vowel is periodic. It repeats each cycle in about 5.7 msec, which is equal to 175 waveforms per second. The fundamental frequency of the speaker's voice is 175 Hz.

quency regions where there is strong resonance are called **formant frequencies**. Figure 10–2C shows that there are several formant frequency regions with stronger energy; however, the scale of the frequency axis is not ideal for determining what those frequencies are. Figure 10–4 shows the frequencies in the range of 0 to 4000 Hz. You can see a low-frequency formant that merges with the fundamental frequency, and another formant frequency below 3000 Hz.

Vowel sounds are characterized by having two prominent formant frequencies. There are often third and forth formant frequencies as well, but vowels can be recognized with only two formants heard.

ACOUSTIC CHARACTERISTICS OF VOWELS

Formant Frequencies Are Created by Resonance of the Vocal Tract

Chapter 5 showed the calculation for the resonant frequency of "closed tube" resonators—resonators such as the vocal tract that are closed at one end (the vocal folds) and open at the other. It was shown that the longer the tube, the lower the resonant frequency. A similar general principle is that the larger the size of the resonating cavity, the lower the resonant frequency. For ex-

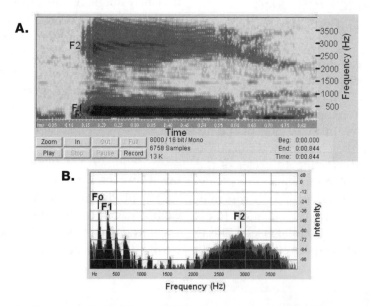

Figure 10–4. A. The same "ee" /i/ vowel is shown with a narrower frequency analysis region. Whereas F2, the second formant frequency, can be seen distinctly (just below 3000 Hz), the first formant frequency, F1, blends with F0, the fundamental frequency. **B.** An FFT spectral analysis provides more detail, though it cannot show how frequency content may change over time. Frequency is along the horizontal axis, intensity in dB is on the vertical scale: more intense components are higher on the figure. The left-most hump in the frequency analysis starting at 0 Hz shows room/instrumentation noise. The next spectral peak is near 175 Hz and shows the fundamental frequency. The second harmonic, about 350 Hz, is emphasized and is the first formant frequency. There is also a peak in the region of the 2800 and 2975 harmonics, which is the second formant frequency region.

ample, if you blow across the top of a nearly full glass Coke bottle, the resonant sound is a high-pitch whistle. The pitch is lowered when the bottle is nearly empty, providing a larger resonant cavity.

The vocal tract can be thought of as having two primary resonant cavities—the portions before and after the place where the tongue creates a narrowing or constriction of the vocal tract. The size of the area behind the point where the tongue comes near the roof of the mouth controls the F1 formant frequency, and the smaller area in front of the tongue controls F2 (Figure 10–5). When the tongue is in a forward position, as it is for the front vowels, the space behind the tongue is larger, and thus F1 will be lower. Meanwhile, F2 is smaller because the tongue coming so far forward makes the area in the front of the mouth smaller. Tongue height will also affect the size of these cavities, and thus the resonant frequencies. If the tongue is low, the F2 resonant cavity is going to be larger. Lowering the tip of the tongue tends to cause the back of the tongue to be a little higher, so that tends to make the F1 cavity smaller, and its resonant frequency higher. Tongue tension has a similar effect—the tense tongue is a little higher in the cavity, so F1 is lower with a lax tongue. Rounding the lips, as for "o͝o" (/ʊ/) in *book*, lengthens the front cavity and drops the F2 frequency further.

F1 and F2 of Vowels

Table 10-1 shows one study's estimate of the average F1 and F2 frequencies of different vowels. Generally speaking, F1 is below 1000 Hz. F2 is below 2000 Hz for the back vowels, but above 2000 Hz for the front vowels. Notice how F1 is lowered for front vowels and for high tongue positions, which is due to the larger size of the cavity behind the point of the tongue reaching toward the roof of the mouth. F2 is highest in front vowels and with high tongue placements, as this creates the smallest space in front of the tongue.

Hearing loss can vary in severity at different frequencies. If the hearing loss is pres-

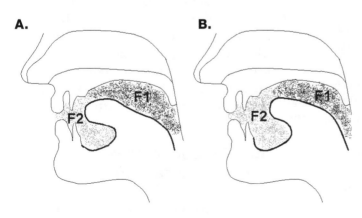

Figure 10–5. The vocal tract is separated into two resonant cavities. **A.** The one in front of the tongue controls the frequency of the second formant (F2), and the one behind the tongue that controls the first formant (F1) frequency. **B.** Moving the tongue back reduces the volume in the rear of the vocal tract and increases F1 frequency, which simultaneously makes the front cavity larger which lowers the F2 resonant frequency. Raising and lowering the tongue also affects the size of these two chambers.

Table 10–1. Average Formant Frequencies for Female Speakers

Tongue Height	Tongue Position	Front			Mid			Back	
		F1	F2		F1	F2		F1	F2
High	/i/ (h**ee**d)	429	2588				/u/ wh**o**'d	430	1755
	/ɪ/ (h**i**d)	522	2161	/ç/ uh	767	1751	/ʊ/ h**oo**d	516	1685
	/ɛ/ (h**ea**d)	586	2144				/ɔ/ h**a**wed	816	1203
Low	/æ/ (h**a**d)	836	2051				/ɑ/ h**o**t	688	1273

Source: From Assmann and Katz (2000).

The IPA symbol for the vowel is shown, followed by a word that contains that vowel. The vowels are arranged by tongue height and position of constriction in the oral cavity. Note that the front vowels tend to have lower F1s and higher F2s than the back vowels. Tongue height also influences the vowel formant frequencies. Vowels with high tongue position have higher F2s, and conversely, lower F1s.

ent only for the highest pitches, and hearing at and below 2000 Hz is relatively good, then vowel sounds should be recognized easily.

Intensity of Vowel Sounds

Most of the energy of speech comes from the vowel sounds. Said another way, vowels are louder than most of the consonant sounds. If a person raises his or her voice, the breath stream is exhaled a bit harder, and the vocal folds vibrate a greater distance. The intensity, especially of voiced sounds (including vowels), is increased.

Low Importance of Vowels for Speech Understanding

Vowels are surprisingly unimportant for understanding conversational speech, at least for those with a good knowledge of the language that is being spoken. A whisper illustrates this. When you whisper, you force your vocal folds to lock in one position, and you are not vibrating your vocal folds at all. The vowels aren't produced (though an aspiration sound is), yet the whispered state-

ment is easily understood. This analogy is somewhat weak: the aspiration sound you make while whispering does change in pitch as you move your mouth. Another reason we know that vowels aren't crucial to speech understanding is that filtering out the lower frequencies (as vowels are made of low frequencies) makes speech sound unusual, but particularly when listening to conversational speech, the message can be understood.

ACOUSTIC CHARACTERISTICS OF CONSONANTS

It's easiest to characterize the acoustic qualities of consonants if analyzed by their manner of production: stops, fricatives, affricatives, nasals, and glides. Within each manner of production, the other major distinctions are whether the sound is voiced or unvoiced, and the place of articulation.

Stop Consonant Burst Energy Is Wideband

Stop consonants have a sudden burst of energy and are short duration—they are transient sounds. Unvoiced sounds (e.g., /t/) can be produced in isolation reasonably well, though as you try, you might find you produce a slight aspiration (/h/) sound as well. Voiced stops (e.g., /d/) can't be made alone, at best they are followed by a neutral vowel, the /ə/ or /ʌ/ "uh" sound. Note in Figure 10–6 that the stop consonant begins with a sudden burst, and notice that the voiced sounds, /b/, /d/ and /g/, tend to be a little longer, and end more gradually because they are coarticulated with the vowel that follows. The spectral view shows the wide-band energy from the stop consonant, and for the voiced sounds, the vowel formants after that wide-spectrum burst of energy.

The spectral content of the unvoiced consonants vary a bit. A generalization is that /p/ has the most low-frequency energy; /t/ has the most high-frequency content, and /k/ the most mid-frequency power. This can be seen in Figure 10–7, which also illustrates that all of these consonants have energy across the spectrum.

Voice Onset Time Distinguishes Voiced and Unvoiced Sounds

The same burst energy is found in the voiced and unvoiced sounds for the same place of articulation, for example, the bilabials /p/ and /b/ (Figure 10–8). What distinguishes

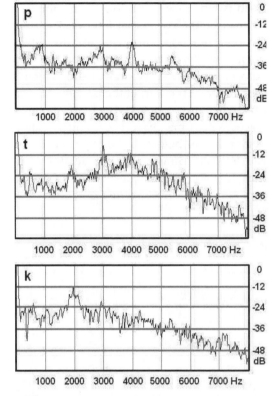

Figure 10–7. The spectral content of plosives vary depending on place of articulation. The phoneme /p/ has a flatter spectrum, with relatively more low-frequency energy. The /t/ has the most high-frequency energy. Note that the concentration of energy is at 3000 to 4000 Hz. The /k/ sound has greatest energy at 2000 Hz, with less energy above and below this point.

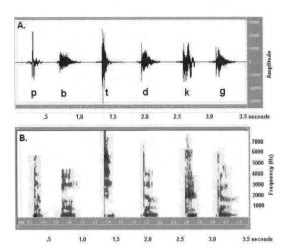

Figure 10–6. **A.** The time waveform shows that stop consonants are brief, and have a sudden onset. The unvoiced sounds are produced in isolation. The voiced sounds, /b/, /d/, and /g/ are produced with the "uh" /ʌ/ vowel afterward, and the time envelope for these sounds trails off more slowly. **B.** The spectral waveform shows the onset, the burst, as having a wide range of frequencies in it.

them is when the vocal folds start vibrating to produce the vowel that follows. The time between the stop consonant and the subsequent vowel is called the "**stop gap**." A related concept is the **voice onset time**, which is the time from the start of the phoneme to the time when the vocal folds begin to vibrate. A voiced sound may have vocal fold vibration beginning just before the burst, or starting as late as about 25 msec after the burst. In contrast, unvoiced consonants have a longer stop gap before the vowel begins.

Formant Frequency Transitions Provide Additional Acoustic Cues

As you know, the size and shape of the vocal tract determines the vowel formant frequencies. When transitioning between a consonant and a vowel while voicing, the shape of the vocal tract is changing. This creates changes in the formant frequencies. Figure 10–9 shows the formant frequency tran-

A.

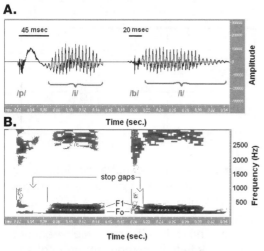

B.

Figure 10–8. The words "pea" and "bee" are shown in the temporal view (**A**) and spectrogram view (**B**). There is a longer time between the burst for an unvoiced consonant, like /p/, and the vowel that follows. **A.** There is 45 msec between the start of the burst for /p/ and the "ee" /i/ vowel that follows, where this voice onset time is only 20 msec between /b/ and "ee" /i/. **B.** The spectral waveform shows the fundamental frequency and first formant bars at the bottom. Note how soon after the burst energy this voicing begins. The time between the consonant and the vowel that follows is the stop gap.

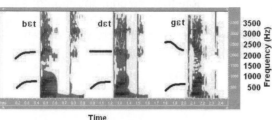

Figure 10–9. Spectrogram view of three words: *bet*, *debt*, and *get*. Each word begins and ends with a stop consonant, and the wide-band energy is visible. All three initial consonants are voiced. The oral cavity is sized differently because the three sounds differ in place of articulation, which affects the spectrum of the formant frequencies of these voiced consonants. The formant frequencies are the dark areas right after the initial consonant burst of energy. The first formant is around 500 to 1000 Hz and F2 is in the region of 2000 to 2500 Hz. In front of each word is a silhouette to show the general shape of the first and second formant transitions from the voiced consonant to the vowel. The second formant frequency is rising over time for /b/, relatively unchanged for /d/, and falls for /g/.

sition for three words: *bet, debt,* and *get.* In each case, the first formant frequency (between 500 and 1000 Hz) rises during the transition from the production of the voiced consonant to the vowel. Note the second formant frequency. For /b/, the second formant is rising across time; it is fairly constant for /d/, but falls after /g/ is produced. There is a different pattern of transition depending on both the consonant produced and the vowel. This make sense, as each consonant/vowel production transitions between different size cavities (as /b/ is bilabial, /d/ is alveolar, and /g/ is palatal, the shape of the cavities start out differently for each phoneme, but in each of these words, the cavity ends up with the tongue in a front position, at a mid height). The direction of the vowel transition is one of the cues the listener can use to identify the consonant. Even if the burst of a stop were not heard, the transition direction of the formants helps to identify which consonant was produced.

Fricatives Have Longer Duration and High-Frequency Energy

The fricatives vary in their spectral content, but all fricatives contain high-frequency energy and are noiselike. The phonemes "s" /s/ and its voiced counterpart "z" /z/ have the highest frequency energy concentration. As shown in Figure 10–10, most of the spectral energy in each of these sounds is above 5000 Hz for this speaker. The "sh" /ʃ/ and voiced "zh" /ʒ/ as in "measure" have strong energy concentration in the 2000 to 6000 Hz range. The other phonemes are less distinct in their energy concentrations. Note the low-frequency energy that is present in all of the voiced sounds (v, ð ,z, ʒ).

Affricatives Have Characteristics of Both Plosives and Fricatives

The affricates, "ch" as in "tea**ch**" /tʃ/, and "**j**" as in "**judge**" /dʒ/, are composed of

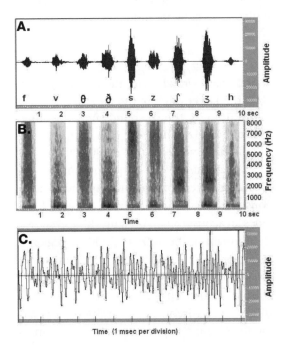

Figure 10–10. A. Time waveforms for the fricatives. Note that each has a somewhat gradual onset and duration of one-quarter to one-half second. **B.** Spectrograms of the fricatives reveal low-frequency voicing energy for the voiced sounds. The voiced and voiceless fricatives for the same place of articulation have similar energy in the mid- to high-frequency regions. The darker bands show the major concentrations of energy, and this figure illustrates that /s/ and /z/ have the most high-frequency energy. **C.** Fricatives are noiselike, as shown by the view of a portion of the time waveform for the unvoiced sound /f/. This unvoiced sound does not have periodically repeating energy. (The sound has been amplified to better illustrate the waveform.)

two sounds made together (coarticulated). The /tʃ/ sound is a combination of "t" /t/ and "sh" /ʃ/, both of which are unvoiced sounds. The /dʒ/ sound is a combination of the voiced /d/ and the voiced "zh" (as in "measure"). The affricates begin with a burst of relatively wide-band energy, and then follow with a longer duration noiselike sound. Figure 10–11 illustrates.

Nasals Have Low-Frequency Energy, Nasal Murmur and Antiresonances

Nasal sounds are classified as sonorant sounds, meaning that they are produced without noiselike friction: they are steady, almost musical sounds. There are two prominent acoustic characteristics of the nasal sounds "m" /m/, "n" /n/ and "ng" /ŋ/: presence of low-frequency energy (sometimes called a **nasal murmur**) and the absence of energy in certain reasons, which are called **antiresonances** or **antiformants** (Figure 10–12). During production of a nasal sound, the breath stream is routed into the nasal cavity, which is lined with mucous membranes and has a complex series of cavities that absorb sound. Nasal sounds have little high-frequency energy, and have one or more low-frequency region where sound is attenuated.

Glides Are Characterized by Vowel Formant Transitions

Sonorants are classified as either being nasals or glides. The glides are "w" /w/, "l" /l/, "r" /r/, and "yuh" as in "yes" /j/. Glides have a lot in common with vowels. They are relatively long in duration (though the "r" /r/ sound is an exception), and produced with a more open vocal tract than other consonant sounds, though the vocal tract is not as open as for vowels.

The sounds /r/ and /l/ can be produced in isolation and sustained, if desired. Both

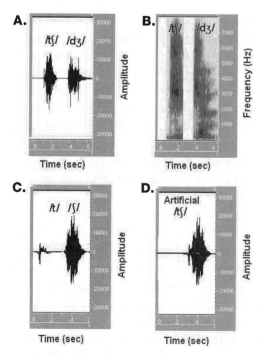

Figure 10–11. A. The time waveform for the affricates /tʃ/ (as in prea**ch**) and /dʒ/ (as in **j**uice). A burst of energy occurs initially, and then there is a prolonged noiselike sound. **B.** Spectrogram view of the unvoiced /tʃ/ and voiced /dʒ/. **C.** The time waveform for /t/ and /ʃ/ are shown for contrast. Note how similar /tʃ/ (in **A**) is to what /t/ and /ʃ/ would look like if placed directly together, as is done in (**D**).

sounds have only low-frequency energy, but /l/ is the lower pitch of the two. As shown in Figure 10–13A, the /r/ sound energy declines above 1500 Hz, where the energy in /l/ starts to fall off in intensity above 500 Hz.

As discussed for stop consonants, the changing pattern of formant frequencies as the consonant is coarticulated with the vowel provides an acoustic cue. As Figure 10–13B shows, the formant in the 1000 to 2000-Hz region is rising for /w/, /l/, and /r/, but it is falling for /j/ ("yuh") as the words *wet, let, Rhett*, and *yet* are spoken. As the "eh" /ɛ/ vowel is initiated, the third formant frequency near 3000 Hz is falling for /l/ but rising for /r/. (The first formant

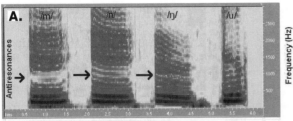

Time (seconds)

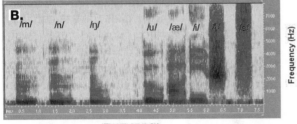

Time (seconds)

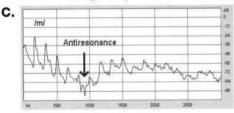

Frequency (Hz)

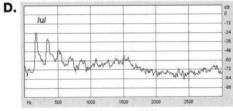

Frequency (Hz)

Figure 10–12. A. The spectrogram of the three nasal sounds, /m/, /n/, and /ŋ/, are shown over a 3000-Hz region to illustrate the frequency region that is almost devoid of energy, that antiresonance, which is near 900 Hz for this speaker. The vowel /u/ is shown for comparison. The low-frequency energy in nasals is sometimes called the nasal murmur. **B.** Another characteristic of nasals is the absence of high-frequency energy, which can be seen in this portion of the figure, which shows the spectrum to 8000 Hz. The sounds "o͞o" /u/, "ah" /æ/, "ee" /i/, "sh" /ʃ/, and "s" /s/ are shown for comparison. The Ling Six Sounds are "m" /m/ plus these sounds. The **Ling Six Sounds** range from low frequency to high frequency, and can be used as an informal test signal. For example, when listening to a hearing aid, these sounds can be spoken to determine if the hearing aid faithfully produces the range of sound. Alternatively, these sounds can be presented to a patient without visual cues as a simplistic test of ability to hear across the frequency range. **C.** The spectral analysis of the nasal /m/ consonant shows an antiresonance near 900 Hz. The energy in that frequency region is 72 dB less than the energy at the fundamental frequency at 175 Hz. **D.** In contrast, for the vowel "o͞o" /u/, the dip at 900 Hz is only about 48 dB less than the intensity of the formant frequency.

frequencies are not easily seen in this figure, as they blend with the fundamental frequency.)

Intensity of Consonants

The sounds recorded for this text were all obtained using microphone close to the speaker's mouth, to show the sound wave-

forms clearly. They are not ideal for showing one very important aspect: consonant sounds, and in general high-frequency sound components of speech, tend to be less intense than the low-frequency components. Consonant sounds tend to be the less intense, high-frequency sounds. The unvoiced consonants are particularly high frequency and low intensity.

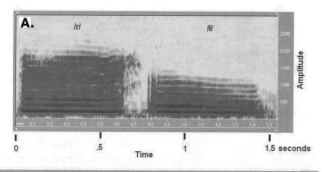

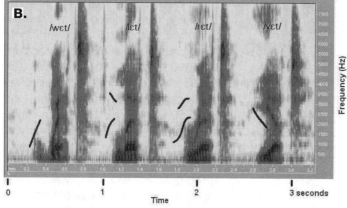

Figure 10–13. A. The phoneme "r" /r/ has more energy above 1000 Hz than does "l" /l/. **B.** The shape of the formant transition is shown with the lines in front of the spectrograms of the words to illustrate that the frequencies transitioned vary across these glide phonemes. The words spoken are "wet," "let," "Rhett," and "yet."

Raising the level of one's voice causes vowels and voiced sounds to increase in intensity. There is some increase in the intensity of stops and fricatives because of the greater volume of air pushing through the vocal tract, so these sounds can be made slightly louder, but only slightly. Try for yourself. Say a vowel quietly, now shout it. Produce the unvoiced "t" /t/ sound quietly, and try to shout it. In quiet conversation, the consonants tend to be less intense than the vowels, and in situations where people raise their voices, the primary impact is to increase vowel intensity.

Importance of Consonants for Speech Understanding

The meaning of speech is conveyed primarily by the consonants. By way of a visu-

al illustration of this, try to interpret the following vowel-free sentence.

"Sp_ch s_nds c_n b_ c_ns_n_ts _r v_w_ ls." Puzzle it out for a while, and you will probably come up with the meaning of this sentence. A similar sentence composed of only vowels is "I _a_ _ea_, _u_ _o_ u_ _ er _ _ a _ _." That will probably leave you scratching your head for a longer period of time. The vowels alone don't provide as much meaning. Furthermore, because there are so many different consonants, an unheard consonant could be one of many different options. This brings us back to that frequently heard complaint of the hearing impaired: "I can hear, but not understand." The loud, low-pitch vowels are detected by the typical person with hearing loss. Most hearing-impaired can detect the low-frequency sounds but have loss of hearing for high frequencies, so the consonant sounds are not distinguished.

Clinical Correlate: Shouting Doesn't Help Most Hearing Impaired

/Most people with hearing loss have worse hearing in the high frequencies, yet often have good hearing in the low frequencies. They report that speech can be heard, but it sounds muffled. When a person with high-frequency hearing loss is not understanding, the speaker may try to be helpful by speaking at a raised voice level. The well-intentioned speaker is often surprised when the hearing-impaired person directs them to stop shouting, saying that it doesn't help. Of course, this makes sense. Speaking louder primarily increases the intensity of the sounds the person with good low-frequency hearing already hears and understands!

SUMMARY

Vowels are distinguished by their formant frequencies, which change depending on the size and shape of the vocal tract. Although vowel sounds carry the loudness of speech, they don't convey the bulk of the meaning. Consonants are less intense, but more important to speech understanding. The voiced consonants will be louder than the unvoiced one, due to the presence of the vocal fold vibration energy. Stop consonants (like *p*, *t*, *b*) are short duration and have energy across the frequency range, though they differ from one another in the frequency pattern of that energy, and in how the energy regions change as one goes from saying the consonant to the next vowel. Fricatives are noiselike sounds. They are longer duration, and like stops, are distinguished within that class of sounds by the energy concentration regions. An affricative is a combination of a stop followed by a fricative. Nasal sounds are unique in that there are parts of the spectrum that are noticeably devoid of sound energy. They have antiresonances. Glides are longer duration speech sounds like /r/ and /w/ that differ again by what frequencies are in them, but also in how the formant frequency energy changes when the consonant-vowel pair is spoken.

You can't understand what you can't hear or see, and as mentioned in the previous chapter, vision doesn't provide all that much information. Hearing loss tends to occur first and worst in the high-frequency regions, so loss of ability to distinguish consonant sounds, especially unvoiced stops and fricatives, is common among the hearing impaired. The presence of the vowel formant transitions, and the duration cues, become important to the person with high-frequency hearing loss.

REFERENCE

Assmann, P., & Katz, W. F. (2000). Time-varying spectral change in the vowels of children and adults. *Journal of the Acoustical Society of America, 108,* 1856–1866.

SECTION THREE

Anatomy and Physiology of the Ear

11

Overview of Anatomy and Physiology of the Ear

In this section of the text, we explore the anatomy (physical structures) and physiology (mechanisms of functioning) for the ear. Introductory chapters are provided first, and are followed by chapters that explore concepts in greater detail. In this chapter, after overviewing the terms used to describe anatomic locations, we begin by providing a brief general overview of the parts of the ear and their physiology.

ANATOMIC TERMS FOR LOCATION

Certain terms are used in locating one structure relative to other structures or planes of the body. The following terms, as they apply to humans, are used in this text and elsewhere.

Anterior	in front of (toward the face)
Ventral	same as anterior
Posterior	behind (toward the back of the head)
Dorsal	same as posterior
Lateral	toward the side of the head
Medial	toward the middle of the head
Superior	above (toward the top of the head)
Inferior	below (toward the feet)
Cephalic	toward the head or superior
Cranial	same as cephalic
Caudal	toward the tail

ANATOMIC VIEWS

Examining internal structures of the body requires that we envision the body as if it were dissected. Just as there are three dimensions to space, there are three basic ways to section the body and describe what is seen. As shown in Figure 11–1, if the head were sliced from vertically ear to ear across the top of the head, a frontal view is exposed. Cutting the head in half down the front of the face creates a sagittal view. Horizontal views can also be shown. The terms axial and transverse are synonyms for horizontal.

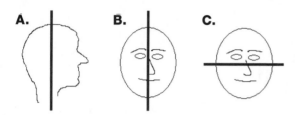

Figure 11–1. The anatomic slices of the head are (**A**) frontal, (**B**) sagittal, and (**C**) horizontal.

GENERAL SECTIONS OF THE EAR

Figure 11–2 illustrates a sketch of a frontal sectioning of the head, showing the right ear. Figure 11–3 provides a more realistic frontal section view on a different scale.

The general sections of the ear are the outer ear, the middle ear, the inner ear, and the retrocochlear pathways. The **outer ear** is composed of the **pinna**, the skin-covered, cartilaginous flap that is also called the **auricle**, and the hole in cartilage and bone that courses (runs) medially, the **ear canal**, more formally called the **external auditory meatus** (or external auditory canal). The area of bone that the ear courses through is called the tympanic portion of the temporal bone.

The **tympanic membrane** separates the outer and the middle ear. The **middle ear** is a cavity in bone containing, among other things, three tiny bones: the **ossicles**. This space is air-filled. Fresh air comes in through the **eustachian tube**, which is connected to the back of the throat in the area called the **nasopharynx.**

The **inner ear** is also a cavity in the temporal bone. It, however, is filled with fluid. There are two major sections to the inner ear—the vestibular system and the cochlea. The **cochlea** is the organ for hearing. Balance-sensing organs are in the **vestibular system**.

Nerve impulses coding hearing and balance information originate in the inner ear. They are interpreted in the brain's cortex. The **retrocochlear pathways** convey the information to the brainstem and brain.

Clinical Correlate: Types of Loss

Damage to any part of the ear can cause a loss of hearing sensitivity. If there is damage to the outer or middle ear, the loss of hearing sensitivity can easily be overcome by just making the sound louder. Damage to the inner ear creates more complicated problems with the encoding of sound, and treatment of cochlear hearing loss is less straightforward. Damage to the retrocochlear pathways very often does not create a major loss of hearing for simple pure tones, as the injury to the nerves frequently allows simple signals to be transmitted, at least under good conditions (such as those used in a hearing test). Retrocochlear pathologies often create a distortion of the signal, and hearing aids are usually not a good treatment.

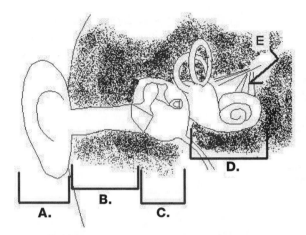

Figure 11–2. Sketch showing the pinna (**A**) and external auditory canal (**B**), which together form the outer ear. The middle ear (**C**) and the inner ear (**D**) are holes in the temporal bone filled with air and fluid, respectively. Nerves conduct the impulses representing the sound to the brainstem and up to the brain for interpretation (**E**).

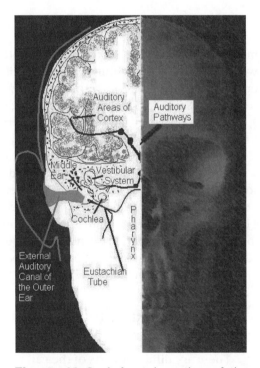

Figure 11–3. A frontal section of the head exposing the auditory structures. At left is a drawing with the anterior tissue removed to show the structures of the ear. The photo to the right helps provide perspective on the relative size and location of these structures. The ear structures are located in the temporal bone of the skull.

THE TEMPORAL BONE

The auditory structures are embedded in the temporal bones, which form the sidewalls of the skull. Figure 11–4 is a lateral view of the temporal bone. The temporal bones can be divided into four portions. There is a thin fanlike superior portion of the temporal bone, which is known as the **squamous portion.** It cradles and protects the temporal lobe of the brain. A thickened extremely hard **petrous portion** forms part of the floor of the cranial cavity (where the brain is located) and surrounds the inner ear. As it is on the inside of the skull, it cannot be seen in this view. The **mastoid portion** posterior to the external auditory meatus and middle ear is said to be "honeycombed" because there are many small air-filled cavities in this part of the temporal bone. The temporal bone also has a **tympanic portion** which forms the floor and parts of the walls of the ear canal. The importance of the temporal bone to us, of course, is that it surrounds or houses part of the external ear as well as all of the middle and inner ear.

OVERVIEW OF PHYSIOLOGY

The outer ear does more than just channel sound to the tympanic membrane. The size and shape of the pinna and external

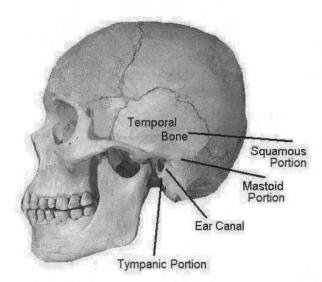

Figure 11–4. Digital photo of the skull showing the temporal bone, sections of the temporal bone, and the location of the ear canal.

auditory meatus increase the amplitude of some mid- to high-frequency sounds. This occurs because sound can **resonate** due to the shape of the cavities of the pinna, and especially the external auditory meatus.

Sound causes vibration of the air molecules in the ear canal, which in turn creates the vibration of the tympanic membrane. That sound energy needs to be conveyed into the fluids of the inner ear. Because fluid is heavier and therefore harder to vibrate than air, for us to hear sound we need to mechanically amplify the sound. The middle ear serves this purpose. The arrangement of the ossicles helps to amplify the force of the sound vibration, and a larger boost comes from the funneling effect of the middle ear. This funneling effect occurs because the tympanic membrane is much larger than the most medial ossicle, the stapes. The tympanic membrane acts as a large sound collector, the stapes transmits the force in a concentrated area, which helps create a larger force vibration of the fluids in the inner ear. Chapter 13 will describe how this occurs.

Once the fluids in the inner ear are vibrating, structures within the cochlea also vibrate. The vibration creates the initiation of nerve impulses. As you will learn in greater detail beginning in Chapter 16, one of the membranes in the inner ear, the basilar membrane, has certain sections that vibrate when high-frequency sounds are present; other locations vibrate in response to low-frequency sounds. The vibration of these specific areas within the inner ear triggers firing of different nerves.

The retrocochlear pathways convey the sound to the brain. They also act to encode some of the properties of the sound, even before the neural signals reach the cortex. The temporal lobe of the brain is the location for the termination of the ascending retrocochlear pathways; it is here that our brains begin to interpret the auditory nerve firings.

SUMMARY

There are different parts of the ear, and thus, different types of loss that are possible. The basic parts of the ear are the outer ear, composed of the pinna and external auditory meatus, the middle ear, which amplifies the sound, and the inner ear, where sound energy in the cochlea is encoded by auditory neurons. The inner ear also houses the balance apparatus. The retrocochlear pathways convey information to the brain. The ear is housed within the temporal bone of the skull. The temporal lobe of the brain receives the auditory information.

12

Introduction to the Conductive Mechanisms

The conductive mechanism is made up of the outer (external) ear, the middle ear, and the soft tissues and bones of the head that surround the outer and middle ear. The term conductive is used as the more peripheral portions of the auditory system conduct sound waves (sound energy) to the sensory receptors.

THE EXTERNAL EAR

The external ear (shown in the previous chapter in Figures 11–2 and 11–3) consists of the **auricle** or **pinna** and the external auditory canal or external meatus. Pinnas come in varying shapes and sizes; however, in humans, they are relatively small and play a minor role in hearing. The pinna has a "funneling" effect, slightly increasing the sound energy entering the canal. This resonance occurs particularly in the 5000- to 6000-Hz range. There is also evidence that, as the pinna is posterior to the opening of the ear canal, it may partially block high-frequency sound waves coming from directly behind the head. This may cause high-frequency sounds (that cannot wrap around the pinna "barrier") to be heard slightly differently when the sound

source is behind the individual. The pinna therefore may aid in locating the source of a sound in the front-back plane.

The external ear canal **(external auditory meatus)** varies considerably from person to person; but, in adults, is usually about 6 to 8 mm (0.25 inch) in diameter and 25 to 35 mm (1 to 1.5 inches) in length. It is usually somewhat oval in shape and forms a slight "S" curve along its length. It terminates medially at the **eardrum** **(tympanic membrane)**, which is usually considered part of the middle ear.

The external auditory meatus is simply an opening or tunnel penetrating the side of the head. It passes through soft tissue at the periphery (skin, fat, muscle, etc.), then through a layer of cartilage, and finally through a portion of the temporal bone. That section of the canal passing through the soft tissue and cartilage is referred to as the **cartilaginous portion**, and the section passing through the temporal bone is referred to as the **bony portion of the external meatus**. The entire canal is lined with skin. Hair follicles located in the skin of the cartilaginous portion of the canal support hairs that tend to point toward the opening of the canal. These hairs are thought to aid in keeping dust, insects, and so forth out of the ear canal.

Also within the skin of the cartilaginous canal are glands, which secrete a waxy substance, called **cerumen**. This cerumen, or earwax, provides a number of benefits. It is mildly antibacterial, it is noxious to insects, and it helps to keep the skin of the canal and eardrum from drying out. Furthermore, cerumen is constantly being produced and there is a "flow" or movement of the wax toward the pinna bringing along with it any dust or debris which may have entered the canal. Thus, cerumen functions to cleanse and to help maintain the health of the external ear canal.

THE MIDDLE EAR

The middle ear forms the second stage of sound conduction. It is a series of spaces and structures. Its responsibility is to transmit the airborne sound of the outer ear to the liquids that fill the inner ear. The surface of the middle ear space is mucosa. Mucous membranes also line the bones in the middle ear.

The middle ear is an irregularly shaped space bordered laterally by the tympanic membrane, and medially by the bony wall that separates the middle ear from the inner ear. The space between the tympanic membrane and the inner ear is spanned by a chain of three bones **(malleus, incus, and stapes)** known collectively as the **ossicles** (Figure 12–1). These bones also go by the less scientific names, the hammer, anvil, and stirrup. Note that the wishbone-shaped stapes has a footplate, which projects onto the medial wall of the middle ear. Posteriorly and superiorly, the middle ear communicates (is open) with the **mastoid air cells**.

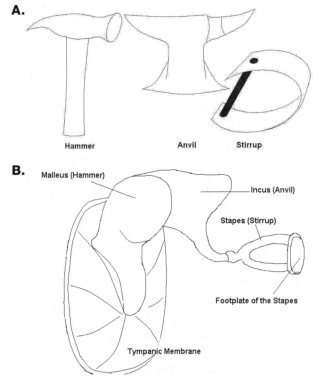

A.

Hammer   Anvil   Stirrup

B.

Malleus (Hammer)

Incus (Anvil)

Stapes (Stirrup)

Footplate of the Stapes

Tympanic Membrane

Figure 12–1. A. The names of the ossicles are derived from the hammer, the blacksmith's anvil, and the horse stirrup. **B.** The three middle ear bones, the malleus, incus, and stapes, are together called the ossicular chain. This figure shows the attachment of the malleus to the tympanic membrane, and how the bones are arranged.

(The mastoid portion of the temporal bone is honeycombed, that is, it contains small air cell spaces, much like the inside of a chicken leg bone.) Anteriorally, the middle ear connects by way of the **eustachian tube** with the back of the throat (**nasopharynx**). The roof of the middle ear is a thin bony plate that forms the floor of the cranial cavity that houses the brain. That is, the roof of the middle ear is the petrous portion of the temporal bone. Figure 12–2 represents the middle ear as if it was a "box," and identifies structures on and in the "walls" of the box. We now turn to a more detailed description of some of the structures found in or adjacent to the middle ear.

The Tympanic Membrane

The eardrum or tympanic membrane is a slightly cone-shaped structure separating the outer and middle ear (see Figures 12–1 and 12-3B). The plane of the membrane is not perpendicular to the external meatus: the lower edge is somewhat medial to the upper edge. A thickened rim (the **annulus**) of the membrane fits into a bony groove (**sulcus**) in the canal wall for much of the circumference of the drum, holding the membrane in place.

Figure 12–3 shows a drawing of a right tympanic membrane. The membrane is divided into two sections based on its physical makeup. Approximately one-fourth to one-third of the membrane (the posterior superior area) consists of two layers of tissue; the skin that is continuous with the lining of the external meatus, and the mucous membrane that is continuous with the lining of the middle ear. This is a rather flaccid (floppy) portion of the membrane known as **pars flaccida.** The remaining two-thirds to three-fourths of the membrane has a third (middle) layer consisting of elastic fibers that lie between the skin and mucous membrane layers. This middle layer consists of radial fibers that run from the midpoint of the eardrum to the periphery, and concentric fibers that follow the contour of the membrane. This creates a "spider web" effect as shown in Figure 12–4. These radial and concentric fibers give the membrane elasticity. This portion of the eardrum is known as **pars tensa**. It is this elastic part of the membrane that is primarily responsible for sound transmission.

Figures 12–1 and 12–3 show that the long process of the malleus, called the manubrium of the malleus, lies against, and is attached to, the tympanic membrane. The manubrium is visible from the outside of the eardrum as a whitish ridge (Figure 12–5). The part that is visible through the eardrum is the **shadow of the manubrium of the malleus,** running downward, and slightly

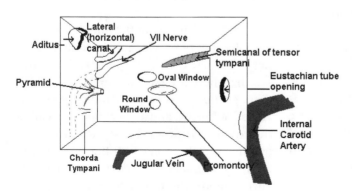

Figure 12–2. A schematic representation of the right middle ear showing the landmarks found on the posterior, medial, and anterior walls. This box view was proposed by Gardner, Gray, and O'Rahilly (1986). See text for a description of the features of the middle ear.

A.

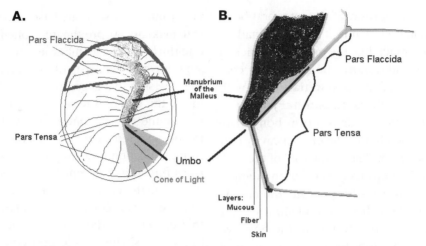

B.

Figure 12–3. A drawing of the right tympanic membrane. **A.** The view as seen when examining the ear with an otoscope. The upper area called pars flaccida is outlined for illustration purposes, but there is no line on the eardrum. The area containing fibers is pars tensa. The center of the eardrum, where the tympanic membrane connects to the manubrium of the malleus, is the umbo. **B.** The eardrum as viewed in frontal cross-section. Medial direction is to the left, the pinna would be to the right. Pars tensa has three layers: skin on the outside, fibers in the middle layer, and mucous membranes on the medial surface. Mucous membranes also coat the ossicles and the middle ear space.

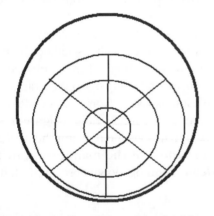

Figure 12–4. Illustration of the "spider web" composition of the fibers in pars tensa.

posteriorly, from about one o'clock for the right ear (from about 11 o'clock for the left ear) to the center of the membrane (Figure 12–3A). The point of attachment of the tip of the long process of the malleus to the most medial point of the membrane is known as the **umbo**. When viewed with an otoscope,

a light reflection, called the **cone of light,** reflects in the lower, anterior quadrant of the ear. The cone of light tip points toward the umbo (Figure 12–3A). Figure 12–3B shows the tympanic membrane in cross-section to show how the umbo is created by pulling the tympanic membrane inward as it attaches to the malleus. Figure 12–5 shows a photograph of an actual eardrum.

Medial Wall Landmarks

The medial wall of the middle ear is the bony boundary between the middle and inner. Refer back to Figure 12–2 and you will see that there are two openings, named for their shapes: a round opening called the **round window**, and an oval opening called the **oval window.** These windows are openings in the bony wall but are not truly "open" as membranes cover each of them. Furthermore, the footplate of the stapes is

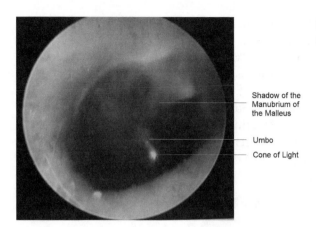

Figure 12–5. A tympanic membrane as seen through a video otoscope.

Shadow of the
Manubrium of
the Malleus

Umbo

Cone of Light

held in the oval window against the oval window membrane by the **annular ligament**. A rounded area called the **promontory** on the bony medial wall anterior and inferior to the oval window forms the base of the cochlea.

The medial wall has three tunnel-like canals or channels. One of these houses the **facial nerve** (cranial nerve VII) which courses around the posterior wall as well. A second houses the **lateral semicircular canal**, one of the inner ear structures for balance, and the third houses the **tensor tympani muscle**. A limitation of the "box" view of the middle ear is that it does not permit an entirely accurate representation of the location of structures, particularly for the semicanal of tensor tympani. This canal is actually curving along the medial/anterior area of the middle ear space.

Posterior Wall Landmarks

In addition to the **aditus**, the opening that connects the middle ear with the mastoid air spaces, and the canal housing the facial nerve, the posterior wall has a small pyramid-shaped projection, the **pyramidal eminence**, which houses the **stapedius muscle**. An additional landmark of the interest on the posterior wall is a small open-

ing to the facial nerve canal through which a branch of the nerve known as the chorda tympani passes. The chorda tympani crosses the middle ear space from posterior to anterior running just behind the eardrum. This will be discussed again, and is illustrated in Figure 15–11. Chorda tympani enters the tissue of the anterior middle ear and follows a course that takes it to the anterior two-thirds of the tongue. Although we have described the nerve as running from the middle ear to the tongue, chorda tympani is actually a sensory nerve that carries information about taste from the anterior part of the tongue to the brain. The remainder of the facial nerve provides both sensory and motor innervations to the face; it does not pass through the middle ear.

The Ossicles

The ossicles are a bridge or chain of three small bones that span the middle ear space from the tympanic membrane to the inner ear, which are sometimes called the ossicular chain. As shown in Figure 12–1, they consist of the **malleus** (hammer), the **incus** (anvil) and the **stapes** (stirrup). The manubrium, or handle, of the malleus is connected to the tympanic membrane whereas the footplate of the stapes is connected to the oval window. In between the malleus and the stapes is the incus, which is attached rather firmly to the malleus so that they tend to act as a unit. On the other hand, the connection between the incus and the stapes, the **incudostapedial joint**, is a rather fragile ball-and-socket arrangement. This permits the stapes to have a somewhat "rocking" movement in the oval window when vibrations are transmitted from the malleus, through the incus and to the stapes.

Overview of How Middle Ear Ossicular Motion Permits Hearing

When the stapes vibrates in the oval window, the cochlear fluids in the inner ear move. It is this motion that permits hearing. The fluids in the cochlea can't be compressed. When the stapes footplate moves in, there will be a corresponding outward movement of the round window to allow for pressure relief. When the stapes footplate rocks outward, toward the middle ear, the round window will move inward. This in/out movement of the stapes footplate happens at the same rate as the sound wave's frequency: a 1000-Hz tone would create a movement of stapes footplate in and out 1000 times per second. Chapter 18 will describe how this fluid motion creates nerve impulses.

Middle Ear Muscles

There are two muscles of the middle ear: the **tensor tympani** and the **stapedius.** Both muscles actually lie outside the middle ear space; however, each has a tendon that enters the middle ear. The tensor tympani tendon emerges from the semicanal of tensor tympani on the medial wall of the middle ear, crosses laterally, and attaches to the manubrium of the malleus. The stapedial tendon emerges from the pyramidal eminence on the posterior wall, crosses medially, and attaches to the neck of the stapes. When these muscles contract, they pull the ossicular chain in opposite directions; the tensor tympani pulls medially and the stapedius pulls laterally. The effect of contracting one or both of these muscles is to "stiffen" the ossicular chain, inhibiting the movement of the ossicles somewhat.

The Eustachian Tube

The eustachian tube is a canal that connects the middle ear with the **nasopharynx** (that part of the throat directly posterior to the nose and above the soft palate). The orifice, or opening, of the tube in the nasopharynx is just above the level of the soft palate and adjacent to the adenoids. The tube is normally in a closed position but it can be opened briefly by contraction of the muscles that elevate and tense the soft palate (the **levator veli palatini** and the **tensor veli palatini**). These muscles contract momentarily when we swallow, yawn, sneeze, or cough. Thus, the eustachian tube stays closed most of the time but opens periodically as a result of the contraction of the palatine muscles.

The eustachian tube serves two functions. First, it is the only source of air for the middle ear. Normal middle ear function requires air pressure to be equal on both sides of the tympanic membrane. In other words, the air pressure in the middle ear must be the same as the air pressure in the outer ear (i.e., atmospheric pressure) for optimal sound energy transfer through the middle ear. As atmospheric pressure changes, and as the tissues of the middle ear absorb air, it is necessary to replenish the air, or to equalize the air pressure in the middle ear, on a periodic basis. The momentary opening of the tube when we swallow, and so forth, provides the opportunity for this equalization to occur.

The second function of the eustachian tube is to provide an exit for mucus or other material that may collect in the middle ear. The lining of the eustachian tube consists of respiratory epithelium that has tiny hairs, or is ciliated, and also contains mucous-secreting glands. The wavelike movement of the cilia tends to move the mucus, along with any foreign matter, including bacteria, down the tube and into the nasopharynx. This also tends to inhibit the spread of infection from the nasopharynx, which usually contains large numbers of bacteria, to the middle ear.

ear contains the malleus, incus, and stapes, which transmit sound from the tympanic membrane to the middle ear. The middle ear also contains two muscles, the tensor tympani and the stapedius, whose contraction attenuates sound transmission through the middle ear. The middle ear is an air-filled space. Fresh air comes into the middle ear via the eustachian tube. The middle ear space is open to cavities in the mastoid portion of the temporal bone, and the entire space and the ossicles are mucous lined.

SUMMARY

This chapter has overviewed the major features of the middle ear. The middle

REFERENCE

Gardner, E, Gray, D. J., & O'Rahilly, R. (1986). *Anatomy: A regional study of human structures.* Philadelphia: W. B. Saunders & Co.

13

Introduction to the Physiology of the Middle Ear

The physiology of the outer ear is relatively simple. The outer ear enhances mid- to high-frequency sound through its resonance characteristics. The middle ear also has some resonant characteristics. The weight and stiffness of the middle ear accentuates some frequency sounds and minimizes transmission of others. However, that is not the primary physiologic action of the middle ear. The middle ear is principally designed to ensure that sound efficiently enters the fluids of the inner ear. There is a loss of sound energy when the sound waves enter the dense cochlear fluids. The ear acts as a mechanical amplifier to boost the sound energy so that this loss is of no consequence.

There are two muscles of the middle ear. Contraction of these muscles lessens the transmission of some frequencies of sound through the middle ear, which protects the ear from some forms of loud sound.

RESONANCES OF THE EXTERNAL EAR

As the external meatus is a closed tube, it resonates. That is, if a series of tones (from low to high frequency) is introduced into the canal, some frequencies will set the air in the canal into vibration more effectively than others. Figure 13–1 (based on Shaw's 1974 data) shows how this resonance produces a "gain" of about 10 dB in the 2000- to 3000-Hz range. Recall that a column of air in a closed tube resonates at the frequency whose wavelength is four times the length of the tube (Chapter 5). If the ear canal is about 1 to 1.5 inches in length, then the resonance of the canal should be to a sound fre-

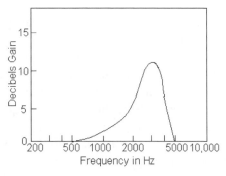

Figure 13–1. Acoustic gain of the external auditory meatus and tympanic membrane. The amount of increase in sound at the eardrum is shown on the vertical scale. Frequency is along the horizontal axis. The data are from Shaw (1974).

quency whose wavelength is 4 to 6 inches long. A 4-inch wavelength would produce a resonant frequency of 3300 Hz and a 6-inch wavelength would produce a resonant frequency of 2200 Hz. Figure 13–1 shows a gain peak in this frequency region: Shaw's data are in general agreement with what our calculations predict the resonant frequency of the external ear canal to be. This gain in the 2000- to 4000-Hz area is one of several factors making the human ear more sensitive to sound in the mid- to high-frequency range.

The outer ear (pinna and external meatus) is a passive system: That is, it does not actively do anything. Its function is simply to provide a pathway for sound waves to enter the head. Except for small changes due to the resonance characteristics of the pinna and ear canal, sound is delivered to the eardrum in much the same form it had in the air surrounding the head.

ENERGY TRANSFER THROUGH THE MIDDLE EAR

Impedance Mismatch Between Air and Cochlear Fluids

The middle ear functions primarily to minimize the energy loss that would occur if sound energy in the air were to impinge directly on the inner ear fluids. The middle ear structures are light and easily moved. In contrast, the fluids of the inner ear require considerably more energy to move; there is greater inertia to fluid than air. This was discussed in Chapter 5. Recall that an **impedance mismatch** occurs when sound is transmitted from air to seawater. Seawater has similar characteristics to cochlear fluids. Because of the mismatch of the impedance of the air of the outer ear and the cochlear fluids, we know that sound would not be

efficiently transmitted to the inner ear if it were not for the middle ear structures. Only a small proportion of the sound energy in air would actually enter the cochlea if the middle ear mechanism were not present. Surgical removal of the middle ear, which creates a direct path for the airborne sound to impinge directly on a membrane-covered window into the inner ear, should result in about 30 dB of hearing loss. As was discussed in Chapter 5, we know that it is harder to move cochlear fluid than it is to move air molecules, because the cochlear fluid has a higher density. It has been estimated that 99.9% of airborne sound bounces off water; only 0.1% is transmitted. You have probably noticed this attenuation of sound when you are swimming under water. The power loss resulting from this is 30 dB. This is calculated by noting that of 1000 power units, only 1 is transmitted through the water. The formula used is:

$$dB = 10 \log 1/1000 = 10 \times -3 = -30 \text{ dB}$$

This loss of power as sound goes from air to fluid is created because of the differences in impedance between air and water, which is termed the middle ear's **impedance mismatch.**

The Middle Ear as an Impedance-Matching Transformer

A major purpose of the middle ear is to overcome this loss of energy that will result when sound strikes cochlear fluid. It is said that the middle ear functions as an **impedance matching transformer**, overcoming the impedance mismatch. There is general agreement on the mechanism by which the impedance matching is accomplished. There appears, however, to be two trains of thought regarding whether the middle ear functions to transmit a sound pressure wave in the air into a sound pressure wave in the inner ear fluids, or whether it functions to convert a sound pressure wave in the air into a displacement of the inner ear fluids. The distinction to be made is whether there is actual compression of fluids or whether the fluids are simply moved without compression occurring.

The middle ear has a mechanical design that increases the force of the vibration of the footplate of the stapes. Two different types of mechanical advantage are used in what amounts to a passive (no battery required), or mechanical, amplification system. These two systems are (a) the lever effect of the ossicular chain, and (b) the areal ratio of the tympanic membrane and the oval window.

Ossicular Lever

The teeter-totter teaches us that a lever can lift a heavy weight; it increases the force that is applied. A child sitting on the long end of the teeter-totter is able to create enough force to lift the adult sitting on the shorter end (Figure 13–2). One of the ways in which the ear overcomes the sound loss that will occur as energy enters cochlear fluid is via a lever action of the malleus and incus. The lever effect of the ossicles occurs because the manubrium of the malleus is longer than the long process of the incus (see Figure 13–2). As already noted, the malleus and the incus are bound rather firmly together by a series of ligaments so that they tend to move as a unit. They are suspended in such a way that their mass tends to be distributed rather evenly around an "axis of rotation" or fulcrum. This centering of mass around the fulcrum results in minimal inertia of the ossicles, meaning that they can be set into motion easily and that they tend to stop moving as soon as the driving force is removed. This is desirable because otherwise there would be an "echo chamber" effect that would cause considerable reverberation of a sound passing through the middle ear.

As seen in Figure 12–1B, and shown schematically in Figure 13–2, the manubrium of the malleus is about 1.3 times as long as the long process of the incus. If these two structures are viewed as a simple lever op-

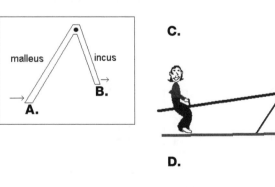

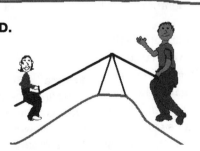

Figure 13–2. A representation of the lever effect of the malleus and incus. The handle of the malleus is about 1.3 times as long as the long process of the incus. Therefore, a force applied to the malleus (**point A**) will be increased 1.3 times at the incus (**point B**). The lever action is exemplified by the teeter-totter (**C**); which would still have a mechanical advantage, even if the levers were bent (**D**).

erating around a fulcrum at the axis of rotation, it is clear that a force applied to the malleus will result in a greater force at the incus. The increase in force will be proportional to the ratio of the two lengths; that is, the pressure at the incus will be 1.3 times as great as the force applied to the malleus.

We can calculate the theoretical dB increase provided, using the formula:

$$\text{dB gain} = 20 \log \text{ malleus length } / \text{ incus length}$$
$$= 20 \log 1.3$$
$$= 20 \times .114$$
$$= 2.3 \text{ dB}$$

Areal Ratio

The areal ratio of the tympanic membrane to the footplate of the stapes (which sits in and fills the oval window) is important in energy transfer. One source cites the average human eardrum as about 66 mm^2 and the average stapes footplate is about 3.2 mm^2. This results in an areal ratio of about 21:1; that is, the eardrum is about 21 times as large an area as the footplate. When one considers, however, that pars flaccida contributes little to sound transmission, plus the fact that the eardrum does not move in and out like a piston, the "effective" size ratio is more debatable. Some will say it is 20:1, others will report that the "effective" areal ratio is about two-thirds of the actual ratio, that is, about 15:1. For the moment, let's use this more conservative figure of 15:1 for the calculation of the advantage attributed to the size between the tympanic membrane and oval window.

The significance of the areal ratio is that energy collected over a relatively large surface is transmitted to a smaller surface. This results not in a total energy gain (the energy at the small surface is approximately the same as the energy at the larger surface), but is an increase in energy per unit area. Fig-

ure 13–3 illustrates this: If one unit of force is applied to each unit of area at the tympanic membrane, the effect at the footplate is 15 units of force per unit of area. This results in a pressure per unit area at the footplate that is 15 times greater than at the eardrum.

The dB increase due to the TM to the oval window ratio is:

$$\text{dB gain} = 20 \log 15/1$$
$$= 20 \times 1.18$$
$$= 23.6 \text{ dB}$$

The ossicular lever and the areal ratio of eardrum to footplate give us two mechanical advantages in series. That is, the energy transferred must pass through both in going from eardrum to oval window. The total advantage for mechanical advantages operating in series is the product of the two. Thus, the total advantage provided by the middle ear is $1.3 \times 15 = 19.5$; that is, the force per unit area applied by the stapes to the oval window of the cochlea is about 20 times greater than that received at the eardrum.

Now, as pressure is equal to force per unit of area, it is possible to determine the effective increase in pressure in decibels by placing the ratio into the decibel formula. Thus:

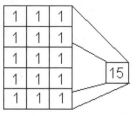

Figure 13–3. Energy transfer from the tympanic membrane to the footplate of the stapes. There are 15 units of energy at both sites; however, energy per unit area is 15 times greater at the stapes.

dB gain = 20 log 20/1
  = 20 log 20
  = 20 × 1.30
  = 26 dB

It appears that the mechanical advantage of the middle ear provides a sound pressure "gain" of about 26 dB. Another way of looking at this is that if there were no mechanical advantage in the middle ear, our hearing would be about 26 dB less sensitive than it is.

However, other estimates of effective size of the tympanic membrane are larger, and may range from 69 to 80 mm². If a larger estimate of the size of the TM is used, then a greater mechanical advantage would be calculated. For example, if the ratio were 70 mm² to 3.2 mm², or a 21.9 size ratio, multiplied by the 1.3 from the lever action, the force increase is 28.5. This would provide a 29 dB increase in sound energy, which would make up for the theoretical loss of energy if 99.9% of sound is reflected off the tympanic membrane.

Regardless of the numbers used, it is clear that the anatomic design of the middle ear creates an impedance matching transformer. The physiologic purpose of the middle ear is to increase sound intensity, so that sound energy is sufficient when it is carried into cochlear fluids.

THE ACOUSTIC REFLEX

The acoustic reflex involves the contraction of one or both of the two muscles that affect middle ear function: the stapedius and the tensor tympani. It is called a reflex because the muscle will contract involuntarily when certain stimulus conditions exist. Most researchers believe that the tensor tympani is not activated by loud sound in humans. This has given rise to the acoustic reflex sometimes being referred to as the **stapedial reflex**. The phenomenon is also called the middle ear reflex.

The acoustic reflex is triggered by a combination of the sound's intensity and bandwidth (range of frequencies present), which the observer perceives as loudness. When an observer perceives the sound at a sufficient loudness level, the reflex is triggered. The lowest level of stimulus intensity that will just trigger the reflex is referred to as the **reflex threshold.** Chapter 3 introduced the concept of decibels hearing level (dB HL, which show how much hearing loss a patient has) and decibels sensation level (dB SL, which describes how loud a signal is above the patient's threshold of hearing). Normal acoustic reflex thresholds, referenced both in dB HL and dB SL, are in the 70 to 100 dB range for pure tones, with thresholds for broadband noise being 10 to 20 dB lower.

When threshold is reached, the muscles receive nerve impulses from the lower brainstem and the contraction occurs. Although in humans there is evidence that the acoustic reflex does not cause a tensor tympani contraction, this muscle may be active when we speak, in order to attenuate the loudness of our own voices.

In normal ears the contraction is bilateral. That is, a loud sound, whether heard in one or both ears, will produce a muscle contraction in both ears.

The effect of contracting one or both of the middle ear muscles is to stiffen the ossicular chain. This, of course, impedes the movement of the ossicles and reduces the efficiency with which sound energy is transmitted to the inner ear. However, as you may remember from the discussion of impedance in an earlier chapter, the stiffness component of impedance primarily affects the transmission of low-frequency sounds. Figure 13–4 shows the average amount that sound reaching the inner ear was reduced (attenuated) in a group of persons who could voluntarily activate the acoustic reflex. Note

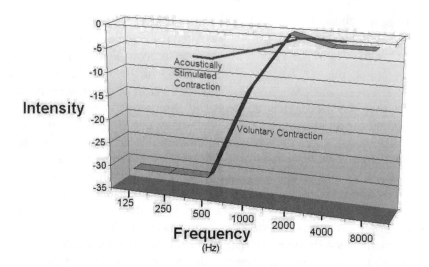

Figure 13–4. Amount by which voluntary contraction of the middle ear muscles reduces sound energy reaching the cochlea. Low-frequency sound is attenuated by over 30 decibels; however, sounds above 1000 Hz are not attenuated as a result of the acoustic reflex contraction. Voluntary muscle contraction data are from Reger (1960). The acoustically stimulated contraction data are from Rabinowitz (1977) as reported by Rosowski and Relkin (2001).

the primary effect is in the low frequencies where about 30 dB of attenuation occurs. There is little or no attenuation for sounds at 1000 Hz. The effect of voluntary contraction is probably not the same as what occurs when sound triggers the reflex. Figure 13–4 shows that the contralaterally triggered reflex from a 105 dB SPL burst of noise creates much less change in sound transmission. However, it shows the same pattern of better attenuation of low-frequency sound.

The primary function of the acoustic reflex is generally considered the protection of the cochlea from high sound energies that could damage the sensitive inner ear structures. However, this protective action has two rather serious limitations. First, as Figure 13–4 shows, contracting the middle ear muscles does not attenuate sound energy that occurs at 1000 Hz and above. Thus, little or no protection is provided from high-frequency sound, and high-frequency sounds are more

damaging to the inner ear than similar intensity low-frequency sounds. These voluntary muscle contractions may overestimate the amount of hearing protection. Those few "gifted" individuals who could voluntary contract the stapedius may also have contracted tensor tympani, or contracted one or both muscles more strongly than occurs for the sound-elicited stimulation, which appears to provide a smaller degree of protection.

The second limitation to how well the reflex serves to protect hearing relates to the time lapse between the sound entering the ear and the contraction beginning: initially all of the high-energy sound reaches the inner ear. Attenuation occurs only after nerve impulses triggered by the onset of the sound reach the brainstem and other impulses are sent back to the muscles. Even though this takes only a fraction of a second, noise initially strikes the inner ear with no attenuation. This can be a serious problem with impulse type noise, such as gunfire or other explosive type noises, where the muscle contractions occur, but only after the noise is over.

Let us return now to the stimulus that triggers the reflex. We have already stated that the muscles contract when the observer perceives the sound at (or above) a threshold loudness level. A point to be made here is that perceived level is the trigger, not intensity per se. It does not matter how intense the sound, if the observer does not perceive the sound at some intensity level, the reflex does not occur. Thus, hearing losses that affect hearing of loud sounds will affect the acoustic reflex. (You will learn in your clinical coursework and later in this text that conductive loss attenuates all sound, but in many cases, cochlear loss prevents hearing for soft sounds, whereas loud sounds are perceived as loud. Therefore, persons with cochlear losses who hear loud sounds as loud may have acoustic reflex thresholds at normal dB HL levels.)

Another point to remember is that the reflex is *triggered* by any loud sound, regardless of frequency. So, a loud, high-frequency sound can trigger the reflex. The middle ear muscle contraction attenuates only the low-frequency sound transmission, however.

SUMMARY

The middle ear functions as an impedance matching transformer, increasing the sound energy about 30 dB as it passes through the middle ear, so that the 30 dB loss of energy that occurs when sound reaches the dense cochlear fluids is of no consequence. The lever action of the malleus and the incus, and the funneling of sound from the larger tympanic membrane to the tiny stapes footplate are the two primary impedance-matching transformer mechanisms.

Although the stapedial reflex is triggered by loud sounds of any frequency, the middle ear reflex only attenuates transmission of low-frequency sound through the middle ear. The acoustic reflex's protective function is limited: it only attenuates low-frequency sound, and there is a brief delay after the sound begins before the reflex can contract. Reflex contraction may serve to attenuate the loudness of our own voices as we speak.

REFERENCES

Reger, S. N. (1960). Effect of middle ear muscle action on certain psycho-physical measurements. *Annals of Otology, Rhinology and Laryngology, 69,* 1179–1198.

Rosowski, J. J., & Relkin, E. M. (2001). Introduction to the analysis of middle ear function. In A. F. Jahn & J. Santos-Sacchi, (Eds.), *Physiology of the ear* (2nd ed.). San Diego, CA: Singular Publishing Group.

Shaw, E. A. (1974). The external ear. *Handbook of Sensory Physiology, 5,* 450–490.

14

Bone Conduction Hearing

Sound is not only sent through the "regular route" of air conduction via the outer ear, through middle ear, to inner ear. It is also sent directly to the inner ear through vibration of the skull, termed "through bone conduction." This has importance for clinical audiology. Measurement of hearing through both routes provides critical insight as to what parts of the ear are creating hearing loss. This chapter discusses how sound becomes bone conducted.

BONE CONDUCTION MECHANISMS

In order for the inner ear to transmit signals that the central nervous system will perceive as sound, it is necessary for cochlear fluids to move, which sets certain sensory structures inside the cochlea into motion. This usually occurs as a result of the ossicles vibrating—waves are produced in the inner ear fluids by movement of the footplate of the stapes in the oval window. Under these conditions, the sound has entered the ear as an airborne sound wave in the outer ear canal, and it is said to be an air-conducted signal. In this case, we are hearing by **air conduction**. However, sound energy may reach the inner ear by another route.

When sound energy in the air reaches 50 to 60 dB HL, it has enough energy to vibrate the entire skull sufficiently to create waves in the inner ear fluids that can stimulate the sensory cells. In other words, the sound being conducted through the bones of the head now reaches the normal hearing person's inner ear at threshold of hearing levels. This is called **bone conduction** hearing. This chapter describes how bone conduction sound transmission occurs.

Skull Vibration

The skull, although a rather rigid sphere of bone, tends to vibrate in different patterns depending on the frequency of the vibrating force. As Figure 14–1 shows, when the vibrating force is applied to the forehead, frequencies of about 200 Hz cause the entire skull to move as a unit, back and forth. At about 800 Hz, the pattern changes and the front and back of the head vibrate in opposite directions. At about 1600 Hz, the pattern of vibration changes again so that the sides of the head are moving toward each other whereas the front and back are moving away from each other on half of the cycle, and in opposite directions on the other half-cycle. The latter two patterns are not only moving the skull but are changing its

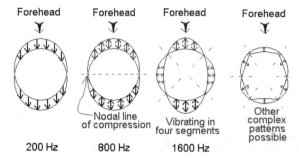

Figure 14–1. Vibrational patterns of the skull, viewed from above, when the vibrating force is applied to the forehead. At frequencies below 200 Hz the skull vibrates as a rigid body, at near 800 Hz a nodal line appears and the front and back of the head move in opposite directions, and at about 1600 Hz there are four independently vibrating segments. Other standing wave vibration patterns are also possible at other frequencies. Adapted from von Bekesy, G., *Experiments in Hearing.* 1960, McGraw-Hill. Reproduced with permission.

shape, producing compressional and flexural forces within the head. As the skull is changing shape, the cochlea inside the temporal bone is also changing shape. This is frequently referred to as "distortion" of the shape of the cochlear shell, and is one mechanism by which bone-conducted sound creates movement of the cochlear fluids.

Inertial Aspects of Bone Conduction

In order to create displacement of the cochlear fluids, it really doesn't matter whether one holds the inner ear still and moves the stapes, or holds the stapes still and moves the inner ear; the resultant inner ear fluid displacement is the same. In bone conduction, the skull is vibrating. Due to the inertia of the stapes footplate sitting in the oval window, the stapes footplate does not vibrate at exactly the same time as the skull, which has the effect of creating additional cochlear fluid displacement.

However, inertial energy is highly dependent on mass and the ossicular chain has very little mass. Thus, inertia of the ossicles would appear to be a relatively minor contributor to bone conduction hearing. This is supported by the observation that an indi-

vidual's threshold of hearing by bone conduction is not dramatically affected when the ossicles are missing or immobilized. In the next chapter (section on **Carhart's notch**), the clinical significance of this will be further explored, as one form of stapes immobilization often does show up with a clinical finding.

Let's consider the importance of the inertial energy contributed by the inner ear fluids. It seems obvious that if one literally "shakes" or vibrates a chamber filled with fluid, waves are going to be created in the fluid. It is not known to what extent fluid inertia contributes to bone conduction hearing, but it would appear to be a significant factor, especially in the lower frequencies.

Compressional Aspects of Bone Conduction

Perhaps at all frequencies, but especially in the higher frequencies where the skull vibrates segmentally, the inner ear contracts and expands to the sound waves. When the inner ear contracts, its volume is decreased and when it expands its volume is increased. As the inner ear is filled with fluid, when it contracts, the excess fluid must go somewhere, and a fluid "flow" occurs in the direction of the round window membrane, the most flexible surface in the otherwise bony walls of the inner ear. The excess fluid simply bulges the round window toward the middle ear. During the phase where the volume of the inner ear expands, fluid flows away from the round window resulting in a retraction of the round window membrane into the inner ear. This flow back and forth in the inner ear is similar to the fluid displacement produced by the in and out movement of the stapes during air-conduction hearing. It provides the necessary movement of the sensory receptors to stimulate a sensation of hearing identical to air conduction hearing. von Bekesy (1960) demonstrated that a sound transmitted by air conduction and one transmitted by bone conduction have the same effect at the cochlea. Thus, there are not separate sensory receptor systems for air- and bone-conducted sounds. The only difference in air-conduction hearing and bone-conduction hearing is the manner in which the acoustic energy reaches the inner ear.

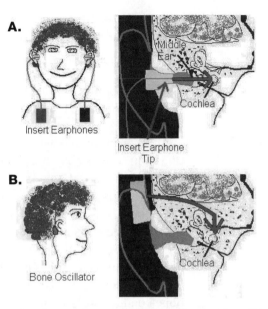

Figure 14–2. In air-conduction testing (**A**) sound is produced by an insert earphone, and transmitted through the outer, middle, and into the inner ear. In bone-conduction testing (**B**), the skull is vibrated by an oscillator placed on the mastoid bone behind the ear. The vibration is transmitted to the cochlea, by-passing the outer and middle ear.

HEARING IS TESTED BY AIR- AND BONE-CONDUCTION

Clinical audiologists will assess hearing both by air- and bone-conduction (Figure 14–2). Earphones placed on the pinnas create air-conducted sound. A more common earphone is the "insert earphone." Sound is routed from a small speaker box, through a tube, and through a hole in a foam earplug. Air-conducted sound travels through all parts of the auditory system.

Bone-conducted sound is transmitted via a **bone oscillator**, also called a **bone vibrator**, which is typically placed on the mastoid behind one ear. Because the skull of an adult is fused, when the skull is vibrated, bone-conducted sound is transmitted to both cochleas. Bone-conducted sound does not travel through the outer or middle ear.

BONE-CONDUCTION BY AIR-CONDUCTION AND THE OCCLUSION EFFECT

If the ear canal of a normal-hearing person is occluded (covered) while the person is listening to a low-frequency bone-conducted sound, the sound will become louder. You can experience this phenomenon for yourself. If you hum, your voice will not only set air waves into motion, but will vibrate the bones of the skull. While humming, tightly press both of your tragus's inward. The tragus is the flap of skin anterior to the pinna (see Figure 15–2). This phenomenon of bone-conducted sound becoming more intense is called the **occlusion effect**. Two factors may be involved in producing the occlusion ef-

Clinical Correlate: Diagnosing Conductive Hearing Loss

Chapter 3 (Figure 3-8) introduced hearing testing via air conduction. Let's consider the information gained by additionally testing by bone conduction.

If a hearing loss is detected when testing by air conduction, but none is found when testing the same frequencies by bone conduction, the patient's loss is coming from the conductive apparatus. The bone conduction results show that the inner ear mechanisms are normal. The loss must therefore be coming from a problem in either the outer or middle ear. This is the case for the right ear for the patient whose audiogram is shown in Figure 14-3. This is termed a **conductive hearing loss.**

In contrast, if the same thresholds are found by both air- and bone-conduction, then the problem is not with the sound conducting system. The left ear in Figure 14-3 shows this type of loss, termed **sensorineural hearing loss.**

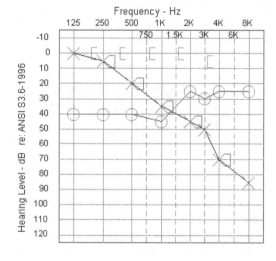

Figure 14–3. Example of how air- and bone-conduction testing gives information about whether the loss is conductive. The right ear air-conduction hearing thresholds are abnormal (*circles*), whereas the right ear bone-conduction hearing (*marked with the [symbols*) show normal hearing. When the sound must travel through the outer and middle ear (air-conduction) there is a loss of hearing; but, there is none by bone conduction, when the sound goes directly to the inner ear. The right ear has normal inner ear hearing—the loss is therefore conductive. In contrast, the left ear does not have a conductive loss. The air-conduction thresholds (*X*'s) and bone conduction thresholds (*marked with the] symbols*) are the same. There was no blockage of sound in the outer or middle ear; all the loss can be attributed to the inner ear (or nerve pathways). Audiogram generated with AuDSim software, used and reproduced with permission courtesy of www.audstudent.com .

fect. First, the mandible, or lower jaw, which is loosely hinged to the skull, may, because of inertia, lag behind the skull when the head is vibrated by bone-conducted sound. The mandible articulates with the skull just in front of the cartilaginous external ear canal (Figure 14–4), the movement of the mandible relative to the skull may produce a slight bulging in and out of the canal wall causing small air pressure changes in the external canal. If the ear canal is open, or uncovered, most of the pressure changes take the path of least resistance and escape into the atmosphere. However, if the ear is covered, or occluded, the path of least resistance is through the eardrum and middle ear. In this case the sound passing through the middle ear adds to the bone conducted sound already reaching the cochlea, producing more intensity and thus appearing louder.

Although mandibular inertia may play some role in the occlusion effect, it is probably not the major factor. It appears that the primary effect is due to energy being radiated from the walls of the external ear canal because these bony walls, being a part of the skull, are also vibrating. The vibration of the canal walls produces pressure changes in the ear canal. The pressure waves pass through the middle ear to the inner ear when the ear canal is occluded (see Figure 14–4).

Clinically, audiologists present sound by both air- and bone-conduction and compare the thresholds of hearing. It is important that the ear canals not be occluded during bone-conduction testing, as they are not closed off when we hear everyday sounds of life. The occlusion effect may improve bone conduction measures by as much as 25 to 30 dB in the low frequencies. There is less effect at higher frequencies. Figure 14–5 shows the

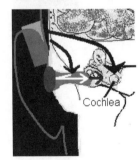

Figure 14–4. Illustration of the occlusion effect. Bone-conducted sound will vibrate the external auditory meatus and create sound in the ear canal. As shown in (**A**), the sound normally escapes the outer ear. If the ear is occluded, (**B**) the sound is channeled through the middle ear to the inner ear.

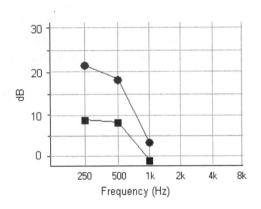

Figure 14–5. Illustration of the size of the occlusion effect: the average decibel amount that bone conduction measures are enhanced by occluding the ears. Data from Dean and Martin (2000), who also reported that there is significant between-subjects differences. Circles are for earphones that rest on top of the ears (supra-aural earphones). Squares represent the average data for insert earphones where the foam tip is deeply inserted into the external auditory meatus.

approximate values of the occlusion effect using the older style supra-aural earphones and deeply inserted insert earphones. The smaller size of the occlusion effect is an advantage of the insert earphones because in one part of hearing testing ("bone-conduction testing using contralateral masking") the nontest ear has to be occluded.

Although bone-conduction measures may be changed by the occlusion effect, the occlusion effect should not be thought of as a change in bone-conduction hearing. Hearing does not change as a result of occluding the ear. What does change is the level of the stimulus reaching the inner ear. Thus, the observed change in threshold is the result of additional energy being delivered to the sensory receptors of the inner ear, not to a change in the sensitivity of the ear itself.

the inner ear in the same manner as occurs during air-conduction testing.

Audiologists test hearing by both air- and bone-conduction, which helps to determine the part, or parts, of the ear creating the hearing loss. Normal hearing by bone conduction in the presence of hearing loss by air conduction points to a problem with the sound conducting mechanism of the ear (a problem with the outer and/or middle ear).

When testing bone-conduction hearing, the audiologist does not want to occlude the ear. Covering the ear prevents the sound created by the vibrating ear canal walls from escaping as it normally does. Ear canal occlusion increases the sound energy transmitted to the cochlea and creates a measurement of an artificially lower threshold for bone-conduction hearing.

SUMMARY

There are a number of variables that contribute to bone-conduction hearing. When the skull vibrates, inertial, compressional, or distortional and displacement forces operate on the inner ear fluids. The bone-conducted sound moves the membranes of

REFERENCES

Dean, M. S., & Martin, F. N. (2000). Insert earphone depth and the occlusion effect. *American Journal of Audiology, 9,* 131–134.

von Bekesy, G. (1960). Bone conduction. In *Experiments in hearing.* Acoustical Society of America/McGraw-Hill Books.

15

Advanced Conductive Anatomy and Physiology

This chapter discusses additional anatomic and physiologic features of the outer and middle ear. Several "clinical correlates," areas where anatomy and physiology have a direct clinical relevance, are noted. This chapter begins with a description of how the pinna develops before discussing anatomic details and physiologic nuances.

PINNA

Embryologic development

Fetal development of the structures of the ear is relatively early, so the features of the pinna are evident for most of the prenatal period. The pinna, or auricle, begins to develop by about 6 weeks gestation. It arises from tissue known as the auricular hillocks, as shown in Figures 15–1A and 15–1B. When the fetus is age 7 to 20 weeks, these small ridges and bumps develop into the features that progressively resemble the adult pinna (Figures 15–1B through 15–1E. The shape of the pinna is adultlike by about 20 weeks, although it grows in size through the preteen years. There are a number of good Web sites providing detailed study of the embryolo-

gy of the ear. Two particularly nice ones are http://www.med.unc.edu/embryo_images/ unit-ear and http://embryology.med.unsw .edu.au/embryo.htm .

Landmarks

The different pinna features are labeled in Figure 15–2. The in-the-ear style hearing aid sits in the **concha**, the bowl or depression closest to the external auditory meatus. The **tragus** is the piece of skin anterior to the concha. The concha is rimmed by the **antihelix**, a ridge of cartilage. In the posterior, superior area of the pinna is a depression called **scaphoid fossa**. The **helix** is the rim of cartilage that runs around the edge of the pinna. It begins at the **crus** (from Latin, anything resembling a leg) **of the helix**. Some hearing aids have a "helix lock," an extension that fits up under the crus of the helix. This ear does not have a pronounced auricular tubercle, or **Darwin's tubercle**. Some people have a more pronounced bump. The **lobule** is, of course, the cartilage-free portion of the pinna.

The characteristics of the resonance of the ear canal can be measured by insert-

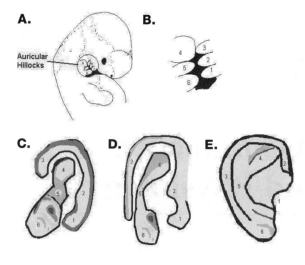

Figure 15–1. The pinna develops from the 6-week-old fetus's auricular hillocks (**A**), which are shown enlarged in (**B**). As these cells grow, these bumps become increasingly defined (**C** and **D**) and the features resemble those of the adult ear (**E**) by 20 weeks gestational age.

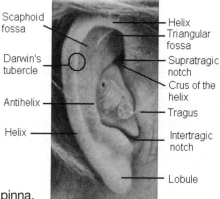

Figure 15–2. Major anatomic features of the pinna.

Clinical Correlate: Defects of the Outer Ear May Signal Middle and Inner Ear Defects

Teratogens are substances in the environment (such as chemicals or drugs a pregnant woman may be exposed to) that adversely affect fetal development and can cause birth defects. Birth defects can also be **genetic** in origin. The outer ear develops from different tissue than the inner ear, so birth defects that affect the outer ear (e.g., having a misshapen or missing pinna) may not signal a genetic defect of the inner ear. However, if the defect is caused by a teratogen, then it is possible that there will be inner ear hearing loss. The inner ear is developing about the same time as the outer ear. A child with a defect of the outer ear has greater risk of having hearing loss.

When fetal developmental abnormality creates an abnormal pinna, with a deformed ear with missing features, it is called a **microtia**. If the pinna is absent entirely, it is an **anotia**.

ing a tube, which is connected to a microphone, into the ear canal (to be discussed below in the physiology section.) **Probe tube measurement** is conducted in hearing aid fitting, and is called, also called "probe microphone measurement" or "**real-ear measurement**." (Also see Chapter 8.) The depth of insertion of this probe can be referenced either to the **intertragic notch**, the notch just below the tragus; or it can be described relative to the notch above the tragus, the **supratragic notch**.

Physiology of the Pinna

Because the high frequencies do not wrap around the head, but bounce off, sound pressure builds up at the side of the head. Figure 15–3 illustrates that, for high frequencies, the sound is about 5 dB louder at the side of the head than it would be if the head were not present. This advantage, or sound gain, is shown in trace (A).

The **pinna** creates **resonances** because of its size and shape. We can measure the amount of sound pressure increase by placing a probe microphone in different areas of the pinna. Shaw (1974) tested the resonances of different areas of the pinna. A probe placed in the scaphoid fossa would measure more sound energy than if the probe were placed on the side of the head. The increase in energy, or gain, caused by the flange of the pinna is shown in Figure 15–3, trace (B). A greater amount of resonance comes if the probe is place in the concha, at the entrance to the meatus, trace (C).

A person with **anotia**, and no other anatomic defect, would not have these normal resonances. His or her hearing would be around 10 dB less sensitive in the high frequencies.

The pinna aids in sound localization and has resonances. As resonances are related to the size of the pinna, the first author's (T.H.) American dingo (Dixi) (Figures 15–4A and 15–4B) has greater resonance than Katie, a poodle (Figure 15–4C), canine companion of the second author of this text (L.P.). Although human ears are said to have muscles, they don't function to move the ears. Other animals, like Dixi, are able to move their two ears independently to aid in sound localization (and to make children giggle).

EXTERNAL AUDITORY MEATUS

Detailed anatomy

As was mentioned in Chapter 12, the external auditory meatus (EAM) is about 25 to 35 mm in length. If measured from the supratragal notch, the length would approximate 25 mm (1 inch). The tragus adds another centimeter of length, so measured from this location, the ear canal is about 35 mm, or 1.4 inches in length. Because the tympanic membrane (TM) is slanted slightly, and is more medial at the lowest point, the TM is about 5 mm greater distance inward at the bottom of the ear canal. The ear ca-

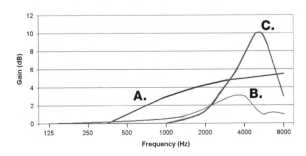

Figure 15–3. Resonances of the pinna and head. (**A**) Head, (**B**) flange of the pinna, and (**C**) concha. Data from Shaw (1974).

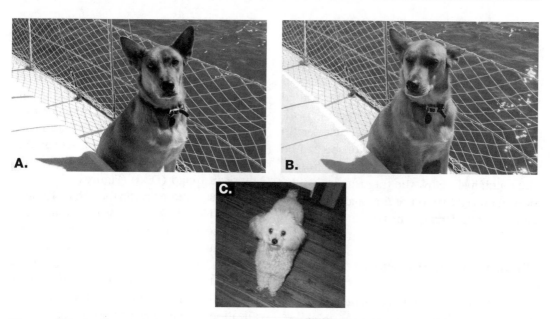

Figure 15–4. A and **B**. Dixi, shown aboard the sailing vessel MoonPuppy, can move each pinna independently. **C**. Katie has less pinna mobility and cute floppy ears. Dixi's erect ears provide for better sound localization and collection ability than Katie's floppy ears.

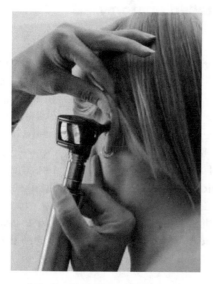

Figure 15–5. To best view the ear canal, pull the pinna up and back.

nal is typically elliptical, being higher than it is wide. The height is about 8 mm, and the width about 6 mm. Children will have shorter and narrower ear canals. The total length of a child's ear canal, including the tragus, would be about 25 cm (1 inch).

The angle of the ear canal changes with age. At birth, the ear canal does not have a very pronounced bend in it. In adults, the external, cartilaginous portion right after the tragus runs slightly upward (superior) and anterior at first, then after the "first bend" the angle changes to posterior (and still superior a bit) as the canal continues medially to the osseocartilaginous junction. The **osseocartilaginous junction** is the narrowest part of the ear canal. It is at this junction where the cartilage portion ends and the bony portion begins. Excessive narrowing of the osseocartilaginous junction is called a **stenosis**. At the osseocartilaginous junction, the ear canal bends anterior and slightly inferior.

Clinical Correlate: Otoscopy and Earmold Impressions

To best view the adult's tympanic membrane with an otoscope, pull the ear canal upward and backward (Figure 15-5). The cartilage before the first bend will deform, straightening the ear canal. When looking in the infant's ear canal with an otoscope, pulling the pinna posteriorly and inferiorly opens and straightens the ear canal best.

Hearing aids typically require "**earmold impressions,**" which are impressions of the concha and ear canal. (In the "old days" the only style of hearing aid was the behind-the-ear hearing aid, which needed to have an earmold made for it. Today, many styles are custom molded to the ear. Although it would be more correct to say you are making an impression for the outside, or shell of the hearing aid, the term earmold impression is more common.) The impression should extend past osseocartilaginous junction, or "second bend" of the ear canal. Failure to do so can mean that the hearing aid or earmold is angled toward the ear canal. That would allow the amplified sound to bounce off the side of the ear canal, rather than being directed toward the tympanic membrane. This is one cause of "feedback," a squealing sound hearing aids make when the amplified sound leaks out of the ear canal and is reamplified.

To safely make an ear impression, the audiologist first inserts a cotton puff or foam block (on a string) into the ear canal. The "**otoblock**" is pushed into the ear with a penlight that has a long, clear, hard plastic tip. Impression material is then inserted in the ear canal with a syringe, and hardens in about 5 minutes. The otoblock seals off the ear canal and prevents the impression material from damaging the TM. The audiologist's knowledge of the length and shape of the ear canal is used when deciding on placement of this otoblock. After the material hardens, the audiologist removes the impression. A forward twist helps remove the impression. If the patient has a stenosis, it is difficult and sometimes impossible to remove the ear impression. The audiologist is alerted to the possibility of a stenosis when the otoblock is tight when inserted at the second bend, but then begins to move freely after that point.

Proximity of the Temporomandibular Joint

As shown in Figure 15-6, the **temporomandibular joint (TMJ)**, the hinged jaw joint, is anterior and inferior to the external auditory meatus. It is located near the lateral, or cartilaginous portion of the ear canal. As this portion of the external canal is cartilaginous, the movement of the jaw alters the shape of the ear canal.

Clinical Correlates: Temporomandibular Joint Pain and the Effect of TMJ Movement on Earmold Impressions

Some patients with disorders of the temporomandibular joint have pain that radiates to the ear. Many times it is difficult for these patients to understand that the source of the pain is their jaw, rather than the ear. To determine if TMJ problems may be the culprit for normal-hearing patients with perceived **otalgia** (pain in the ear), place your fingers on the jaw joint. Ask the patient to open and close the jaw. If you feel a clicking sound, and/or the patient hears a clicking or describes discomfort, TMJ disorder is probable, and a referral to a dentist for evaluation and management is appropriate.

When removing earmold impressions, it is sometimes helpful to have the patient open his or her jaw. This expands the size of the opening, easing removal. Some patients open their jaw when inserting and removing hearing aids, as well.

Some patients have considerably differently shaped ear canals when the jaw is open versus when it is closed. If these patients wear hearing aids, they may experience feedback when chewing, as the opening creates a pathway for amplified sound to leak out of the ear canal. Some audiologists routinely make two ear impressions, one with the jaw open, and one with the jaw closed, to facilitate the laboratory's fabrication of the hearing aid shell (or earmold, if a behind-the-ear hearing aid is prescribed). Digital hearing aids with advanced feedback cancellation algorithms offer a significant advantage for these patients.

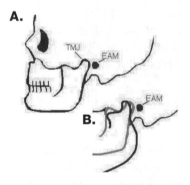

Figure 15–6. Illustration of the proximity of the external auditory meatus and the temporomandibular joint (**A**), and of the change in this proximity with opening of the jaw (**B**).

Proximity of Nerves to the External Auditory Meatus

Cranial nerve X, the vagus nerve, runs underneath the posterior and inferior ear canal. Some persons can have this nerve stimulated with irritation of the ear canal (as when making an ear impression, for example). This causes a cough reflex in affected persons. The articulotemporal nerve (sensory nerve for the skin of the pinna) and one of the sensory branches of the VII nerve (facial nerve) are also in proximity to the ear canal.

Skin of the External Auditory Meatus

The outer layer of the tympanic membrane is skin and, of course, so is the lining of the ear canal. The skin growth is from the umbo outward, so there is a natural outward migration of old skin cells which takes place at a rate about as fast as your fingernails grow. The skin is thicker in the cartilaginous portion of the EAM; it is about 1.0-mm thick in the bony portion, but 2.0-mm thick more laterally.

Cerumen

Cerumen, or ear wax, is formed by secretions coming from the base of the tiny hairs in the cartilaginous portion of the EAM. The secretions of the **apocrine** and **sebaceous** glands combine to form cerumen. Sebum is high in lipids, a type of fat. Apocrine glands are a type of sweat gland.

Excessive stimulation of the hairs in the ear canals, such as via use of **Q-tips**, is said to stimulate the production of wax, as well as increasing the potential for **cerumen impaction**. Q-tip users typically push wax inward with the Q-tip, as well as removing some of the material. When wax is pushed inward, it has a longer time to oxidize and dry, making removal more difficult. Skin growth normally helps push wax outward. The motion of the TMJ also helps debris to move laterally.

Cerumen ranges in color from pale yellow to dark reddish brown. It grows darker in color as it ages and oxidizes. Although most Blacks and Caucasians have a wet and sticky wax texture, a drier, ricelike textured wax is typical of Orientals.

Detailed Physiology of the External Auditory Meatus

The resonance of the pinna was introduced in Chapter 12 (Figure 12-1), and was elaborated on earlier in this chapter (see Figure 15–3). The resonance of the external auditory meatus adds another 10 dB to the effect. The frequency of the peak resonance varies from person to person, and is larger in some individuals, smaller in others. Figure 15–7 shows all the resonances of the average external ear, and their total.

Clinical Correlate: Cerumen Management

Cerumen removal, also called **cerumen management,** is within the scope of practice of audiologists, although we are typically not reimbursed by insurance carriers for performing this procedure. Wax, sufficient to create difficulty in either making earmold impressions or in performing hearing testing, has been reported in up to 40% of adults, and 10% of children. Patients with cognitive impairments also have a high incidence of wax impaction. To permit the audiologist to remove cerumen safely requires that the audiologist have knowledge of the anatomy of the ear canal, as well as recognition of the pathologic conditions that would make cerumen removal unsafe.

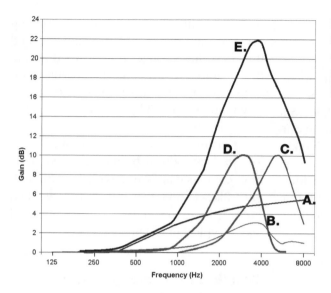

Figure 15–7. Resonance of the (**A**) head, (**B**) flange of the pinna, (**C**) concha, (**D**) external auditory meatus, and of the total external ear (**E**). Data from Shaw (1974).

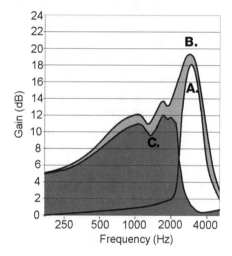

Figure 15–8. Example real-ear measurement. **A**. The real-ear measurement of the natural resonances of the ear, termed real-ear unaided gain. **B**. Real-ear aided gain, showing the amplification the hearing aid provides, as measured in the ear canal. The shaded area shows the difference between the two measures. The amount of this difference, the real-ear insertion gain, is shown in curve (**C**).

The location of the microphone in the external auditory meatus is critical to the accuracy of the resonance measurements made. The ear canal is a tube, closed at one end. Figure 4-8D had shown how two sound waves, identical in frequency, can cancel each other out. This can happen if the sound reflecting off the eardrum is opposite in phase (180 degrees out of phase) relative to the sound wave striking the TM. When the reflection is 180 degrees out of phase, **standing waves** are created, which creates "dead spots" (decreased SPL) in the canal. "Hot spots" where the sound intensity doubles can also occur. The closer the probe microphone is to the TM, the more accurate the measurement because the standing waves won't be measured except at a much higher frequencies. (Only frequencies with very short wavelengths could be canceled or summed if the measurement takes place close to the TM.)

Clinical Correlate: Real Ear Measurement

Real-ear measurement was introduced in Chapter 8. Although less popular in the original form today, clinical measurement of the patient's ear canal acoustics can be made, using a probe microphone "real-ear" system. The individual's ear canal length and shape creates unique resonances. When a hearing aid is inserted into the ear canal, these resonances are destroyed. The hearing aid in the ear removes the natural resonances and makes the hearing loss worse. The hearing aid needs to make up for the loss coming from the destruction of the natural resonances and then supply the needed amplification to treat the hearing loss.

In clinical real-ear measurement, a probe microphone is placed near the tympanic membrane. As the length of the ear canal, plus the tragus, is about 35 mm, if the probe is placed 29 mm from the intertragal notch, the tip of the probe is about 6 mm from the TM. This permits accurate measurement (without standing wave problems) for frequencies up to about 6 kHz. The hearing aid is placed in the ear, and the measurement of the amplification, or gain, across frequencies is again made. In this way, we can determine how much louder the sound is when the aid is in the ear (**real-ear aided gain**), and if we subtract the unaided resonances, we measure the amount of improvement the hearing aid provides (**real-ear insertion gain**). This is shown in Figure 15–8.

As discussed in Chapter 8, more recent real-ear technology does not directly measure the original resonances (the real-ear unaided response) or the insertion gain. Instead, speech sounds are produced, and the spectrum of the speech is measured in the ear canal. Calculations of the desired intensity of the amplified speech sounds are made based on the patient's hearing loss, and the hearing aid controls are adjusted until the hearing aid creates the desired amplification. This still allows for customization based on the patient's unique ear canal resonances, and the unique ways in which the hearing aid destroys this natural amplifier.

TYMPANIC MEMBRANE

Slant and Cone Depth

The tympanic membrane is not oriented straight up and down, but slants inward at the bottom, as illustrated in Figure 15–9. It is more medial at the lowest point by about 5 mm (0.5 cm, or about 0.2 inches). The angle of the tilt has been described as being from 40 to 55 degrees. The manubrium of the malleus is attached to the mid-

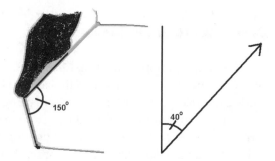

Figure 15–9. Illustration of the approximately 150-degree cone angle of the tympanic membrane, shown here in side view. The TM is not straight up and down, but slants so that the bottom is more medial. A line from the bottom of the TM to the top runs at about a 40 to 55-degree angle.

Clinical Correlate: Cone of Light

When learning otoscopic inspection, it is helpful to first locate the cone of light (see Figure 12-5). Look from the bright reflection to its tip, which is the umbo of the eardrum. The manubrium of the malleus will be superior and anterior. That means when viewing a right ear, the malleus runs from the center to about the 1 o'clock position. When viewing the left ear, it runs to about 11 o'clock.

dle fiber layer of the tympanic membrane, and the malleus is pulled in toward the middle ear space by ligaments. The TM center is therefore drawn inward, too. The TM forms a very shallow cone, which has about 140 to 150 degrees of angle.

Also, the cone is tilted in the anterior/posterior aspect. The posterior side is slightly more lateral. The cone of light seen on otoscopic inspection results from the cone being tilted in this arrangement (anterior/posterior plus superior/inferior). As illustrated in Figure 15-10A, light waves that strike the TM do not bounce straight back out. They collect in one area of the tympan-

ic membrane, specifically the inferior, anterior area.

DETAILED STUDY OF THE OSSICULAR CHAIN

Figure 15-11 highlights some of the parts of the ossicular chain. The **head of the malleus** is the largest part of the malleus. Extending below it is the **manubrium of the malleus**. The shadow of this part of the bone (which actually appears white even though it is called a "shadow") can be seen through the tympanic membrane on otoscopic in-

A.

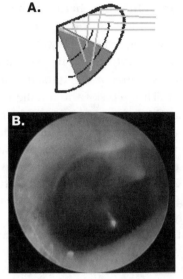

B.

Figure 15–10. Reflections of the light from the otoscope off the cone-shaped and slanted TM gather in an area that reflects back brightly. This is called the cone of light. **A.** The cone is created by the tilt of the tympanic membrane in the up and down, and front to back directions. **B.** The cone of light is the reflection to the lower right in this photograph of the tympanic membrane of this right ear.

spection. The **lateral process of the malleus** protrudes toward the tympanic membrane. It is visible on otoscopic examination as a bright white bump on most TMs. There is also an **anterior process,** which is sometimes called the **malleolar prominence**. A ligament attaches here to help hold the ossicular chain in place. The malleus attaches firmly to the incus's body at the **malleoincudal joint**. The balance of the incus is maintained by it having two arms, or processes. The shorter, fatter top process is conveniently called the **short process of the incus**. Extending inferiorly is the **long process of the incus**, which terminates at the **lenticular process**. The **head of the stapes** and the lenticular process meet at the **incudostapedial joint**. The wishbone-shaped crurae (plural of **crus**) extend medially to the **footplate of the stapes**, which you may recall sits in the oval window to the cochlea.

As mentioned previously, **chorda tympani**, a branch of the VII nerve, crosses between malleus and incus. Chorda tympani controls taste to the anterior portion of the tongue. Damage to this nerve can cause patients to perceive a "tinny" taste.

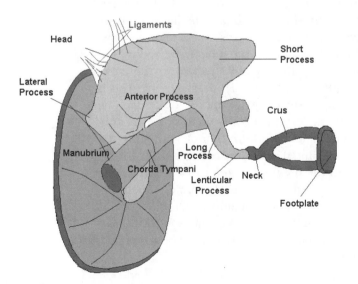

Figure 15–11. Parts of the ossicular chain and some of the ligaments holding the chain in place. The chorda tympani runs between malleus and incus.

RESONANCE OF THE MIDDLE EAR

Mass and Stiffness of the Middle Ear Affect Sound Transmission Differently at Different Frequencies

The middle ear ossicles, though lightweight, do have mass. The air inside the middle ear also has some mass. The middle ear system is stiffened by the ossicles and by the ligaments that hold the ossicles to the walls of the middle ear space. Any vibrating object that has mass and stiffness has a preferred frequency of vibration (a resonant frequency), and the middle ear is no exception. Another way to think of resonance is to examine the frequencies that would be attenuated as they pass through the system. Very low frequencies will not pass through the middle ear efficiently because the system has some stiffness. Stiff things don't vibrate well at low frequencies. However, the middle ear is not extremely stiff, so very high frequencies will not be transmitted readily either. The mass of the middle ear also keeps the high frequencies from being efficiently transferred through the middle ear.

In Chapter 13, you read about the middle ear transformer. Recall that it gives about 26 to 29 dB of mechanical advantage as sound goes from airborne to pressure changes within the cochlear fluids. The actual amount of advantage is not equal at each frequency. This is expected, as the middle ear doesn't pass very low and very high frequencies as effectively. Above 2000 Hz, the middle ear system attenuates the sound transmission. Various investigators have reported that the best sound transmission is at about 1000 Hz, which could be considered the middle ear resonant frequency.

Clinical Correlate: Carhart's Notch

In Chapter 14, the mechanisms of bone conduction were overviewed. The inertial component was described as the lagging behind of the stapes footplate when the cochlear shell vibrates. Figure 15–12 asks you to consider how this could happen. If you attached a rubber membrane to the side of a roll of masking tape, then placed a weight in the center of the membrane and moved the roll of tape side to side, the weight attached to the membrane would take a slight amount of time to start moving. This is the **inertial lag**. When you stop moving the roll of tape in one direction, and start moving it in the other side-to-side direction, the weight on the membrane would, for a brief time, have the membrane continue in its initial direction.

You also learned in the previous chapter that when testing by bone conduction, the walls of the EAM vibrate, which creates a sound wave. If the ear is not occluded, then most of this sound escapes the ear canal, though some sound will still travel through the middle ear space, and is part of the bone-conduction hearing mechanism.

If you have a fixation of the stapes in the oval window, you will have a conductive hearing loss—you don't hear well by air-conduction. Bone conduction should be normal. However, if you have a stapes fixation, you are deprived of both the bone-by-air conduction mechanism of hearing, and importantly, the inertial lag mechanism. As a result, your hearing by bone conduction is depressed. This doesn't happen at all frequencies, it is most noticeable around 2000 Hz. This is called a **Carhart's notch**, named after Raymond Carhart who described this clinical phenomenon often associated with **otosclerosis**, a fixation of the stapes footplate in oval window. The best frequency for this inertial lag is 2000 Hz, and this has been used to explain the frequency at which the notch, or decrease in bone conduction hearing, occurs. To restate, as the ossicular chain has greatest inertial lag at 2000 Hz, it is theorized that removing the vibration of the ossicular chain, and its contribution to bone conduction hearing, will affect 2000-Hz bone-conduction thresholds the most.

Transmission of Sound Through the Tympanic Membrane Is Affected by Mass and Stiffness

The acoustic impedance of the middle ear system is the degree to which sound striking the eardrum bounces off. This can be measured clinically (Chapter 8, middle ear analyzer). The percentage of sound bouncing off is typically not measured; the measurement is more complex. Before discussing the measurement process in the clinical correlate sections, let us consider conditions which would make more sound bounce off the eardrum. If the middle ear system had more stiffness, the resonant frequency of the middle ear would shift higher, as the low frequencies aren't transmitted through a stiff system very well. The added stiffness would lower the overall sound transmission, but would show up most when assessing low-frequency sound reflection off the eardrum. Adding mass won't hurt low-frequency sound transmission as much as it does high-frequency transmission, so adding mass has the effect of lowering the middle ear resonant frequency.

The middle ear space is normally air filled. The eustachian tube is responsible for clearing fluid accumulation (mucous membranes secrete mucus into the middle ear space) and for providing fresh air when the mucosa naturally absorbs some of the air in the middle ear space. If the eustachian tube does not open frequently enough, a pressure difference can occur between the air in the middle ear space and the air outside. The difference in air pressure creates an impedance mismatch. Just as airborne sound doesn't transmit to fluid readily because fluid has a higher density and stiffness, sound won't travel through the TM as well when air in the middle ear has a different air pressure. The difference in pressure creates additional TM stiffness. You likely have noticed that when ascending or descending in an airplane; your ears are "stuffy" and you don't hear well until you "pop" your ears (open your eustachian tubes).

Clinical Correlate: Measuring Middle Ear Resonance

Although not widely done, middle ear resonant frequency can be measured clinically as a part of the test called **tympanometry**. This measurement may add information about what is creating a middle ear pathology. Too high a resonant frequency means the ear is either too stiff or has loss of mass. Too low a resonant frequency indicates excessive middle ear mass or loss of stiffness.

Clinical Correlate: Measuring Middle Ear Pressure

Tympanometry was introduced in Chapter 8. Audiologists measure how well the middle ear receives sound by presenting a low-frequency (220 Hz) tone to a sealed ear canal. While the tone is being presented, the air pressure is changed in the ear canal. When the air pressure in the ear canal is made to be the same as the air pressure in the middle ear space, the sound will be transmitted through the tympanic membrane with greatest ease. This test, called **tympanometry**, is used to determine whether the eustachian tube is opening frequently enough, or whether the mucosa in the middle ear has absorbed the air. Tympanometry can also detect if fluid has accumulated in the space, because in that case there is poor sound transmission no matter what pressure is applied to the outer ear. The impedance mismatch is occurring between the air in the outer ear and the fluid in the middle ear.

Tympanometry also gives information about stiffness pathologies. It is one of the routine tests. In conjunction with testing of the acoustic reflex, tympanometry gives the audiologist valuable information about the **site of lesion**, that is, the anatomic location of the hearing problem.

ACOUSTIC REFLEX PHYSIOLOGY

Reflex Latency

As introduced in Chapter 13, the acoustic reflex is triggered by the perception of loud sound. When the reflex occurs, the stiffening of the ossicular chain reduces the transmission of low-frequency sound. The reflex does not occur instantaneously. The sound must be heard, and a signal must ascend the reflex path, then descend to the VIIth nerve. The **latency** of the reflex is the amount of time between the sound being presented to the ear, and the reflex contracting. Not all sounds create the same latency of contraction. Low-frequency sounds tend to have ear-

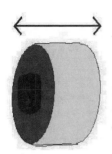

Figure 15–12. Visual to assist you in thinking about the inertial lag of the stapes. This sketch illustrates a roll of masking tape with a rubber membrane attached on one side, and a weight glued to that membrane. If you move the roll of tape side to side, do you see that the membrane would move back and forth slightly later than the tape does? The weight on the membrane creates this inertial lag.

Clinical Correlate: Measuring Acoustic Reflex Latency

Because the acoustic reflex has a pathway through the internal auditory meatus, researchers examined whether persons with tumors of the VIIIth nerve, which runs through the internal auditory meatus, would have a longer latency reflex. Although in general they do, other reflex abnormalities also occur, and are more commonly measured.

---

lier latency reflexes. Later in your studies this may seem surprising. You will see in Chapter 18 that it takes longer for low-frequency sounds to travel up the cochlea to the place where it will create a nerve impulse.

The louder a sound is, the shorter the latency. The literature says that reflex latency can be as short as 10 msec. However, if latency is measured clinically, it is measured at 10 decibels above the reflex threshold (often called 10 dB SL). Measured in this way, it takes about 100 msec for the reflex to reach 10% of its maximum. Full contraction would take about another 100 msec.

Reflex Adaptation

The acoustic reflex, when it occurs, will not remain indefinitely. The duration of the reflex, even when the sound remains on, can sometimes be quite short. High-frequency sounds yield the shortest contrac-

tions of the reflex—the reflex "adapts" or "decays" rapidly. For example, if presented with a steady 4000-Hz tone 10 dB above the reflex threshold, the muscle contraction would have decayed to about one-quarter of its original strength within 30 seconds. A 500-Hz tone at this same intensity would keep the reflex at nearly full strength for over 2 minutes.

In clinical testing and in research, the tones that elicit the acoustic reflex can be kept at a steady intensity. In real-life noise exposure, however, sounds change frequency and intensity over time, and these changes cause a renewed strengthening of the reflex.

Reflex Threshold

As described in Chapter 13, the acoustic reflex threshold occurs for normal hearing persons at 70 to 100 dB HL. As the nor-

Clinical Correlate: Measuring Acoustic Reflex Decay

Tumors of the VIIIth nerve can reveal themselves by the presence of inordinately fast decay of the acoustic reflex. The audiologist testing **reflex decay** will keep the tone on for 10 seconds, but typically only measure the decay for the first 5 seconds. If the reflex went to half contraction strength in under 5 seconds, that would be "positive" for abnormal reflex decay. Reflex decay is not clinically tested at frequencies above 1000 Hz, because people with normal neural functioning can have reflex decay in the first 5 seconds if the signal is a high-frequency tone.

Clinical Correlate: Reflex Threshold Testing May Reveal Type of Hearing Loss

Interestingly, many persons with damage to the cochlea also have reflex thresholds in the 70 to 100 dB HL range. This is due to a phenomenon called **recruitment**, the phenomenon where soft sounds are not perceived, but loud sounds sound loud. Recruitment is a hallmark of cochlear loss. In contrast, persons with lesions to the nerves characteristically have reflexes that come in at elevated levels, or are absent entirely. Persons with a disorder of the conductive system also have reflex thresholds that are present at an elevated intensity level or are absent. This is partially due to the conductive loss reducing the intensity of the sound. If the conductive pathology adds mass or stiffness to the ear, the second reason that the reflex may not occur until a louder than normal ("elevated") level (or may not occur at all) is that the pathology creates a situation where the relatively small effort the muscle contraction creates can't move the stiff or heavy middle ear system.

The combination of tympanometry and acoustic reflex testing provides powerful information. Not only do these tests assess the conductive apparatus, but they also help differentiate cochlear and retrocochlear losses.

mal hearing person has a threshold of 0 dB HL or near that level, then the sensation level of the reflex will also be in the range of 70 to 100 dB HL. (Sensation level is the intensity above threshold—see Figure 3-7.) Recall that it is not the physical intensity of the sound that triggers the reflex, but the fact that the sound that reaches the brainstem level is at a loud perceptual level.

SUMMARY

This chapter discussed some of the more advanced features of middle ear anatomy and physiology including pinna embryology, detailed examination of parts of the pinna, the resonances of the outer and middle ear, how cerumen is produced, and why the cone of light appears on the tympanic membrane. We reviewed the detailed parts of the ossicles and also the nerves that run in and near the middle ear, and examined the properties of the acoustic reflex. Many of these anatomy and physiology notes have direct clinical importance, as highlighted in this chapter.

REFERENCES

Shaw, E. A. (1974). The external ear. *Handbook of Sensory Physiology, 5,* 450-490.

16

Introduction to the Sensory Mechanics

The inner ear is a complex system of spaces and structures within the skull's temporal bone. It houses two sensory systems: the **cochlea**, containing the organs of hearing, and the **vestibular system**, containing the organs that sense motion. Chapter 11 presented the major features of the inner ear, which is nestled in temporal bone below the base of the brain. This chapter will further describe the major structures within the cochlea, and introduce the nerves that send the information toward the brain.

THE BONY LABYRINTH

The term **bony labyrinth** is used to label or describe the series of channels and cavities in the temporal bone that contain both the auditory and balance systems. As was seen in Figure 11–2, and is shown more accurately in Figure 16–1, the bony labyrinth consists of a central chamber called the **vestibule**, a spiral or snail-shaped tunnel called the **cochlea**, and three nearly circular tubes called **semicircular canals**.

Figure 16–1 illustrates the space as if it were a freestanding structure. It is important to remember that the inner ear is actu-

ally a hole in the temporal bone. The space is filled with a fluid called **perilymph**.

The **oval window**, into which the footplate of the stapes sits, is located in the bony wall of the vestibule. The **round window** is inferior to the oval window. Both windows "look out" toward the middle ear space and are covered with membranes.

THE MEMBRANOUS LABYRINTH

Within the bony labyrinth is a series of membranous tubes and pouches: the membranous labyrinth. As seen in Figure 16–2,

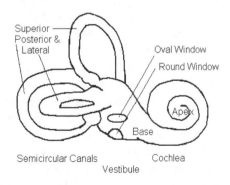

Figure 16–1. Illustration of the cochlea, vestibule, semicircular canals, and the location of the windows into the cochlea.

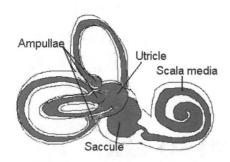

Figure 16–2. Illustration of the membranous labyrinth within the bony labyrinth. The fluid called endolymph is inside the membranous labyrinth (shown here as the shaded region); perilymph is outside it.

the membranous labyrinth has two pouches, the **utricle** and **saccule**, located in the vestibule; three canals, one in each of the **superior, posterior,** and **lateral** semicircular canals; and the **cochlear duct** or **scala media** of the cochlea. The entire membranous labyrinth is filled with a fluid called **endolymph**. The membranous labyrinth is surrounded by **perilymph.**

The Vestibular System

The part of the inner ear that involves balance or equilibrium is called the vestibular system. The membranous portion of each ear's vestibular system contains five sensory receptors: one each in the three semicircular canals, one in the **utricle,** and the other in the **saccule.** The sense organs of the semicircular canals are in the enlarged area near the juncture on the canals with the vestibule—each of these bulges is called an **ampulla**. (The plural of ampulla is ampullae.)

The sensory receptors in the utricle and saccule are gravity sensitive and respond to linear acceleration. That is, they inform the brain when the head is moving in a straight line (or stopping if the head is already in motion.) The sensory receptors in the ampullae of the semicircular canals are sensitive to angular (or rotary) acceleration.

This means that they inform the brain when the head is turned from side to side or tilted up and down. The three semicircular canals on each side of the head are arranged in different planes so that horizontal and vertical head movement stimulates different canals to different degrees. This will be discussed in detail in Chapter 24.

The hearing and balance portions of the inner ear are interconnected. The endolymph and perilymph are common to both systems. Thus, disorders that affect the inner ear may affect both sensory systems, that is, may produce equilibrium problems as well as hearing loss.

The Cochlea

The cochlea is often drawn as a freestanding structure; however, as previously mentioned, the outline of the cochlea, shown in Figure 16–1, is actually the outline of where a hole begins. Figure 16–1 is an illustration of what might be seen if the inner ear were filled with cement, and then the bone that surrounds the inner ear were chipped away. This concept is further illustrated in Figure 16–3. The cochlea here is shown in cross-section. The bone surrounding the cochlea can be seen; the sections of the cochlea are the large holes in bone. The arrows illustrate that the actual cochlea spirals. Although not illustrated in Figure 16–3, at the very apex of the cochlea, the membranous labyrinth ends just before the very top. This is called the **helicotrema**

STRUCTURES WITHIN THE COCHLEA

Gross Structures

Figures 16–4 and 16–5 show a cross-section view of just one coil of the cochlea. Note the relationship of these figures to Fig-

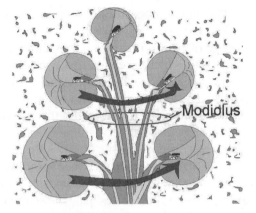

Figure 16–3. The cochlea spirals. This illustrates a cross-section through the snail shell-shaped structure and shows that the cochlea is embedded in bone. There is a central space, the modiolus, through which the nerves run. The middle section of each cross-section is the membranous labyrinth, filled with endolymph. The darker gray sections contain the fluid called perilymph.

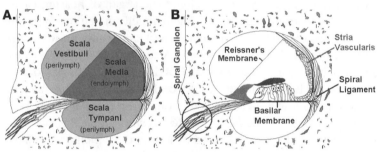

Figure 16–4. A. The three scala of the cochlea. **B**. Membranes and ligament within the cochlea, and spiral ganglion nerve cells are shown, as well as other cells found within the cochlea.

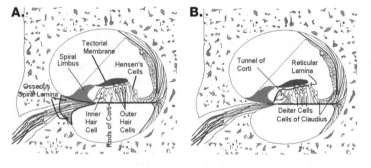

Figure 16–5. The organ of Corti within the cochlea. Different features are labeled in (**A**) and (**B**).

ure 16–3. Figure 16–4B shows the two membranes, the **basilar membrane** and **Reissner's membrane**, that divide the bony labyrinth into three chambers, or **scala**. **Scala vestibuli** communicates (connects) directly with the vestibule. **Scala tympani** communicates with scala vestibuli at the apex of the cochlea, at the helicotrema. These two membranes, basilar and Reissner's, delineate **scala media** and come together near the apex of the cochlea to create a closed tube. Thus, the perilymph of the bony labyrinth (in scala vestibule and scala

tympani) is separated from the endolymph of the membranous labyrinth (in scala media). Endolymph and perilymph are chemically different fluids, so it is important that the membranes keep them separated.

At the bottom end of the cochlea, at the base, scala tympani dead ends at the bony wall separating the inner ear from the middle ear. This area is called the **promontory**. This bony wall juts out into the middle ear space. The **round window** between the middle ear and inner ear is also in this wall. It is important to note that scala media is between the oval window into the vestibule and the round window from the middle ear into scala tympani.

Stria vascularis is an important structure located in scala media. It lies along the bony radial side of scala media. (As the cochlea spirals, this structure is on the outside wall of the cochlea shell.) Stria vascularis coils throughout the cochlea, from base to apex. Stria vascularis is a dense layer of tissue with a rich capillary network. The stria vascularis appears to be the source of endolymph—it secretes endolymph into scala media. Figure 16-4B illustrates the location of this structure. Radial to stria vascularis (even more toward the outside of the shell) lies **spiral ligament,** which attaches basilar membrane to the shell of the cochlea. We further discuss spiral ligament below. When examining Figure 16-4B, please note that there are nerve cells coming from the cochlea. They exit in groups, and have cell nuclei that clump together to form a **spiral ganglion.**

Fine Details of Features in the Cochlea

Figure 16-5 highlights the features of the part of the cochlea known as the **organ of Corti.** Chapter 17 will describe some of the ways that the organ of Corti varies from base to apex, but it should be noted that the same general features would be present in a cross-sectional view at any level of the cochlea from base to apex (except at the helicotrema of course, where there is no scala media and no organ of Corti.)

Note in Figure 16-5A that the thickened layer of periosteum (tissue of the same type that covers bones) called the **spiral limbus** rests on the bony shelf known as the bony or **osseous spiral lamina**. The nerve cells exiting the cochlea go through holes in the osseous spiral lamina. These holes are called **habenulae perforata.**

The upper edge or lip of the limbus provides the point of attachment for the inner edge of a third membrane, the **tectorial membrane**, which extends out into scala media. The outer edge of the tectorial membrane appears to be loosely attached to some of the supporting cells (**Hensen's cells**) that sit on basilar membrane. The tectorial membrane is gelatinous; it is made mostly of water. Resting on the basilar membrane, between it and the tectorial membrane, are several layers of supporting cells and structures, plus the sensory receptor cells of the organ of hearing called **hair cells**. The hair cells in one row, adjacent to the osseous spiral lamina, are known as **inner hair cells** A supporting structure called the **rods of Corti** (or pillar cells of Corti or the **arch of Corti**) separates this row of inner hair cells from three rows of **outer hair cells**. Figure 16-5B shows that the hair cells are covered by a protective membrane called **reticular lamina**. The perilymph from scala tympani is found under reticular lamina. This figure points out the space beneath the arch of Corti, called the **tunnel of Corti**.

The complexity of the cochlea is particularly amazing given its small size. Even though the human cochlea spirals through about two and three-quarter turns from **base** to **apex**, the length of the cochlea is only about 30 mm (1.2 inches). Furthermore, the width of the cochlea, as indicated by the width of the basilar membrane, that is, the distance from the edge of the bony or osseous spiral lamina to the spiral ligament, which connects it to the bony wall of scala media, is less than 1 mm.

Inner hair cells tend to be somewhat rounder than the outer hair cells (Figure 16-6). As one can tell by seeing a nucleus illustrated in Figure 16-6, we are examining structures at the single-cell level.

Generally, there are three rows of outer hair cells near the base of the cochlea with one or two additional rows toward the apex. There are a total of about 3,500 inner hair cells and 12,000 outer hair cells.

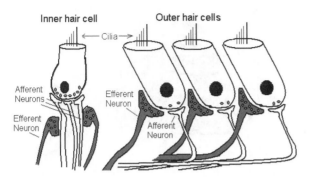

Figure 16–6. Illustration of inner and outer hair cells. Both have cilia on top, and both have afferent (sensory) nerves below. Hair cells differ in shape: the inner hair cell is more bulbous. The outer hair cells are shaped more like a test tube. Also, the location of the efferent (descending) neurons differs on outer and inner hair cells. Efferent neurons connect to outer hair cells directly, but to inner hair cell first-order (first sensory) neurons.

The upper surface of each hair cell contains hairlike projections called **cilia** or **stereocilia** (the terms are synonymous). The cilia on the outer hair cells are attached to the underside of the tectorial membrane. The cilia of the inner hair cells are not embedded in tectorial membrane. **Reticular lamina** covers the top of the hair cells and keeps the endolymph of scala media from coming in direct contact with the hair cells.

The rods of Corti shown in Figure 16-5A come together at the upper surface to form the **tunnel of Corti**, shown in Figure 16-5B. This structure appears to give rigidity to the organ of Corti. The top surface of the rods also becomes a part of the surface of the reticular lamina. Other supporting cells in the vicinity are **Deiter cells** below the outer hair cells, and a group of cells radial to the outer hair cells called the **Hensen's cells**, and more radial still are the **cells of Claudius**. The hair cells and associated structures resting on the basilar membrane are known collectively as the **organ of Corti**—the sense organ of hearing.

Mass and Stiffness Differences Along Basilar Membrane

One final look at Figures 16-3 and 16-4 shows the connective tissue called spiral ligament that connects the basilar membrane to the bony wall of scala media. The cochlea,

from the tip of osseous spiral lamina to the radial wall of the cochlea, then, is spanned by the width of the basilar membrane plus the width of the spiral ligament. As one goes base to apex, the width of the basilar membrane increases whereas the width of the spiral ligament decreases. In fact, the basilar membrane is about 5 times as wide at the apex as at the base of the cochlea. The wider the membrane, the greater its mass, so this increase in width is one of the causes of the increase in mass as the basilar membrane coils toward the apex. Figure 16-7 and Figure 16-3 illustrate the concept of the change in basilar membrane width.

In addition to the **mass gradient** along the basilar membrane, there is also a stiffness gradient. However, the **stiffness gradient** is in the opposite direction from the mass gradient. The basilar membrane is about 100 times stiffer at its base than at its apex. Thus, we have a membrane that has little mass and considerable stiffness at its base, but with progressively more mass and less stiffness going up the cochlea toward the apex.

Review of How the Detailed Features Fit Within the Larger Picture

The earliest figures in this chapter illustrated the larger view of the cochlea. It

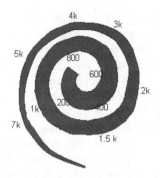

Figure 16–7. A drawing showing that the width of the basilar membrane increases from base to apex to the cochlea and indicating how frequency (in Hz) is distributed along the membrane. As will be discussed in Chapter 17, different regions of the cochlea respond to different frequencies. In actuality, the basilar membrane is about 0.5-mm wide at the apex, and 0.1-mm wide at the base.

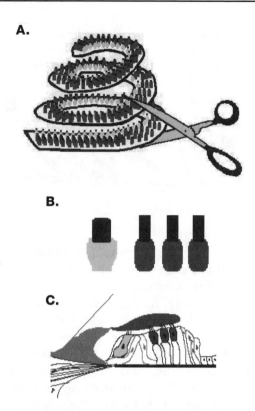

Figure 16–8. A. Sketch of the arrangement of the outer and inner hair cells on the spiraling basilar membrane. Typically, the hair cells are seen in cross-section, as illustrated in cartoon fashion in (**B**) and with the sketch (**C**).

is worthwhile to return to the "big picture" view to ensure that the reader remains comfortable with what is being illustrated in the cross-sections. Figure 16–8A is a cartoon sketch of the basilar membrane, coiling from base to apex. On this "basilar membrane" rests the rows of outer hair cells (in darker gray) and the single inner hair cells (in lighter gray.) In actuality, the hair cells are tightly packed together, rather than standing freely as shown in this figure. Cross-sectioning of Figure 16–8A would result in the features shown in Figure 16–8B which contrasts with the sketch of a cross-section of the cochlea shown in Figure 16–8C. Figures such as Figure 16–4 and 16–5 illustrate the features seen in cross-section, as if the cochlea had been cut to expose its structures.

COCHLEAR BLOOD SUPPLY

The organ of Corti does not have a direct blood supply: there are no capillaries within the structure itself. Oxygen and nutrients reach the organ in two ways. First,

the stria vascularis is richly supplied by a branch of the cochlear artery. This permits oxygen and nutrients to be delivered to the organ of Corti via endolymph.

The second source of arterial blood is by way of a spiral branch of the cochlear artery that runs the length of the cochlea under the basilar membrane. The organ of Corti has a high metabolic rate and a rich supply of oxygen is critical for normal function.

INNERVATION OF THE COCHLEA

The auditory nerve will be further discussed in Chapter 20; however, it is desirable at this point to provide a brief description of the innervation by the sensory receptors, namely, the hair cells. The inner ear is innervated by the VIIIth cranial nerve. Although the VIIIth nerve is sometimes called the "auditory" nerve, there are two major branches of this nerve: the cochlear branch, which innervates the organ of Corti, and the vestibular branch, which innervates the sensory receptors in the vestibular system. Both branches pass through an opening in the temporal bone called the **internal auditory meatus**, which separates the inner ear from the brainstem (see Figure 11–2, white space where the nerves will go). Before reaching the internal auditory meatus, the cochlear nerves pass through the **modiolus,** or center core, of the cochlea. Recall that the nerves enter the osseous spiral lamina by way of small openings called **habenulae perforata** in the bony spiral lamina. Points where nerve cell bodies are bunched together are called ganglia. The **spiral ganglia** of the auditory nerve are illustrated in Figures 16–4B and 16–9.

Figure 16–9 is a sketch of the basilar membrane and afferent (sensory) nerves. This figure illustrates that the nerves exiting the cochlea cluster together so they can exit the habenulae perforata, and that the nerves that come from the apex of the cochlea will

remain toward the inside of the nerve bundle in the modiolus.

Neurons have different parts. The dendrites connect to the hair cell. The cell bodies will cluster together to form the spiral ganglion in the cochlea's modiolus. The axon will send a neural pulse down to the terminal buttons at the very end of the nerve where neurotransmitters will be released. The dendrites of the next neuron will pick up the neurotransmitter and, in turn, cause that next neuron to fire.

The hair cells have both **afferent** and **efferent** innervation. That is, **neurons** (nerve fibers) that carry impulses from the sensory receptors to the brain (afferent), and neurons that carry impulses from the brain to the sensory receptors (efferent) are both present in the cochlea.

SUMMARY

The inner ear is a fluid-filled hole in bone. Within it is a membranous chamber that courses between the vestibular system and the cochlea. A different fluid is within the membranous labyrinth (endolymph) and outside it (perilymph).

The balance system structures are in the vestibule and semicircular canals. The utricle and saccule of the vestibule sense straight-line motion; the semicircular canals tell us when we rotate or tilt our heads.

The cochlea contains inner and outer hair cells that rest on supporting structures on the basilar membrane. The basilar membrane is widest and floppiest at the apical coil; near the oval and round windows at the base it is narrow and stiff.

The organ of Corti includes the hair cells, the supporting arch of Corti, and other supporting cells. The hair cells are covered by reticular lamina, which keeps the endolymph of scala media off the hair cells, which are bathed in perilymph coming from the scala tympani below.

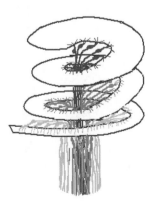

Figure 16–9. Illustration of the arrangement of the afferent neurons from the cochlea.

Both inner and outer hair cells have cilia on top. The outer hair cell stereocilia embed in the gelatinous tectorial membrane; the inner hair cell stereocilia do not.

Both inner and outer hair cells have afferent (ascending) and efferent (descending) neural connections. The nerve cells exit/enter the cochlea via holes in the osseous spiral lamina (habenulae perforata). The sensory nerve cell bodies clump together in spiral ganglia in the modiolus. The nerve fibers then ascend via the internal auditory meatus, and synapse in the brainstem.

17

Advanced Study of the Anatomy of the Cochlea

Chapter 16 discussed the major anatomic features of the cochlea. This chapter provides more detail, focusing on the hair cells, and providing some information on physiology. Most of the "how it works" information will be discussed in Chapter 18.

HAIR CELL HEIGHT AND NUMBER

As described in the previous chapter, the outer hair cells are more numerous than the inner hair cells: three to four (though sometimes as many as five) outer hair cells sit side by side when the basilar membrane spiral is viewed in cross-section. Outer hair cells are on the radial side, that is, located closer to stria vascularis. Inner hair cells are on the other side of the arch of Corti, and are closer to the modiolus.

In total, there are about 12,000 outer hair cells in each cochlea and about 3,500 inner hair cells. The outer hair cells are shaped like a column or test tube. However, not all outer hair cells are identical. The outer hair cells at the apex of the cochlea are taller than those at the base (Figure 17–1). This adds to the mass on the basilar membrane. Recall

that at the apex, basilar membrane is wider, and therefore more massive. The taller hair cells add further to the increased mass of the basilar membrane toward the apex. This mass/stiffness difference will become an important physiologic feature, as you will learn in the next chapter. Whereas the outer hair cells are taller at the apex, inner hair cells stay the same height from base to apex. The inner hair cells are pear-shaped, in contrast to the straighter outer hair cells. In Figure 17–1, individual cells are shown. The nuclei of the hair cells and arch of Corti pillar cells (also called rod cells) can be seen.

STEREOCILIA AND THEIR TIP LINKS AND SIDE LINKS

The terms stereocilia or cilia refer to the tiny hairlike projections that reach through reticular lamina (the covering on top of the cochlea) and into scala media. Figure 17–1 illustrates that the tallest cilia of the outer hair cells embed in the gelatinous tectorial membrane. The cilia on inner hair cells do not embed.

Figure 17–1 also illustrates that stereocilia change height depending on location.

Outer hair cell stereocilia are about 2.5 μm at the base, and 7.2 μm at the apex. (7.2 μm is equal to about 0.0003 inches.) Inner hair cell stereocilia are about 4.2 μm in height at the base of the cochlea, and about 7.2 μm at the apex. Therefore, at the base, the inner hair cell stereocilia are taller than the outer hair cell stereocilia. However, at the apex of the cochlea, the outer and inner hair cell stereocilia are about the same height.

There are more stereocilia on an outer hair cell (about 150) than on an inner hair cell (about 60), and this is due to the way the rows of stereocilia curve. Figure 17–2 illustrates that the rows of inner hair cell stereocilia are in a nearly straight line. The outer hair cell stereocilia, in contrast, form a W shape. Both outer and inner hair cell stereocilia have about three rows on each hair cell and both have the tallest stereocilia toward stria vascularis. We will return to this important anatomic concept when we discuss tip links.

Later, this book will cover the vestibular system hair cells. Vestibular system hair cells have a tall, stiff special cilium, called a kinocilium. Cochlear hair cells don't have kinocilium per se, but do have a rudimentary little bud of a kinocilium, located even more radially than the tallest stereocilium. The kinocilium is rooted directly into the hair cells, whereas the stereocilia are rooted in the **cuticular plate** (Figure 17–3).

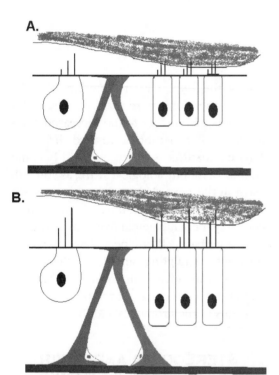

Figure 17–1. Illustration of the differences in hair cells at the base (**A**) and apex (**B**) of the cochlea. Outer hair cells are twice as tall at the apex. Both the outer and inner hair cell cilia are taller toward the apex. Note also that the stereocilia on individual hair cells are tallest radially, that is, toward stria vascularis, which would be on the right-hand side in this figure. This illustration does not include the surrounding, supporting cells. Note that some of the cilia of the outer hair cells are embedded in tectorial membrane.

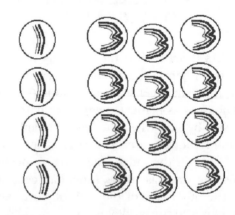

Figure 17–2. Illustration of the hair cells from above. The individual cilia are so close together the rows appear to be lines. The inner hair cells (to the left) have stereocilia that align in nearly straight rows. Outer hair cell stereocilia rows form a W-shaped pattern. Both types of hair cells have the shortest stereocilia (illustrated with the thinnest line) toward the modiolus.

The stereocilia are connected to one another (see Figure 17-3) by **side links,** also called **cross-links,** from the taller cilia to the shorter neighbor. This ensures that if you bend the tallest of the cilia, all of the cilia will bend. Not illustrated is the fact that cilia are connected side to side along one row—that is, between neighboring cilia of the same height. In addition to the side links, cilia have **tip links**. Tip links run from the tip on one cilia to the side of the taller stereocilium next to it.

Inside the stereocilia are **microchannels** that allow the passage of certain ions (chemically charged particles) from the endolymph of scala media into the body of the hair cell. The tip links connect to **insertion plaques** at the opening of the microchannels. The insertion plaques ride on **elastin**, a type of protein filament, so the location of the insertion plaques can be higher or lower. As will be discussed in Chapter 19 on advanced cochlear physiology, movement of the cilia side to side will allow the tip links to control the opening of the insertion plaques. This allows a chemical within the endolymph to come into the microchan-

nels and then enter the hair cell. (You can look ahead to Figure 19-1 for another view.)

SUPPORTING CELLS

Outer hair cells sit on **Deiter cells**. Deiter cells have a projection on them that reaches upward and becomes part of reticular lamina, which forms the protective covering over the surface of the hair cells to prevent endolymph from freely coming in contact with the hair cells (Figure 17-4). These projections or "processes" are called **phalangeal processes of the Deiter cells.** Note that the sides of the outer hair cells do not have any other cells directly in contact with them. In contrast, the inner hair cells are nestled within **inner phalangeal cells**.

CHEMICAL COMPOSITION OF ENDOLYMPH AND PERILYMPH

Endolymph, the fluid within scala media, is high in **potassium**, which has the chemical abbreviation **K+.** The amount of

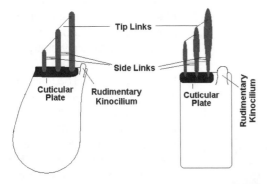

Figure 17–3. Side view of an outer (*left*) and inner (*right*) hair cell. Kinocilium do not rest in the cuticular plate, whereas the rootlets of the stereocilium do. Stereocilia are connected by side links and by tip links.

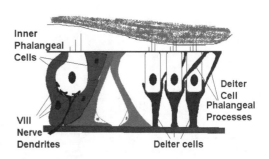

Figure 17–4. Illustration of the supporting cells: the inner phalangeal cells, and the Deiter cells. Additionally, note that the nerve cell dendritic processes are in contact with the hair cells. Here, only the more numerous connections to the inner hair cells are illustrated.

sodium (Na+) in this fluid is relatively low. This relative density of potassium and sodium makes endolymph's chemical composition similar to that of fluids found within many cells. Both potassium and sodium are positively charged ions. (They have fewer electrons than protons, so their charge is positive.) Stria vascularis is the source of endolymph—it is able to secrete this fluid and nourish it with oxygen and other nutrients.

Perilymph has the inverse balance of potassium and sodium. It is high in sodium, and relatively low in potassium. This chemical balance is similar to cerebrospinal fluid (CSF), the fluid that surrounds the brain cavity and the spinal cord. Interestingly, there is a connection between the brain cavity and the inner ear. As will be shown in Chapter 24 (Figure 24-1), there is a small aqueduct, or membrane-lined channel, between the subarachnoid space (the web-filled area inside the cranium between the brain itself and the skull) and the vestibule. The subarachnoid space contains CSF. However, it is thought that the cochlear perilymph probably is produced by spiral ligament, which extends into both scala vestibuli and scala tympani, because the **cochlear aqueduct** is not patent (open) in adults, and the chemistry of CSF and perilymph are not identical.

COMPARATIVE ELECTRICAL CHARGES OF FLUIDS IN THE COCHLEA

Chapter 6 reviewed the concept of "potential difference," the idea that a surplus of electrons has the potential to flow, creating an electrical current. That chapter mentioned that if ion concentrations are different, potentials also occur. This is the case within the cochlea. Different fluids within the cochlea have different concentration of ions, and so they have different electrical charges. Whenever discussing a chemical charge as positive or negative, we have to compare the charge to some standard or reference. For example, if we compare sodium-rich perilymph's charge to water, we would see that potassium is positively charged (Figure 17-5A). That is, water molecules have equal numbers of protons and electrons and do not have any polarity; sodium is more positively charged than water. Endolymph has an even higher concentration of positively charged ions than

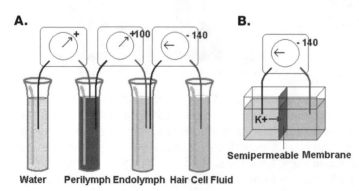

A.

Water   Perilymph Endolymph Hair Cell Fluid

B.

Semipermeable Membrane

Figure 17–5. A. Perilymph has an ionic charge more positive than water. Endolymph is even more positively charged; it has a charge of +100 mV relative to perilymph. The inside of hair cells is negative relative to endolymph, by about 140 mV. **B.** Reticular lamina across the tops of the hair cells is a semipermeable membrane. This semipermeable membrane maintains a potential voltage of 140 mV between the hair cell and the endolymph, with the inside of the hair cell being more negative.

does perilymph. If the endolymph's potential were compared to that of perilymph, we would find that endolymph is about 100 mV more positive than perilymph.

The inside of hair cells is negatively charged relative to endolymph. To a lesser extent, hair cell fluid is negatively charged relative to the perilymph that it is bathed in—basilar membrane does not keep perilymph off the hair cells the way that reticular lamina keeps endolymph separated from the hair cells. It should be noted that some sources state that the fluid bathing the hair cells is not perilymph, but a similar fluid called **cortilymph.**

Reticular lamina, a semipermeable membrane, separates the potassium-rich endolymph from the hair cells. The positively charged ions attempt to pass through this resistive barrier in order to equalize the charge across the membrane. To use the terminology of Chapter 6, there is a -140 mV *potential* for ion flow between the inside of the hair cell and the perilymph above it (Figure 17–5B).

Without sound being present, reticular lamina allows only a little endolymph to reach the hair cells. As will be discussed in Chapter 19, moving the cilia side to side opens the insertion plaques and allows potassium into the microchannel of the cilia, making the hair cell less negatively charged. The amount of side-to-side motion of the cilia determines the width of the opening in the microchannels and, therefore, how much potassium can enter. The analogy will be made that the cilia act as a variable resistor, controlling the ion flow rate.

POTASSIUM INFLUX REGULATES CALCIUM COMING INTO HAIR CELLS

Recall that the inside of the hair cell is negatively charged. Opening microchannels will allow positively charged potassium to enter the hair cell, partially depolarizing the cell. Additionally, calcium (Ca^{++}) enters via the microchannels. The depolarization of the hair cell (the hair cell becoming less negative when potassium and calcium enter) triggers another chemical change within the hair cells. Channels on the side of the hair cell open, allowing calcium to enter the hair cell in this manner as well. As calcium is also positively charged, it further depolarizes the negatively charged inside of the hair cell.

CIRCULATION OF IONS

The body of a hair cell has special channels that allow the hair cell to get rid of excess calcium and potassium. These are called **calcium channels** and **potassium channels.** Potassium channels are also called **potassium pumps.** The calcium, as noted above, comes in the sides of the hair cells. The potassium coming into the cell triggers the opening of the calcium channels. Calcium channels on the sides of the cell also serve to get rid of the excess calcium, which is put back into the perilymph surrounding the cell.

The chemical changes inside the hair cell trigger movement of the chloride molecule that is located in proteins of the outer hair cells. The movement of the chloride molecule is going to trigger a change in the shape of the outer hair cell. This is of great significance to the physiology of hearing, and Chapter 19 will explore this in greater depth.

When potassium is pumped out of the body of the hair cells, these chemicals are transported through the supporting cells back to stria vascularis. **Gap junctions** are small channels between cells that allow these ions to move from cell to cell. The stria vascularis then renourishes the endolymph.

Clinical Correlate: Gap Junctions and Deafness

Gap junctions are important to proper functioning of the cochlea. A defect of the connexin 26 gene disrupts the cycling of potassium through gap junctions, membrane channels that are also called connexin. Depending on the degree to which these gap junctions are abnormal, hearing loss will progress at different rates. Connexin 26-related deafness is recessively inherited (both parents have an affected gene in order for the offspring to potentially have this defect). It is an increasingly common form of deafness. The tendency for deaf persons to marry each other is cited as one reason for the increase in prevalence of this cause of genetic hearing impairment.

NEUROTRANSMITTER RELEASE

Movement of potassium and calcium into hair cells depolarizes the hair cell (makes the charge of the hair cell less negative.) The cell depolarization stimulates the release of **neurotransmitters** from the base of the hair cells. The neurotransmitters are absorbed by the dendrites of the VIII nerve cells and excite the cells, causing them to fire.

SUMMARY

The inside of the hair cell is negatively charged relative to the endolymph above reticular lamina. There are microchannels in the stereocilia of the hair cells that allow some of the potassium from the endolymph to enter the hair cells when the cilia are deflected toward the stria vascularis. This sets off a chemical change in the hair cell. Calcium is also brought into the hair cell, which further reduces the negative polarization of the hair cell. The depolarization of the hair cell triggers the release of neurotransmitters at the base of the cell.

We have seen that inner and outer hair cells have different anatomic features. The outer hair cells are not supported along their sides, and have stereocilia that embed in tectorial membrane. The shapes of the inner and outer hair cells also differ.

18

Introduction to Cochlear Physiology

The physiology of the cochlea is truly amazing. Georg von Bekesy won the 1961 Nobel Prize in Medicine for his discoveries about cochlear mechanics. In the last several decades much more has been discovered about cochlear physiology and our knowledge continues to grow. In this chapter, the reader is guided through the different steps from fluid motion, created by the vibration of stapes footplate, to the generation of a neural impulse. We begin with a brief review of the major anatomic points that relate to physiology.

ARRANGEMENT OF THE CILIA RELATIVE TO TECTORIAL MEMBRANE

Recall that both the outer and the inner hair cells are on top of basilar membrane (with supporting cells beneath them). Both types of hair cells have cilia, but only the cilia of the outer hair cells embed in the gelatinous layer above: the tectorial membrane. The cilia of the inner hair cells reach toward, but don't actually touch, tectorial membrane. Also, please note that tectorial membrane is attached at the spiral limbus

rather firmly. Figure 18–1A schematically illustrates.

You will soon read about how the basilar membrane moves up and down in response to sound. At this point, let's focus on what happens to the hair cell cilia when this up and down vibration of basilar membrane occurs. When basilar membrane is moved upward or downward, the cilia on the hair cells will bend sideways, which is termed **shearing of the cilia**. Figures 18–1B and 18-1C illustrate this process. A deflection of basilar membrane downward creates a movement of the cilia sideways, specifically, toward the modiolus. That is, if you look at the angle of the cilia relative to the reticular lamina on top of the hair cells, the cilia are deflected sideways, toward the central core of the cochlea. When basilar membrane moves upward, the cilia shear in the other direction—toward stria vascularis.

You can demonstrate this shearing to yourself by placing rubber bands around a binder. Place the rubber bands across the binder running up and down. Hold the binder with one hand on the spine, and the other hand on the edge, with the binder partially opened with that hand. Watch the apparent side-to-side motion of the rubber

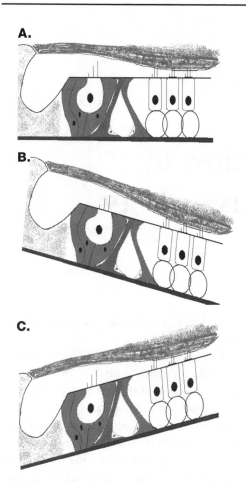

Figure 18–1. A. Illustration of the relative position of the structures of the organ of Corti in the absence of sound. **B**. When basilar membrane moves down, the cilia on the hair cells are deflected toward the modiolus. **C**. Movement upward creates a ciliary deflection toward the stria vascularis.

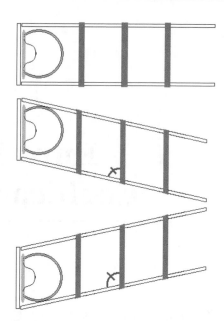

Figure 18–2. The side-to-side shearing of the hair cell cilia occurs in a way that can be visualized if you put rubber bands across a binder, and flex the open end up and down.

bands as you move the edge of the binder up and down, as illustrated in Figure 18-2. Note that the angle of the rubber bands, relative to the binder's lower edge, changes.

MASS/STIFFNESS GRADIENT OF THE BASILAR MEMBRANE

The next anatomic relationship to review is the relative width of the basilar membrane as it winds around from base to apex. Although the outside shell of the basilar membrane is widest at the base (look back at Figure 16-3), the basilar membrane is actually widest at the apex. At the base, the osseous spiral lamina and spiral ligament will span a larger distance than at the apex. The relative size arrangement is shown schematically in Figure 18-3, which shows the cochlea as if it were uncoiled. Figure 16-7 also illustrated the change in basilar membrane width.

Because basilar membrane is wider at the apex, it is more massive. At the base, the narrow basilar membrane is also stiffer. The basilar membrane is progressively floppier as it coils upward to the apex. The progressive, gradual change in mass and stiffness of basilar membrane is termed the **mass/stiffness gradient.**

The change in mass and stiffness will affect how well any one location on the basilar membrane vibrates. Just as heavy objects, like a larger tuning fork, vibrate at lower frequencies (Figure 18–4); the wide, heavier apical basilar membrane will vibrate best to low frequencies. As described in Chapter 5, if mass remains the same, adding stiffness increases the resonant frequency. You can demonstrate this to yourself by taking a rubber band and plucking it as you stretch the band tighter and tighter.

If the cochlear fluids are vibrating slowly, in response to low-frequency stimulation, then the heavy, floppy apical end of the basilar membrane would be free to vibrate. Conversely, if the sound is high frequency, then the vibration will take place at the light, stiff base. Before describing exactly how the wave is propagated to these specific places on the basilar membrane, we review the sections of the cochlea.

REVIEW OF DIVISIONS AND MEMBRANES WITHIN THE COCHLEA

As was discussed in Chapter 16, the cochlea is divided into three compartments, with Reissner's membrane and basilar membrane serving as the dividers. As shown schematically in Figure 18-5, the oval window is continuous with the upper chamber,

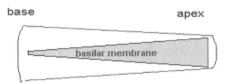

Figure 18–3. Illustration of the relative size of the cochlea shell and basilar membrane. Here, the cochlea is shown as if it were uncoiled and lying flat.

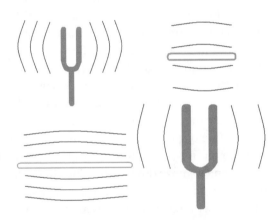

Figure 18–4. Illustration of the fact that the lighter tuning fork and the stretched-tight rubber band vibrate at higher frequencies.

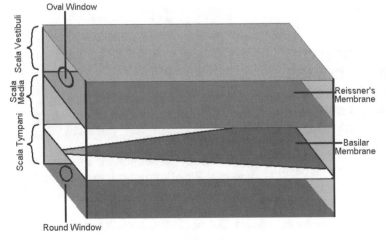

Figure 18–5. Schematic illustration of the uncoiled cochlea, showing that the cochlea is divided into three chambers (scala). Oval window is in scala vestibuli, round window is in scala tympani. Basilar membrane changes its width as it goes from base to apex.

scala vestibuli. Round window "looks out" toward the tympanic membrane from scala tympani.

Basilar membrane increases its size as it extends from base to apex. (Osseous spiral lamina and spiral ligament take up the rest of the side-to-side area so that the endolymph remains in scala media.)

When stapes footplate moves inward toward scala vestibuli, the fluid in the cochlea must move, because the cochlear fluids can't be compressed. The only opening to relieve the pressure is at the round window. There are two membranes between round and oval windows: Reissner's and basilar. Reissner's membrane is easy to deflect downward. It is not particularly massive, nor particularly stiff, and it does not change its mass or stiffness as it coils from base to apex. Therefore, Reissner's membrane can be deflected along any location in the cochlea. When Reissner's membrane moves, for example, downward when the stapes footplate moves inward, the largely incompressible fluid of scala media must be displaced. The movement of the endolymph in scala media will cause basilar membrane to move downward. This, in turn, will move the perilymph of scala tympani, and cause a budging of round window. When stapes footplate moves outward, during the rarefaction phase of the sound, Reissner's and basilar membranes will move up, and round window would be sucked inward.

THE IN-AND-OUT MOTION OF STAPES FOOTPLATE BECOMES AN UP-AND-DOWN MOTION OF BASILAR MEMBRANE, CALLED THE TRAVELING WAVE

von Bekesy described the fact that basilar membrane does not move up and down equally at all locations. It will only deflect optimally in one location, and that location is dependent on how fast stapes footplate moves inward and outward. Figure 18–6A illustrates that, rather than pushing all of basilar membrane downward, a specific area of the membrane will deflect as the stapes footplate moves in, and when stapes footplate moves outward, the opposite deflection occurs (Figure 18–6B). Figures 18–6A and 18–6B illustrate two snapshots in time. If the basilar membrane is observed as the footplate oscillates in and out, a wavelike motion, that appears to travel up the basilar membrane, can be viewed.

Figures 18–6A and 18-6B are inaccurate in one important aspect. They show the entire width of basilar membrane deflecting. In actuality, one side of the membrane is held in place firmly at spiral ligament, and the opposite edge is held at osseous spiral lamina; therefore, these outer edges are not free to move. The classic figure by Dallos (1988)

A.

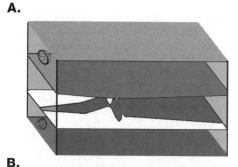

B.

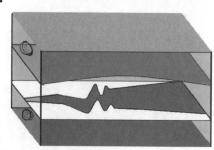

Figure 18–6. Deflection of basilar membrane in a wavelike motion with stapes footplate moving inward (**A**) and outward (**B**). Reissner's membrane also deflects up and down, but not in the wavelike motion.

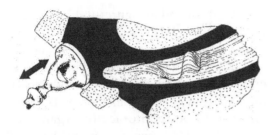

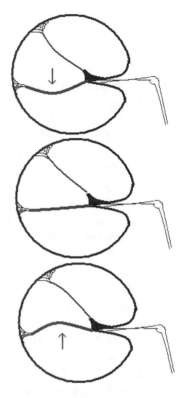

Figure 18–7. From Dallos (1988), an illustration of the motion of basilar membrane in response to stapes footplate vibration. Note that the edges of basilar membrane near osseous spiral lamina and spiral ligament do not vibrate as much as the center-most part. Dallos, P. Cochlear Neurobiology, June/July 1988, *ASHA*. Reprinted with permission.

(Figure 18-7) more properly illustrates the wavelike motion of basilar membrane.

The figures shown above represent the cochlea as viewed from the side. Figure 18–8 provides a different view, from a cross-section of the cochlea. Assume that this cross-section is from a point at or near where the greatest vibration of basilar membrane occurs. Note that the middle part of the basilar membrane is vibrating more than the edges. The outer hair cells are located near this point of maximum motion.

THE LOCATION OF THE MAXIMUM PLACE OF MOVEMENT ON BASILAR MEMBRANE IS DETERMINED BY THE SOUND FREQUENCY

If the stapes footplate is moving in and out rapidly (as occurs when hearing high-frequency sounds), then basilar membrane is going to deflect readily at the base of the cochlea. At the base of the cochlea, basilar membrane is relatively stiff and light. Just as a light tuning fork vibrates at high frequencies, the light, stiff end of basilar membrane will move best with high frequencies. If the

Figure 18–8. Illustration of the movement of the cochlear membranes as sound is present at the ear. This figure illustrates a single coil of the cochlea at three moments in time. Note that this is a drawing of a cross-section of the cochlea on the left-hand side. The mirror image, flipped left to right, has been shown in most of the other figures in this text. At the top, we see the movement of the membranes as they would occur when stapes footplate moves inward. In the middle, the basilar membrane is back at its position of rest, as occurs when the stapes footplate is midway through its cycle and is even with the oval window. When the stapes footplate moves away from the cochlea, toward the middle ear, the basilar membrane deflects upward, as shown in the bottom figure. Note that the maximum movement of the membrane is at the center point, as was also noted in Figure 18-7.

sound frequency is lower, then the stiffness of the basal coil of the basilar membrane limits its vibration. An area farther up on basilar membrane will move best. For example, a 1000-Hz tone will create the greatest up-and-down movement of basilar membrane at a middle point up the cochlea. The area of basilar membrane just a little bit higher up will not vibrate well at all. The mass of the basilar membrane at this slightly more apical area is not matched to the 1000-Hz vibration frequency, and so the mass dampens the motion very readily. If the frequency is lower, for example, 200 Hz, then some wave motion will still be seen at the middle of the cochlea, but the maximum motion will occur farther up the cochlea, toward the apex (where the basilar membrane is massive and floppy).

Nobel laureate Georg von Bekesy described the motion pattern of the basilar membrane. He observed that the basilar membrane appears to move in waves, as would occur if you attached one end of a bed sheet to a wall, pulled the sheet out away from the wall until it was hanging loosely, then whipped the end you are holding up and down. That wave would travel down the entire length of the bed sheet, although, of course, the movement of any one cotton thread is up and down. The wave in the bed sheet will travel the full length because the sheet has no change in mass or stiffness. The cochlea's **traveling wave** appears to grow as the wave moves apically, then diminishes very quickly and won't vibrate the basilar membrane farther up (that is, more toward the apex and away from the point of maximum up and down displacement) because of the **mass/stiffness gradient** of basilar membrane.

The louder the sound is, the more displacement up and down occurs in the traveling wave. A soft sound creates a small ripple, a loud sound a larger (taller) amplitude wave.

If the basilar membrane were viewed in time-lapsed photography, one would see a blur of motion on basilar membrane in a defined area. This area is called the **envelope of the traveling wave.** Figure 18–9 illustrates this.

As illustrated in Figure 18–10, different frequency sounds create different locations of the traveling wave peak. Low-frequency sounds create the maximum vibration closer to the apex; high-frequency sounds closer to the base. The basilar membrane is therefore said to be **tonotopically organized**; that is, there is a different anatomic location for encoding different frequency sounds.

THE HEIGHT OF THE TRAVELING WAVE ENVELOPE IS RELATED TO SOUND INTENSITY

If the sound is loud, the stapes footplate vibrates in and out a farther distance. This will create a larger displacement of basilar

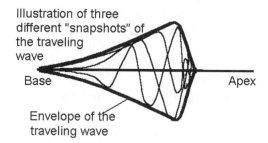

Illustration of three different "snapshots" of the traveling wave

Base   Apex

Envelope of the traveling wave

Figure 18–9. The basilar membrane continues to move up and down in a wavelike pattern as the stimulus continues. The motion is always within a defined area, called the envelope of the traveling wave, if the sound remains at the same frequency and intensity.

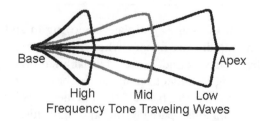

Base   Apex

High   Mid   Low
Frequency Tone Traveling Waves

Figure 18–10. Traveling wave envelopes for low-frequency, mid-frequency, and high-frequency sounds.

membrane. As illustrated in Figure 18–11, the height of the traveling wave reflects the intensity of the sound.

CILIARY SHEARING

Returning to the Concept That the Up-and-Down Basilar Membrane Motion Creates Side-to-Side Shearing of the Hair Cell Cilia

As was shown in Figure 18–1, when the basilar membrane moves up and down, the cilia of the outer hair cells move side to side, that is, toward and away from stria vascularis. The attachment of the cilia in tectorial membrane creates this **shearing**, or sideways motion. As the fluid in scala media moves with the up-and-down motion of basilar membrane, currents are created in the space between the reticular lamina (covering above the hair cells) and the tectorial membrane (this area is also called the subtectorial space). This fluid motion allows the cilia of the inner hair cells to move, so they too will shear sideways in synchrony with the up and down motion of basilar membrane. However, if we were observing the cochlea of a dead mammal, we would see that the currents in the subtectorial space

would not be enough to shear the cilia of the inner hair cells if the basilar membrane up-and-down movement is slight, as it is for soft sounds. In this case, the fluid movement in the space below tectorial membrane is only sufficient to shear the inner hair cell cilia if the sound is about 50 or 60 dB SPL or louder.

Shearing of Cilia Opens Microchannels in the Cilia and Creates Chemical Changes in the Hair Cell Body

Microchannels, tiny channels in the cilia, open when the cilia move side to side in the direction toward stria vascularis (Figure 18–12). These channels allow potassium (K^+) and calcium (Ca^{++}), positively charged ions, to go from the endolymph into the body of the hair cell. The inside of the hair cell itself is negatively charged, so these positively charged ions make the hair cell less

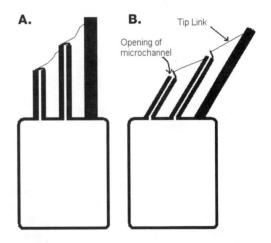

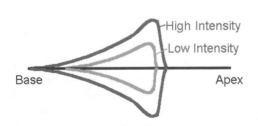

Figure 18–11. Illustration of the traveling wave occurring in response to a low-intensity (mid-frequency) sound and the traveling wave for the same frequency sound, at a higher intensity.

Figure 18–12. The tip link that runs from the top of one cilia to the side of the adjacent, taller cilia, is thought to open a microchannel in the cilia. Here, the opening is greatly exaggerated, as if a trap door were being pulled open.

negative. The hair cell is **depolarized**. This chemical change in the hair cell triggers another change. Special channels in the side of the hair cells open, allowing more calcium to enter the hair cells. This creates even greater depolarization of the hair cell which creates two effects. First, it will allow the hair cell to release a **neurotransmitter**, a chemical that will cause the neurons to fire.

Outer hair cells have an additional change that takes place when potassium and calcium enter the hair cell—the cell itself changes its shape. The hair cell shrinks and becomes fatter as the cilia move toward stria vascularis (as potassium enters the cell), and then the outer hair cells become taller and thinner when the cilia move the opposite direction, toward the modiolus. This tall/thin change in the shape of the cell body happens when the outer hair cell body is pumping out the potassium and calcium, which occurs at the time when the cilia shear toward the modiolus, firmly shutting the opening in the cilia. (These pumps are on the sides of the hair cells.) The motion of the outer hair cells, becoming tall-

er and shorter in response to the rarefaction and compression cycles of the sound wave, is called the **active mechanism of the outer hair cells**. Also related to this concept, you will hear that outer hair cells are **motile.** There is no active mechanism for the inner hair cells.

THE ACTIVE MECHANISM ENHANCES THE MOTION OF THE INNER HAIR CELL CILIA

The outer hair cell cilia are embedded in tectorial membrane, whereas the inner hair cell cilia are not. When basilar membrane moves, tectorial membrane will move with it, because of the attachment of the outer hair cell cilia to tectorial membrane. When the outer hair cells contract, shortening, and then grow taller, this accentuates the motion of tectorial membrane. (An analogy is provided in Figure 18–13). Because the motion of tectorial membrane relative to basilar membrane is increased by the shortening of the outer hair cells, there is more fluid flow

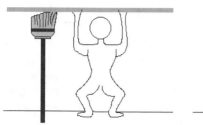
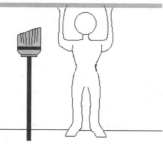

Figure 18–13. An analogy of what happens when the outer hair cells contract and lengthen. When the person holding a board above head level squats, the board hits the broom straws and causes them to deflect. Similarly, when the outer hair cells (which indirectly rest on basilar membrane and have their cilia embedded in tectorial membrane) shorten, then tectorial membrane is pulled downward. The tectorial membrane can then deflect the cilia of the inner hair cells.

in the subtectorial space and therefore the inner hair cells' cilia will be deflected, even if the sound is low intensity. If the active mechanism of the outer hair cells creates enough motion, then the inner hair cell cilia may even touch tectorial membrane and be mechanically deflected. When the motion of basilar membrane is extreme, as it is for loud sounds, then the up-and-down motion of the basilar membrane will be sufficient to deflect the cilia of the inner hair cells, even if there isn't an active mechanism. With loud sound, the inner hair cell cilia either directly contact the tectorial membrane or move because the fluid flow in the space above the inner hair cells shears the cilia. The importance of the active mechanism is that it creates movement of the inner hair cell cilia when low-intensity sound is present at the ear. Without the active mechanism, the person would not hear low-intensity sound, but would still detect moderate and loud intensity sound.

In Figure 18–13, the illustration suggests that only tectorial membrane is moved by the active mechanism; however, basilar membrane also moves. Basilar membrane would be pulled upward when tectorial membrane is pulled downward because basilar membrane is not like a rigid floor, it is able to deflect. Increasing the motion of basilar membrane's vibration has the net effect of increasing the amplitude of the traveling wave. However, this increase in amplitude attributable to the active mechanism occurs only at the peak of the traveling wave, not all along the traveling wave. Figure 18–14 illustrates this.

HEARING REQUIRES INNER HAIR CELL STIMULATION

Because 95% of the sensory (afferent) neurons are connected to inner hair cells, we presume that they are primarily the ones responsible for encoding sound. The active mechanism of the outer hair cells allows for the enhancement of the inner hair cell ciliary shearing so that even soft sounds create sufficient movement of inner hair cell cilia to allow the channels in the inner hair cell cilia to open. When potassium enters the inner hair cells, chemical changes in the inner hair cell create a release of neurotransmitter at the bottom of the inner hair cell. Again, inner hair cells do not have an active mechanism.

SUMMARY

In review, this chapter has described that the basilar membrane moves up and down in response to sound. The size of the up-and-down wave that appears to travel up the basilar membrane depends on the intensity of the sound. The location of the peak of the traveling wave is determined by the frequency of the sound; low-frequency sounds cause more apical peaks of the traveling wave. When basilar membrane moves up and down, the cilia will move side to side, called shearing. The shearing of the cilia of the outer hair cells starts a chemical chain reaction inside the outer hair cell that makes the outer hair cell shrink and stretch as the sound wave cycles through compression and

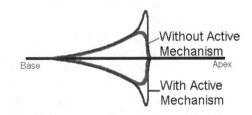

Figure 18–14. The active mechanism of the outer hair cells increases the amplitude of the traveling wave near the traveling wave peak because it increases the movement of basilar membrane.

rarefaction phases of vibration. This active mechanism creates an enhancement of the motion of basilar membrane relative to tectorial membrane, which enhances the flow of the fluid surrounding the inner hair cell cilia. Said another way, hearing soft sounds is made possible because of the active mechanism of the outer hair cells—the inner hair cell cilia will shear farther because of the ac-

tive mechanism. However, the active mechanism does not cause a net increase in basilar membrane vibration when the sound intensity is loud. Figure 18-15 reviews this graphically.

Figure 18-16 provides another view of how the movement of the cilia of the inner

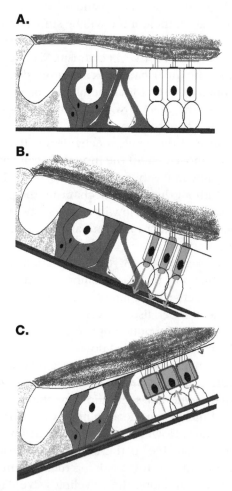

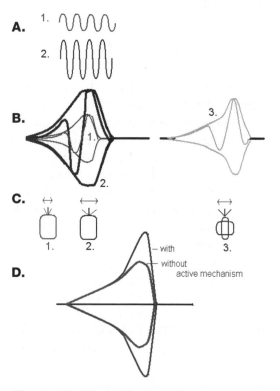

Figure 18–15. A. The same frequency pure tone at a low *(1)* and high *(2)* intensity. **B.** The traveling wave peak grows taller as the sound increases from low intensity *(1)* to high intensity *(2)*. The traveling wave peaks more apically when the frequency is lower *(3)*. **C.** The cilia will shear more for a loud sound *(2)* than a soft sound *(1)*. The active mechanism enhances the amount of side-to-side ciliary shearing for low-intensity sounds. **D.** The active mechanism creates greater amplitude basilar membrane movement and a higher peak to the traveling wave.

Figure 18–16. Relative to the position of rest **(A)**, basilar membrane is moved downward (and reticular lamina upward) when the outer hair cells elongate **(B)**. When the outer hair cells shrink, becoming fatter when the cilia shear toward stria vascularis, basilar membrane moves upward and reticular lamina downward **(C)**. Note that the cilia of the inner hair cells would physically deflect because of the proximity of reticular lamina.

hair cells is enhanced because of the active mechanism of the outer hair cells. Inner hair cell stimulation is critical because the vast majority of the afferent neurons are connected to the inner hair cells.

REFERENCE

Dallos, P. (1988, June/July). Cochlear neurobiology: Revolutionary developments. *ASHA*, pp. 50-56.

19

More Hair Cell Physiology

This chapter provides an overview of the fascinating mechanics of hair cells. It is awe inspiring to realize what we understand about the features of these single cells; however, some of what is reported in this chapter is still speculative.

CALCIUM CHANNELS, POTASSIUM PUMPS, AND THE ACTIVE MECHANISM

Review of Cellular Chemistry Changes

In Chapters 17 and 18 you read about the process by which positively charged ions enter the hair cells. To review, the movement of the stereocilia toward stria vascularis causes a stretching of the tip links, which opens microchannels in the stereocilia. These channels are sometimes called **transduction pores**. As illustrated in Figure 19–1, this allows potassium to enter. Calcium is also entering via the cilia. When these two positively charged chemicals enter the negatively charged hair cell, the hair cell is depolarized. The **depolarization** opens calcium channels in the sides of the hair cells, in

a region called the **basolateral surface** (toward the base of the hair cells, on their lateral surface). This allows more calcium to enter the hair cell, further depolarizing it.

There are channels that function to remove the excess calcium and potassium.

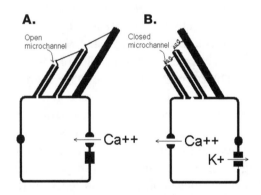

Figure 19–1. A. During depolarization, as the cilia shear toward stria vascularis, the negatively charged hair cell depolarizes as the positively charged ions enter. Calcium channels on the basolateral surface open, further depolarizing the cell. **B**. During the phase of sound that causes the shearing of the stereocilia toward the modiolus, the calcium channels are extruding calcium, and the potassium pumps are removing potassium; the hair cell is hyperpolarizing (becoming even more negative with the removal of the positively charged ions).

They are also located on the basolateral surface of the hair cell membrane. A channel that removes potassium is called a **potassium pump**. When the cilia shear toward the modiolus, the transduction pores close and little potassium is able to enter the hair cell. During this time the potassium pumps effectively repolarize the hair cell. The calcium channels on the basolateral surfaces simultaneously work to remove calcium from the inside of the hair cells, which also repolarizes the hair cell to its negative state. Another term to describe the increasingly negative charge during this phase of cilia vibration is **hyperpolarization**—the hair cell is becoming even more negatively charged than it would be in a resting state.

Prestin Protein Contraction Creates the Active Mechanism

Recall that the active mechanism causes outer hair cells to elongate and contract. A protein is located in the surface of the outer hair cells that is responsible for the hair cells ability to change shape. The changes in polarization of the outer hair cells trigger the stretching/contracting of this protein. A chloride molecule changes its position within the protein, which is thought to trigger the protein molecules shape change. However, these contractile proteins on the cell membranes are not always triggered. For the proteins to create this stretch/contract, the influx/outflow of potassium and calcium must be at the proper rate for that hair cell. For example, a hair cell located at the place where the 1000-Hz traveling wave peaks will contract and elongate 1000 times per second if there is a 1000-Hz tone present. However, if the basilar membrane were being moved by a 300-Hz tone, peaking farther up basilar membrane, then we do not see the contraction/elongation.

The name of the protein found in the outer hair cells that permits the active mechanism is **prestin.** (Some books capitalize Prestin.) The name is based on the musical term, presto, meaning a rapid tempo. The rates of contraction are very rapid compared to that normally seen in proteins that create muscle movement, as the contraction occurs at the rate of the sound frequency, which can be up to 20,000 Hz in the human ear.

Let's elaborate on the idea that outer hair cells' active mechanisms are "tuned" to respond only to a certain frequency range. A normal outer hair cell has the ability to be motile in response to a limited range of stimulus frequencies. For example, a hair cell located at the 2000-Hz "place" on the basilar membrane can readily contract/elongate 2000 times per second. It would be able to contract/elongate at similar rates, too, for example, 1900 Hz. If the cilia were sheared by an 800-Hz tone, the prestin would not contract. The 2000-Hz hair cell would not be "active" in response to that frequency. Of course, a hair cell located farther up the cochlea, at the place where 800 Hz is encoded, would contract in response to the 800 Hz stimulation.

OTOACOUSTIC EMISSIONS ARE SOUNDS THAT COME FROM THE COCHLEA AS A RESULT OF THE ACTIVE MECHANISM OF THE OUTER HAIR CELLS

When the active mechanism occurs, fluid motion is enhanced. The contraction of the outer hair cells pulls basilar membrane up and tectorial membrane down; the subsequent elongation forces those two membranes farther apart. Remember that fluids are not compressible, so if the fluid moves, there has to be a change in the position of oval and round window. When the basilar membrane/tectorial membrane and Reissner's membranes are moved additionally because of the active mechanism of the outer hair cells, it is going to create another pressure wave in the cochlear fluids. This pressure wave will be propagated back outward—that is, out toward the stapes footplate. This movement is not at the exact same time as the start of the sound entering the cochlea. It takes several milliseconds for the sound wave to travel to its peak place and trigger the active mechanism.

Because sound is traveling outward from the cochlea, the ossicles will vibrate in reverse direction, creating a movement of the tympanic membrane. The impedance matching transformer now works in reverse, allowing the energy to efficiently go from the high-impedance cochlea to the low-impedance air of the outer ear. A sound is therefore present in the outer ear, which is termed an **otoacoustic emission.** Otoacoustic emissions are low-intensity sounds that are found in the outer ear canal as a result of the active mechanism of the outer hair cells. They are a byproduct of the healthy inner ear, and will be absent if there is damage to the outer hair cells. Otoacoustic emissions testing is used clinically in order to evaluate the health of the outer hair cells, and can be used in screening for hearing loss, because almost all types of hearing loss create damage to the outer hair cells.

There are various types of otoacoustic emissions (OAEs). OAEs can be categorized as **evoked** or **spontaneous otoacoustic emissions.** Evoked otoacoustic emissions are measured in response to a sound being placed into the ear canal. We can further differentiate the types of evoked otoacoustic emissions as distortion-product OAEs or transient (click-evoked) OAEs. **Transient evoked OAEs** are elicited by brief sound pulses. If the ear is healthy, after a time delay, an emission (sound transmitted outward from the cochlea to the outer ear) will be present in the ear canal. The time delay results from the time required for the sound to travel to the place of stimulation on the basilar membrane and then be transmitted back to the outer ear. **Distortion-product OAEs** are created when two continuous pure tones are presented together to the ear. The ear creates otoacoustic emissions at these same two frequencies, but these emissions can't be measured because the tones evoking the emission are still present and at the same frequency as the emission. You would not be able to tell if the sound measured is the one being produced or emitted. However, the ear also creates otoacoustic emissions at frequencies other than just the stimulus frequencies, because the normal ear creates some distortion of the sounds. We measure the presence of the emission at one of these distortion frequencies. The most commonly measured distortion frequency is the **cubic difference tone** frequency, which is calculated as the frequency that is two times the lower frequency, minus the higher frequency. For example, if the stimulus frequencies were 1000 Hz and 1212 Hz, the distortion product would be at 788 Hz (2000 Hz – 1212 Hz).

In addition to evoked otoacoustic emissions, another class of otoacoustic emission is the **spontaneous** OAE. For over half of normal hearers, a region or regions of outer hair cells is/are contracting and elongating, even without sound being present. The person doesn't typically perceive the spontaneous OAE, as the brain learns to tune out the neural activity coming from the spontaneous OAE. As not all normal hearers have spontaneous OAEs, there is limited clinical use for testing of this type of response.

TIP LINKS AND INSERTION PLAQUES

Both outer and inner hair cells have tip links, which open the microchannels or mi-

Clinical Correlate: Use of Otoacoustic Emissions Testing in Neonatal Testing

Transient and distortion product otoacoustic emission testing is commonplace in audiology. This technology is used by some hospitals to screen the hearing of newborn infants. A limitation to this application is that neonates often have debris in the outer ear, and can have some fluid in their middle ears. Either of these problems could prevent the measurement of the otoacoustic emission in the normal hearing neonate, especially if the infant is recently born.

Otoacoustic emissions are also used within the diagnostic audiology clinic. The sounds that produce the otoacoustic emission have been set to intensity levels that help to distinguish between normal and not-normal outer hair cell function. Said another way, the signal intensities are low enough that with even minor hair cell damage, the otoacoustic emission should be absent. This allows OAEs to be used as a screening test for cochlear damage. Even mild cochlear hearing loss (damage to the active mechanism) is detected.

Although the otoacoustic emission is not detected using clinical OAE tests in an ear with mild cochlear damage, the ear with mild hearing loss may still have some hair cells with a functioning active mechanism. Once hearing loss exceeds about 50 dB HL, the active mechanism is entirely absent. If the loss is less than 50 dB HL, if the signal intensities were increased, you might then be able to measure the otoacoustic emission. Testing to try to find out when the OAE is first present has not been very helpful. It doesn't let us predict how much cochlear loss is present with any real accuracy. The screening version of the testing is the most powerful use. Even a mild (e.g., 20 to 30 dB hearing loss) typically will cause the test to be abnormal. The screening test, though, does not let you know the extent of loss: the screening test typically shows an absent otoacoustic emission as soon as there is even relatively mild damage to the active mechanism.

Hearing loss up to 50 dB HL is associated with damage to outer hair cells and the loss of the active mechanism. When inner hair cells also are damaged, then the loss becomes greater than 50 dB HL. As otoacoustic emissions testing measures the outer hair cell active mechanism only, OAE testing will not tell the audiologist about the inner hair cell damage, and therefore does not tell the audiologist if the loss is mild or profound.

OAE testing is considered "frequency specific." A pair of distortion product tones stimulates a given region of the basilar membrane, so the cochlear function can be examined frequency by frequency. The transient (click) signal stimulates the entire basilar membrane, but the response coming from different regions of the cochlea have different characteristics. The response coming from the apex of the cochlea has a greater delay in being emitted due to the longer traveling wave time. The response from the apex of the cochlea also is a different frequency emission than a response coming from the base of the cochlea. Both distortion product and transient otoacoustic hearing screening tests are able to differentiate which regions of the cochlea are normal and which are abnormal.

Otoacoustic emissions testing does not reveal hearing loss coming from nerve pathway problems. A child who has **auditory neuropathy** might have no connection between the hair cell and the auditory nerve, or might have damage at one of the auditory nerve centers. This child would have normal otoacoustic emissions and would not be identified as hearing-impaired using just otoacoustic emissions testing.

cropores on the cilia. The site where the transduction pores are located on the cilia—the location of the insertion plaque—moves up and down on the cilia. These insertion plaques may rest on little filaments. It is theorized that they move up and down under the control of a protein called myosin I. As illustrated in Figure 19–2, movement of the insertion plaques would have the effect of allowing either more or less potassium to enter the cells.

Calcium is probably the substance that triggers the movement of these insertion plaques. If the hair cell does not fully repolarize, because sound is present, and the hair cell calcium channels on the basolateral surface of the hair cell bodies are not able to fully return the hair cell to its normal state, there is an excess of calcium. In the presence of this calcium within the hair cell, the insertion plaque will slowly slip downward. This downward motion makes the channels open less wide (Figure 19–2C). When the

sound is no longer present, and calcium is fully pumped out of the cell, the insertion plaque is moved upward by the myosin I protein. This allows the transduction pore to open wider, letting in more potassium. The hair cell is more sensitive as a result.

Figure 19–2 is a gross exaggeration of the location and movement of the insertion plaques. The true anatomic location is very close to the tip of the stereocilia, and the amount of movement up and down is not large.

The movement of the insertion plaques up and down does not occur as fast as the contraction of the hair cell bodies. The **adaptation motor** is a slower form of motion, which is thought to keep the tension on the tip links at the ideal level. When the sound is quiet, the adaptation motor allows the hair cell to be more sensitive because the transduction pores can open wider. When sound is loud, the transduction pores open less. Potentially, this mechanism could control the

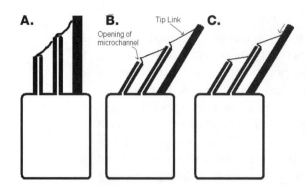

A.

B. Tip Link

Opening of microchannel

C.

Figure 19–2. The position of the insertion plaque controls the amount of opening of the micropores. In this illustration, moving the insertion plaque upward creates a greater opening of the micropores (**B**) than when the insertion plaque is moved downward (**C**).

Clinical Correlate: Temporary Threshold Shift

Persons who are exposed to loud sound may experience a temporary loss of hearing sensitivity, called a **temporary threshold shift**. There are many mechanisms that may explain the phenomenon. Breakage of the tip links is just one. Loud sounds create an influx of the salt potassium, and with it, calcium. The calcium channels and potassium pumps cannot remove these chemicals fast enough to fully repolarize the hair cell, and the hair cells will swell. The active mechanism will not work properly in a swollen hair cell. Other changes take place as a result of loud sound. As noted above, the tip links may break, temporarily stopping cell function. Additionally, cilia can be fused and damaged—a physiologic change that is considered permanent, yet the ear is able to retain function, though not at the level previously enjoyed. Further noise exposure can rupture the cell membrane, killing hair cells, creating a **permanent threshold shift**, also called a **noise-induced hearing loss**. Depending on the type of noise, whether it is steady-state or very sudden (impact or impulse noise), the type of damage in the cochlea differs. Longer duration noises destroy outer hair cells, and with it, the active mechanism. Very loud impulse noise can mechanically damage inner hair cells as well as outer hair cells.

amount of the active mechanism of the outer hair cell, and thereby indirectly control the amount of neurotransmitter released from inner hair cells. When sound exposure is loud, if there is depolarization of the hair cells, and not enough time to fully repolarize the cells, the insertion plaques move downward, which will minimize further depolarization.

Tip links are evidently fragile. Exposure to loud sounds can break these very thin filaments. Some research is suggesting that they repair themselves within about 12 hours. Rupture of the tip link might help to preserve hearing by preventing microchannel opening, limiting the amount of potassium that enters the hair cells.

SUMMARY

The active mechanism of the outer hair cells appears to be triggered by the depolarization of the outer hair cells. Hair cells are "tuned" to have a contractile response if the rate at which calcium is coming into, and being pumped out of, the cell is at about the right rate for that hair cell. A hair cell stimulated at a frequency that is significantly different from what the hair cell is tuned to respond to will not trigger the active mechanism.

The active mechanism response is measured via otoacoustic emissions testing. This technique is a good screening tool of cochlear function. It can usually detect even mild cochlear damage, and is frequency specific: it identifies which areas of the cochlea are and are not normal.

The normal active mechanism, and therefore the sensitivity of the inner hair cell, is somewhat self-regulating. The location of the insertion plaques can move up and down. This changes how much potassium can enter the transduction pores. When the hair cells are stimulated by loud sounds, the insertion plaques move down the cilia, creating less stimulation from the same sound.

20

Overview of Cochlear Potentials and the Auditory Nervous System

The side-to-side shearing of the cilia of the hair cells changes the internal chemistry of the hair cells. We can measure and record the electrochemical changes. This chapter introduces two potentials that arise from the hair cells: the cochlear microphonic and the summating potential.

This chapter also examines how the hair cell changes lead to release of **neurotransmitters** at the base of the hair cells, triggering the firing of the auditory neurons. The firing of the auditory neurons encodes the sound; the signal is carried up the VIIIth nerve. The VIIIth nerve fibers will synapse with other neurons in the brainstem. Some processing of sound occurs in the brainstem, as the signal is transmitted up toward the cortex, where the signal is interpreted.

The primary pathway is ascending, or **afferent**; however, there are also descending (or **efferent**) pathways from the brain and brainstem to the ear. These pathways are also overviewed in this chapter.

CHEMICAL CHANGES IN THE HAIR CELLS AND NEURONS

Chapter 18 described how the up-and-down motion of basilar membrane creates the side-to-side shearing movement of the cilia. As you recall, normally functioning outer hair cells respond to the incoming potassium by changing their size and shape. The active mechanism of the outer hair cell created a larger motion of basilar membrane relative to the location of tectorial membrane. That created greater movement of the inner hair cell cilia. Therefore, even low-intensity sounds are able to move the cilia of the inner hair cells enough to open transduction pores in the inner hair cell cilia and begin the "hearing" process.

The Cochlear Microphonic

Recall that shearing of the cilia toward stria vascularis allows potassium into the hair cell. As potassium, K+, is positively charged, this results in the negative charge of the inside of the hair cells lessening—the hair cells **depolarize.** When the cilia deflect in the opposite direction, toward the modiolus, the microchannels that bring potassium into the hair cells are effectively shut off. The hair cell is able to excrete the potassium (and other depolarizing chemicals that entered the hair cell). The hair cell voltages return to their normal, negative polarity.

The depolarization and repolarization changes can be measured. The response that is recorded mimics the stimulus. For example, if a hair cell located near the middle turn of the cochlea were stimulated by a mid-frequency sound, such as a 1000-Hz pure tone, the hair cell would be seen to grow more and less negative 1000 times each second. This chemical change in the hair cell polarity is called the **cochlear microphonic.** The name's origin is interesting. In some of the earliest experiments measuring the cochlear microphonic, an electrode was placed on the round window in order to measure the hair cell polarity indirectly. The voltage fluctuation (relative to a "ground" electrode placed somewhere else in the body) was fed into an amplifier and a speaker. When 1000 Hz was presented to the ear, the sound coming out of the speaker was 1000 Hz. The ear was acting like a microphone, picking up the signal that could be heard by the experimenters, thus the name "cochlear microphonic."

The Summating Potential

While sound is present, the inner and outer hair cells change in a second way, in addition to having the alternating current changes recorded as a cochlear microphonic. The hair cells also become in general a bit less negatively charged overall—even when the hair cell cilia are sheared toward the modiolus. (Actually, the change is not always positive—that point will be elaborated on in the next chapter. Furthermore, whether you call it a negative or positive charge depends on how you measure it. The important concept is that, for a given measurement system, the potential will always be in the same direction, either positive or negative.)

The overall change in the hair cell voltage is always in the one direction—as described here, the hair cell is more positive during stimulation. The louder the sound, the

greater the effect. This change in the voltage of the hair cells is called the **summating potential.** Whereas the cochlear microphonic was an alternating more positive/more negative change in the hair cell polarity (an **AC** event, that is, alternating current), the summating potential is a change in just one direction, so it is described as a **DC signal**—a "direct" or unidirectional current change.

The hair cells that are more positive while a sound is present are the ones that are releasing the excitatory neurotransmitter that will stimulate the firing of the VIIIth nerve fibers. The summating potential is sometimes referred to as a "distortion" of the cochlea. As it is related to the firing of the auditory nerves, it is an important distortion! However, there is a disease that creates hearing loss, **Ménière's disease**, which also causes the summating potential to become excessively large, which reinforces considering the summating potential a distortion potential.

Action Potentials

When the summating potential is occurring, **neurotransmitters** are released from the bottom (base) of the hair cell. As was mentioned in Chapter 16, the dendrites of the auditory nerve are located under the hair cells. The neurotransmitters released by the hair cell are absorbed by the afferent nerve fibers. (Figure 20–1 presents a pictorial view of the parts of a nerve fiber.) When sufficient amounts of neurotransmitters are absorbed, the neuron will create a spike of electrical activity that travels down the axon of the nerve. This spike is called the **action potential**.

As you know from earlier reading, the frequency of the sound determines the maximum point of basilar membrane displacement. That is—basilar membrane is **tonotopically organized**. Different locations are

A. **B.**

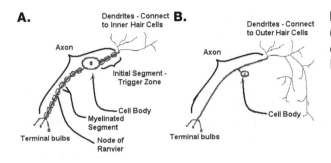

Figure 20–1. Type I (**A**) and type II (**B**) auditory first-order neurons. (Cochlear Neurobiology: Revolutionary Developments. *ASHA.*)

Clinical Correlate: VIIIth Nerve Tumors Cause High-Frequency Hearing Loss

Tumors of the VIIIth nerve can grow either on the auditory or vestibular branch of the VIIIth nerve within the internal auditory meatus. Vestibular tumors are more common than ones that originate on the auditory branch. Both branches traverse the very small space of the internal auditory meatus, so regardless of which branch the tumor grows from, both nerves can be affected. Compression of the nerve created by the growing tumor will generally harm the outside of the auditory branch first. High-frequency hearing loss is typical as a result, as the high-frequency nerves are on the outside of the nerve bundle. Balance problems can also occur because of the compression to the vestibular nerve portion.

---

responsible for sound encoding for different frequencies, as was shown in Figure 16–7. The nerve fibers connecting to the hair cells are also tonotopically organized, as can be seen in Figure 16-9. Nerves that arise from the base of the cochlea, encoding high-frequency sounds, will be on the outside of the nerve bundle.

PATTERN OF NEURAL FIRING ENCODES FREQUENCY AND INTENSITY

The location of the nerve is one of the keys to encoding frequency; however, it is not the most important way that sound fre-

quency is encoded. As you know, the traveling wave grows as it moves base to apex, so a hair cell can be stimulated by the sound that peaks at its location, or its cilia could shear in response to a traveling wave that peaks a bit more apically (coming from a lower frequency sound.) The auditory nerve's *pattern* of firing has to be examined to understand how the ear encodes frequency, as a neuron can respond to more than just one sound frequency. You might expect that the neuron fires in response to each cycle of the sound wave; however, in most cases, a neuron can't fire that often. We will return to the discussion the pattern of firing soon, but first, it's helpful to consider what happens as intensity increases.

The more intense the sound, the more neurotransmitter is released from hair cells, and the more often the nerves fire. Also, a larger number of nerves fire when the signal intensity increases. But higher frequency of stimulation causes nerves to fire faster, too. How, then, does the auditory nerve encode both frequency and intensity when the signal frequency and intensity will both affect firing rate? Let's examine this conundrum further.

Neurotransmitter release is time-linked to the cilia shearing. The neurotransmitter is released in response to the cilia shearing toward stria vascularis. Therefore, a neuron, if it is going to fire, is going to fire about at the time when the tip links are open, due to the sheared cilia.

However, the neuron is not able to fire to each cycle of the sound wave. Neurons simply can't fire that rapidly—they have a recovery period, also called a **neural refractory period** or refractory time. So, no matter how loud the sound, there will be a maximum firing rate for any given nerve. We know that the nerve is not going to fire to each cycle of the sound wave, but that when it fires; it tends to fire in synch with the excitation of the hair cell. For low-intensity sounds, the neuron fires infrequently—many cycles of the pure tone would have been present before the nerve fires again. The small amount of neurotransmitter released with each wave cycle is absorbed by the nerve dendrite. When enough of these little doses, each delivered one cycle at a time, have accumulated, the nerve will fire. If the sound is louder, the amount of neurotransmitter released is larger, so the nerve will require fewer cycles before it fires. Let's think about it another way. If we examine 100 neurons stimulated by a continuous, low-intensity pure tone, perhaps on average 2% of them would fire with each wave cycle. Increasing the intensity of the tone will cause more of the nerves to fire to each wave cycle, perhaps 5% of them. In both the case of the low-intensity and louder sound, one or more neuron fired to each wave peak. In this example, if 2% of the 100 neurons fire, then there are two neurons firing to the peak of each cycle. That increases to 5/100 neurons when the intensity increases. The ear therefore can determine the sound frequency from the firing pattern of the *group* of neurons' firing rate. The intensity can be determined from how many neurons in the group fired per wave peak. This simple explanation is relatively accurate; however, it is not fully detailed. Chapter 21 provides a more complete explanation.

THE PRIMARY AFFERENT AUDITORY PATHWAY

Location of Afferent Neuron Dendrites

The VIIIth nerve fiber dendrites come in contact with the base of the hair cells. There are two types of auditory sensory (afferent) neurons: type I and type II.

A **type I neuron** is illustrated in Figure 20–1A. The type I auditory **first-order neuron** (first neuron in the sequence from cochlea to cortex) is **bipolar**. That means that the axon is on both sides of the cell body. Although the dendrites are under the inner hair cells themselves, within the cochlea, the initial part of the axon of these neurons exit the cochlea via holes in the osseous spiral lamina. Those holes are called **habenulae perforata**. About 90 to 95% of the 30,000 neurons are of this type. The dendrites of about 20 type I neurons will connect to a single inner hair cell. Type I neurons are also called **radial nerves** because they radiate out to the inner hair cells. The axons of type I neurons are myelinated. These fatty myelin sheaths form segments around the axon. The neural impulse will jump across these myelinated sheaths and the neural spike will be conducted faster, as it jumps from one **node of Ranvier** (area without myelin) to the next node of Ranvier.

Type II neurons connect to outer hair cells. The cells themselves look different; the cell body, rather than being in line, is off to the side (see Figure 20–1B). They are sometimes described as pseudomono-polar neurons. The axons of type II neurons are not myelinated, so the nerve conduction time is slower. A single type II neuron's dendrites will connect to many outer hair cells. As there are almost 12,000 outer hair cells and only about 1500 of these spiraling type II fibers, in order to innervate all of the outer hair cells, the dendrites of the **spiral nerve fibers** branch profusely and run to as many as 10 different outer hair cells. The term spiral fiber is applicable because each of the nerve dendrites spirals apical-ward for up to one-third of a turn of the cochlea. A spiral fiber follows the outermost row of outer hair cells for some distance, then dropping back to the middle row and finally to the innermost row of outer hair cells. They give off dendritic branches that innervate a number of hair cells as they go. Figure 20–2 illustrates the difference in the connection of neurons to outer and inner hair cells.

Both type I and type II neurons end with **terminal buttons**. This enlargement at the end of the axon has vesicles that release neurotransmitter. The dendrite of the **second order neuron** (second neuron in the sequence from cochlea to cortex) will synapse with the terminal button. The second order neuron will absorb the neurotransmitter, and then it too can fire. All neurons have the same basic components: dendrite, cell body, axon, and terminal button.

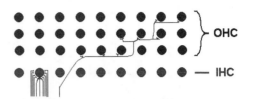

Figure 20–2. Afferent innervation pattern of an inner hair cells (IHC) and a few of the outer hair cells (OHC). This view is from above the basilar membrane, with the inner hair cells located on the bottom row. Dallos, P. Cochlear Neurobiology. June/July 1988, *ASHA*. Adapted with permission.

exit the cochlea through small holes or perforations in the osseous spiral lamina: the habenulae perforata. The neurons will cluster together to exit via these holes, and will remain grouped together as the axons run toward the core—the modiolus. Because groups of neurons are clustered together, leaving via the habenulae perforata, the cell bodies also cluster together, forming **spiral ganglia** (see Figures 16–9 and 20–3). (The singular form is spiral ganglion.)

Vestibular afferent nerve fibers arise from the balance structures and form two branches: superior and inferior sections of the vestibular portion of the VIIIth nerve. The cell bodies cluster near the internal auditory meatus in ganglia. The auditory and vestibular branches of the VIIIth nerve then together course medially through the internal auditory canal. As they make their way toward the brainstem, the two branches twist. The facial nerve (cranial nerve VII) and the anterior inferior cerebellar artery are also in the internal auditory canal. The internal auditory meatus is about 8-mm (just under 1/3 inch) long and about 4-mm wide.

Course of the VIIIth Nerve

The dendrites of the VIIIth nerve are in the cochlea, below the hair cells. The axons

Cerebellopontine Angle

The VIIIth nerve enters the brainstem at the area called the **cerebellopontine an-**

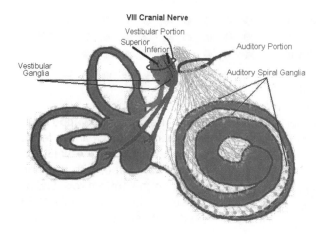

VIII Cranial Nerve
Vestibular Portion
Superior
Inferior
Auditory Portion
Vestibular
Ganglia
Auditory Spiral Ganglia

Figure 20–3. Sketch illustrating the membranous labyrinth, the location of the auditory and vestibular ganglia, and nerve branches.

gle (CPA). As the name implies, this is the area where the cerebellum and pons join. As seen in Figure 20-4, the VIIIth nerve takes a bend, thus the "angle" portion of this anatomic location.

Nuclei

Nuclei are distinct groups or hubs of neurons, specifically the gray matter portion made up mostly of cell bodies (rather than the white matter, which is mostly axons). The primary auditory pathway has several well-defined nuclei, which are illustrated in Figure 20-4.

Cochlear nucleus is the first nucleus in the auditory system. All the VIIIth nerve fibers will synapse on neurons of the cochlear nucleus. About two-thirds of the neurons then **decussate**, or cross to the other side of the brainstem. A major pathway for this decussation is the **trapezoid body**, which has a nucleus. The next major nucleus is the **superior olive**, also called the **superior olivary complex.** A small nucleus is superior to the superior olive: **lateral lemniscus**. Though small in size, it creates a rather large electrical potential that is one of the main ones that can be recorded with electrodes placed on the skin. The **inferior colliculus** and **medial geniculate body** are the oth-

er major nuclei. As shown in Figure 20-4, there are multiple points of decussation of the auditory pathway. However, the strongest pathway is between one ear and the opposite side of the brainstem: More fibers decussate to the contralateral side of the brainstem than remain ipsilateral.

In the brainstem, several different neurons will synapse with the next higher order neuron. For example, the neurons in the superior olivary complex receive input from the right and left ears. This allows for encoding of the direction of the sound signal. Also, it appears that some neurons encode different features of sound, for example, some encode the onset and offset of a sound, which could encode the duration of a phoneme. It appears that the brainstem structures are, in essence, doing preprocessing of sound.

Primary Auditory Cortex

The auditory pathway leads to the primary auditory cortex, located in Heschl's gyrus of the temporal lobe. This is an area within a fold of the temporal lobe. It cannot be seen looking at the outside of the brain. Heschl's gyrus is tonotopically organized. Just as the cochlea has specific areas for specific frequencies, the cortex has pitch-spe-

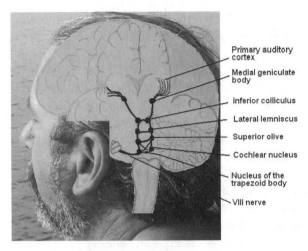

Primary auditory cortex

Medial geniculate body

Inferior colliculus

Lateral lemniscus

Superior olive

Cochlear nucleus

Nucleus of the trapezoid body

VIII nerve

Figure 20–4. Illustration of the location of the major structures of the ascending auditory pathway. Half of the cerebellum, the occipital lobes, and much of the temporal lobes are removed. The VIIIth nerve enters the brainstem at the cerebellopontine angle, and then synapses at cochlear nucleus. The sketch shows the extensive decussation of the pathways, and illustrates that not all nerve pathways synapse at each nucleus. Only the left ear pathway is illustrated.

Clinical Correlate: ABR Testing Measures Synchronous Neural Discharge

Audiologists measure the auditory nervous system activity when conducting **auditory evoked potentials testing.** The most common form of this testing is the **auditory brainstem response** (ABR) test. ABR testing allows us to assess the health of the primary auditory pathway, which can be affected by tumors of the VIIIth nerve and cerebellopontine angle, and neural demyelinization (e.g., multiple sclerosis). ABR testing shows the activity of the auditory nervous system after stimulation. A visual display shows a waveform with multiple peaks. The different peaks are generated by neurons at different levels in the auditory system—for example, an early wave comes from the VIIIth nerve, whereas a later wave comes primarily from lateral lemniscus. ABR is a test of neural synchrony, but it can also be used to estimate hearing sensitivity. Sound intensity is reduced to determine the lowest level that creates a response, which allows the audiologist to predict the hearing threshold in those who cannot participate in behavioral testing (e.g., infants).

cific areas. The auditory pathway nuclei are also tonotopically organized.

Neural pathways lead from the primary auditory cortex to association areas of the brain, which permit interpretation of the signal. Linguistic information is interpreted by the left hemisphere, whereas features such as tonality and rhythm are interpreted by the right hemisphere. The **corpus collosum** is a nerve tract between hemispheres; information received by each temporal lobe is shared.

Clinical Correlate: Right Ear Advantage

The pathway from the right ear to the left hemisphere of the brain, where language information is processed, is stronger and more direct. As a result, listening to speech in difficult noise situations is easier with the right ear. This **right-ear advantage** is most noticeable in young children. They will have a better speech-understanding-in-noise score for the right ear. Some children do not have age-appropriate maturation and development of the auditory nervous system and are said to have **auditory processing disorders**. These children (and adults) typically have a larger right-ear advantage (or left-ear deficit) than usually seen at that age. There are other deficits associated with auditory processing disorders as well. Sequencing of sound information may be problematic, and auditory memory may be deficit. Audiologists assess auditory processing disorders using various behavioral tests, and using auditory evoked potentials testing.

INTRODUCTION TO EFFERENT NEURONS

Whereas afferent (sensory) neurons' dendrites are at the hair cells, and convey the information toward the brainstem, **efferent neurons'** terminal buttons synapse in the cochlea. They send information down from the brainstem (and brain) to the cochlea.

The overwhelming preponderance of the approximately 30,000 auditory neurons (all but about 500) are afferent. There are two types of efferent neurons, just as there are two types of afferent neurons. The efferent neurons that contact the type I sensory neurons (those coming from the inner hair cells) synapse on the neuron itself (see Figure 16–6). They affect the ability of the first-order sensory neuron to absorb the excitatory neurotransmitter from the hair cells. Type II efferent neurons connect directly to the side of the outer hair cells. As will be discussed in Chapter 23, these neurons will influence the outer hair cell's ability to change shape—they inhibit the active mechanism.

SUMMARY

The influx of potassium, a positively charged chemical, and the removal of this chemical from the hair cells, occur in perfect synchrony with the sound. This creates a change in the hair cell potential called the cochlear microphonic. The depolarization of the negatively charged inner hair cell during the presence of sound creates a general change in the hair cell polarity—as long as the sound is on, the hair cell is a little less negative than if there were silence. This change in hair cell polarity during sound stimulation is the summating potential. The hair cells with a summating potential are the ones that are releasing neurotransmitter.

The neurotransmitter is absorbed by the dendrite of the neuron below the hair cells. Most of the afferent neurons are of type I: they connect to the inner hair cells.

Not all neurons are firing at the same time. At any given time, some fraction of the neurons are firing, and that firing is time-linked to the cilia shearing toward stria vascularis, depolarizing the hair cells. Increase in intensity causes more neurons, overall, to fire to each sound wave peak. Because some neurons are firing to each wave peak, the neural signal encodes the timing of the wave peaks. Furthermore, because the auditory nerve is tonotopically organized, knowing which nerve is firing also provides a cue to the sound's frequency. More neurons fire to each sound wave peak as intensity is increased.

The first-order auditory neuron synapses multiple times in the brainstem. About two-thirds of the neurons will decussate across the brainstem, creating a stronger neural path from one ear to the contralateral primary auditory cortex.

Although the vast majority of the neurons are afferent, there are some descending nerve fibers. This provides a means for the higher brain centers to affect how readily the first-order neuron absorbs neurotransmitter, and provides a way for the hair cell active mechanism to be attenuated.

REFERENCE

Dallos, P. (1988, June/July). Cochlear neurobiology: Revolutionary developments. *ASHA,* pp. 50–56.

21

Advanced Study of Cochlear and VIIIth Nerve Potentials

This chapter discusses electrochemical changes in hair cells and neurons, and how they are measured and analyzed. Ions flowing into hair cells create chemical changes. These physical changes in the chemistry of the hair cells can be recorded and analyzed. The neurotransmitters stimulating the VIIIth nerve fibers trigger chemical changes in the neurons, which also can be recorded. This chapter reviews the resting potentials of the cochlea and describes the **graded**, or stimulus-evoked potentials, which are also called **receptor potentials**.

The firing of the first-order neurons, the VIIIth nerve fibers, is also described. One individual first-order neuron would fire most readily to a specific frequency. That neuron can fire to other frequencies, but the intensity of the pure tone will have to be increased. A graph of the intensity needed for different frequencies to stimulate a neuron is called a **neural tuning curve.** The differential sensitivity of a neuron to different stimulus frequencies is related to the traveling wave envelope. This concept, relating the traveling wave to the tuning curve, is discussed in detail.

CHARACTERISTIC FREQUENCY

Before discussing the potentials, two new terms are defined: **cochlear tuning** and characteristic frequency. An outer hair cell's active mechanisms will only occur if the stimulus is at or near a given frequency. The frequency that elicits the best motile response of an outer hair cell is the frequency to which the hair cell is "tuned." Inner hair cells are also "tuned," even though they don't have a motile response. An inner hair cell will release the greatest amount of neurotransmitter to a stimulus of a certain frequency, because the basilar membrane is tuned, and because the outer hair cells enhance that tuning. A related term is **characteristic frequency**. The frequency that elicits the maximal response from a hair cell or from a nerve fiber is its characteristic frequency.

COCHLEAR RESTING POTENTIALS

Chapter 17 explained that the ionic concentrations inside and outside of hair cells creates different electrochemical charges. There is the possibility ("potential") for equalization of these differences in electrochemical charges (for example, if the hair cell ruptured, or if hair cell cilia shear.) Thus, these cellular charges are called potentials. The cell membrane acts to maintain these differences in charge, and to allow the potentials to change. The static chemical charge differences, those that exist even when sound is not present, are referred to as **resting potential differences**, or the **resting potentials** of the cochlea.

Endocochlear Potential

As described in Chapter 17, potentials have to be measured relative to another substance. If you compare the charge of endolymph to that of perilymph, you are measuring the endocochlear potential, which is about +100 mV. Another name for **endocochlear potential** is **endolymphatic potential**.

Intracellular Potentials

The outer hair cells are about –70 mV in polarity, compared to the perilymph in which they are bathed (recall that the basilar membrane allows the perilymph to come into the area below reticular lamina.) The inner hair cells are not as negatively charged. It is estimated that they are about –40 mV, relative to perilymph. The potential between endolymph and the hair cells is of interest to us. Some authors describe the difference in charge from endolymph to the hair cells as a "voltage drop" of about 170 mV for the outer hair cells, and 140 mV for the inner hair cells. The term "voltage drop" reflects the fact that the inside of hair cells is negative relative to the endolymph. Figure 21–1 provides a visual aid.

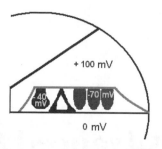

Figure 21–1. Endolymph is 100 mV more positive than perilymph. Inner hair cells are about 40 mV more negative than perilymph and outer hair cells about –70 mV. The hair cells are therefore 140 (inner) and 170 (outer) negative relative to endolymph.

COCHLEAR RECEPTOR POTENTIALS

There are two **receptor potentials** in the cochlea, that is, potentials that change in response to auditory stimulation. Receptor potentials are also called **generator potentials**. The first, the **cochlear microphonic**, is better understood and easier to understand than the summating potential. A review of the difference between alternating current and direct current might help the reader understand this next section (see Chapter 6, specifically Figure 6–3.)

Cochlear Microphonic

Perhaps it is worth one more restatement: when the cilia shear toward stria vascularis, the microchannels in the cilia open, allowing potassium to enter the cell. This triggers an influx of calcium as well. Both of these are positively charged ions, so the hair cell becomes less negative. The potassium pumps and calcium channels will work to remove these positively charged ions, and will do so more effectively when the cilia are deflected toward the modiolus, firmly shutting the micropores. Thus, in response to a pure tone (a sound with air molecules vibrating in simple harmonic motion), the voltage in a hair cell that is tuned to that frequency (has that characteristic frequency) will cycle less negative then more negative again, and the course of this voltage change will follow the signal. As shown in Figure 21-2, the voltage inside the hair cell mimics the stimulus wave.

Sensitive electrical recording devices can be placed either inside a hair cell or near

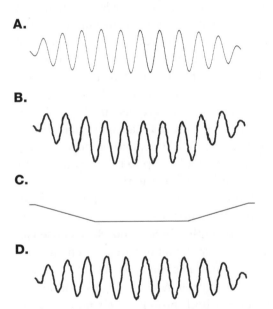

A.

B.

C.

D.

Figure 21–2. If a sinusoidal signal (here, one that turns on and off gradually) is put into the cochlea (**A**), a recording of the activity in scala media near the hair cells shows a similar pattern (**B**), though it is degraded slightly by noise introduced by imperfect recording techniques. The response also is shifted away from baseline as the signal gets progressively more intense, and returns to baseline when the sound goes off. The tracing shown in (**B**) is composed of two parts: a shift in the baseline (**C**), and the sinusoidal part (**D**). The alternating portion (**D**) is the cochlear microphonic. The portion that is the offset (**C**) is the summating potential, which is a graded DC potential.

hair cells in order to pick up these electrical changes. Wever and Bray conducted this type of experiment in the late 1920s. They placed an electrode on the round window, and could visualize the changes in voltages using an oscilloscope, or they could hook up the electrode to an amplifier and speaker and listen to the sound, which they termed the **cochlear microphonic**.

The cochlear microphonic alternates negative and positive, just like a sine wave does. Thus, the cochlear microphonic is an **AC potential** (an alternating current.)

We now understand that the cochlear microphonic is coming from the variations in the intracellular potentials of the hair cells. As discussed below, you will not always see a cochlear microphonic, but if it is present in the healthy ear, the cochlear microphonic will be generated by both outer and inner hair cells.

Early studies of the cochlear microphonic helped to validate the traveling wave theory. If the electrode is placed in the base of the cochlea, all different frequencies will create a cochlear microphonic, as the basilar membrane's traveling wave moves base to apex. However, electrodes monitoring hair cells at the apex of the cochlea show cochlear microphonics only for low-frequency sounds.

According to Santos-Sacchi (2001), the cochlear microphonic is not always evident. Cochlear microphonics are seen in response to low-frequency stimuli. As the stimulus gets higher and higher in frequency, the cochlear microphonic becomes smaller. Hair cells with characteristic frequencies above 2 kHz or 3 kHz will not show evidence of a cochlear microphonic for frequencies near and above their characteristic frequency. This makes some sense physiologically. The potassium pump and the calcium channels cannot get rid of the chemicals fast enough to allow full repolarization if the stimulus is very high frequency. However, this does not mean that the active mechanism doesn't occur for high frequencies. The contractile properties do occur, even at the high frequencies, and even though the hair cell is not able to fully cycle through depolarization/repolarization.

The cochlear microphonic's size generally increases as the sound intensity increases. However, it will reach a point where it is at its maximum. This happens at approximately 100 dB SPL. When the sound intensity exceeds 100 dB SPL, the size of the cochlear microphonic actually decreases. When this occurs, the waveform will also be distorted.

Summating Potential

When measuring the voltage change in a hair cell that is responding to sound, the output from the hair cells is not *only* the sinusoidal signal that mimics the input (the cochlear microphonic), but consists of a form of distortion as well (Figure 21–2B). The distortion portion is called the **summating potential** (Figure 21–2C). The distortion is a deflection of the entire waveform—it shifts either up or down.

As the amplitude of the signal grows, the summating potential generally gets larger. As shown in Figures 21–2B and 21–2C, as the signal increases in amplitude, the polarity gets more negative. As the signal decreases in intensity, the summating potential magnitude reduces. Note that the summating potential illustrated is negative or zero. It does not cycle negative to positive. Any single recording of a summating potential will show either a gradual negative or gradual positive potential—here it is always negative. As the voltage at any one location to any single sound doesn't alternate between positive and negative, the summating potential is described as a **DC** (direct current) **potential**.

In this chapter, when the summating potential is said to be negative, it means that the voltage measured in the *endolymph* of scala media is growing more negative. This

means that the positively charged ions in the endolymph are entering the hair cells. (This may be referred to as AVE SP in some texts, meaning we are viewing the change in the endolymph relative to the average polarity of the perilymph in scala tympani and scala vestibuli.) The influx of positively charged ions into hair cells occurs when the hair cells are becoming depolarized—less negatively charged—during excitation. Use caution when reading other texts. The location of the electrodes (hair cell/scala media/scala tympani. . .) affects the polarity. If examining the polarity inside the hair cell, the summating potential would be positive during sound stimulation. When doing testing using electrodes that are not in the cochlea, but on the round window or in the ear canal, if you compare that voltage to a reference somewhere else in the body, the summating potential can be either positive or negative. It will depend on how the electrodes are hooked up to the recording unit. The important idea is that the summating potential is related to a general depolarization of the hair cells.

Currently, there is no clear consensus on whether the summating potential originates from inner hair cells or both inner and outer hair cells. A recent investigation suggests that both produce the summating potential, though the inner hair cells are the larger contributor.

The summating potential is not always negative, however. If you were to place a needle electrode in the endolymph near the peak of the traveling wave (near a cell "tuned" to respond to that frequency), the summating potential would be negative. The closer you are to the exact tuning frequency for that cell, the larger the summating potential becomes. However, if you are measuring a cell's response to a sound that is not at or near its characteristic frequency, then the summating potential is positive in polarity. This has an important implication. We can determine if the sound is near the hair cell's characteristic frequency by seeing if the summating potential is negative. Negative summating potentials (measured in the endolymph) are associated with nearby inner hair cells that are releasing neurotransmitters, and stimulating the auditory nerve.

Comparison of the Tuning of the Cochlear Microphonic and the Summating Potential

The cochlear microphonic seems to indicate whether a traveling wave has stimulated the cell (although sometimes the cochlear microphonic can't be accurately recorded). A hair cell located toward the base will provide a cochlear microphonic to essentially any sound, even low frequencies. The cochlear microphonic is not selectively tuned. The cochlear microphonic will not be an accurate indicator of whether or not a given hair cell is generating release of neurotransmitters. (Determining whether or not a hair cell [inner or outer] has a cochlear microphonic doesn't tell us much about whether the inner hair cell is releasing neurotransmitter and encoding the sound.)

In contrast, there is only a limited range of frequencies where a negative summating potential (measured in the endolymph near the hair cells) is seen. This suggests that the presence of a summating potential is related to neurotransmitter release and neural encoding.

Summary of Cochlear Microphonic and Summating Potential

Both the cochlear microphonic and summating potential are stimulus-related or graded receptor potentials. The cochlear microphonic gives us evidence of the fact that the cilia shearing causes fluctuation in the

---

Clinical Correlate: Ménière's Disease and Enhanced Summating Potentials

Ménière's disease is a disorder where too much endolymph is produced or too little endolymph is reabsorbed. In either case, the endolymphatic pressure is too high. As you might expect, this allows for excessive flow of ions from the endolymph into the hair cells. The patient may experience a sensation of aural fullness. Hearing loss, tinnitus, and dizziness can result.

One of the clinical findings of Ménière's disease is that the summating potential increases in size. If the summating potential reflects hair cells not fully repolarizing, but staying somewhat depolarized during the presence of an ongoing sound (and creating neurotransmitter release), this makes sense. The excess fluid pressure creates too much depolarization. In this case, it's not healthy for the ear, and is not associated with good hearing, but the opposite.

intracellular potentials. It appears that the general depolarization of the hair cells, specifically the inner hair cells, which is reflected by the summating potential, is an important indicator of whether or not an action potential will be generated by the VIIIth nerve.

ACTION POTENTIALS

Electrical Potentials in Neurons

Neurons function electrochemically. The inside of the neuron is electrically charged relative to the outside. This charge is due to the ionic difference between the chemicals inside the cell and those outside the cell. The inside of the neuron contains a concentration of potassium that is 20 to 50 times higher than the outside of the cell. The outside of the neuron, on the other hand, has high concentration of sodium and chloride relative to the inside. These chemical differences across the cell membrane produce an electrical charge, or **resting potential**, of 50 to 90 mV with the inside being negative relative to the outside. By changing the chemical relationship, primarily by increasing or decreasing the sodium inside the cell, the magnitude of this potential can increase or decrease. When a potential, whether negative or positive, moves toward zero (i.e., no potential) **depolarization** or **hypopolarization** is said to occur. When the potential moves away from zero, (i.e., becomes more negative) **hyperpolarization** is said to occur.

The resting potential in the neuron is maintained because the cell membrane is largely impermeable to the passage of sodium and potassium. That is, the membrane blocks the passage of sodium into the cell and of potassium out of the cell. However, applying certain chemicals to the neuron can change the permeability of the cell

membrane. In the human auditory system, the hair cells release the **neurotransmitter glutamate**, which reduces the opposition of the membrane to sodium flow. As sodium moves into the cell, the magnitude of the polarity drops toward zero. Chemicals that create the depolarizing change in the neuron are said to be **excitatory** in nature as hypopolarizing the cell causes it to respond by sending a nerve impulse down the axon.

There are other chemicals that are **inhibitory** in nature. That is, they increase the opposition of the cell membrane to sodium flow and the polarity across the membrane increases. The cell becomes hyperpolarized; that is, it is moved further from the depolarized condition that results in the axon transmitting an impulse. A neuron in a hyperpolarized state would thus be inhibited, or more difficult to excite into activity.

Depolarization, the excitatory process in neurons, normally begins in the dendrites or cell bodies where it is a relatively gradual and graded response to incoming stimulation. That is, the cell's potential will vary up and down depending on the excitatory or inhibitory signal it receives. This change in the resting potential in the dendrites and cell body (soma) is called the **generator potential**. The portion of the curve labeled *GP* in Figure 21–3, where the polarity changes from about negative 70 mV to negative 40 mV, is the generator potential.

If the depolarization in the cell body reaches some **threshold** criteria (the dashed line in Figure 21–3 labeled *T*), it triggers an instantaneous and total depolarization of the axon. This total depolarization, followed immediately by a repolarization, travels the length of the axon. Thus, we have an electrical event that has the appearance of a "spike" which runs the length of the axon from the soma to the terminal buttons at the end of the axon. This event is variously known as an **action potential**, **spike potential**, or **nerve impulse**.

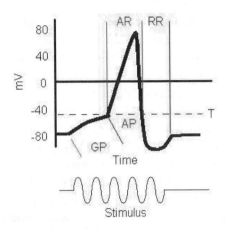

Figure 21–3. A graphic representation of the electrical activity associated with a nerve action potential. When a stimulus is presented, the neuron begins depolarizing. This activity called the generator potential (GP) continues until threshold (T) is reached. At this point an action potential (AP) occurs with its absolute refractory (AR) period followed by its relative refractory (RR) period. Adapted from Durrant and Lovrinic's (1984) adaptation of B. Katz (1966) from *Nerve, Muscle and Synapse*.

As the action potential is the result of a total depolarization and repolarization of the axon, it is an **all-or-none response**. That is, when an action potential occurs, it occurs to its maximum capability. An action potential is like a one-bit digital signal—either you have an action potential or it is not present. A neuron's action potential does not change size—it either travels down the axon or it does not. There are no "large" action potentials versus "small" amplitude ones. Figure 21-3 shows what an action potential looks like when recorded on a graph.

Refractory Period

When threshold of response in the axon is reached and an action potential is generated, some time elapses before the axon is repolarized to its resting state. This period of time between depolarization and repolarization is called **refractory** time. A neuron's refractory time is divided into two segments. Initially, there is an **absolute refractory** period (that portion labeled *AR* in Figure 21-3) when the neuron is in such a depolarized state that is cannot respond again no matter how strong the stimulus applied to it. This period lasts until the neuron's polarity goes below the trigger threshold level. This followed by a period when the axon is hyperpolarized. The channels repolarizing the cell temporarily overwork, further lowering the cell voltage. If a sufficiently strong stimulus is applied to it, the cell could fire. As the repolarization process continues toward the normal resting state, the stimulus intensity required to initiate a second response is less and less. The period of time when the neuron will respond again, but only if the stimulus strength is increased, is called the **relative refractory period**. This is the portion of the curve labeled *RR* in Figure 21-3.

If a signal that is just barely loud enough to stimulate the neuron is continuously present, the neuron will respond repeatedly, but at a relatively slow rate of fire. That is, after firing the first time, it will not fire again until it has fully recovered at the end of the relative refractory period. The low stimulus level will create a more gradual increase in the generator potential; it will take a longer time for the action potential trigger level to be reached. On the other hand, if an intense stimulus is continuously applied, the neuron will fire at a faster rate as the cell's potential builds toward the firing threshold more quickly and because it does not have to be fully recovered to respond; it may respond during the relative refractory period.

Spontaneous Discharge Rates

Even when there is no sound present, neurons will fire, on average, at some rate.

This is called the neuron's **spontaneous discharge rate** or **spontaneous firing rate**. An auditory neuron may fire spontaneously as seldom as once per second, or as often as 100 times per second. Some scientists classify auditory neurons into two groups by their spontaneous discharge rate: high and low. Others use three classifications: low, medium, and high spontaneous firing rates.

When a neuron is firing spontaneously, it is probably because some neurotransmitter (i.e., glutamate) is being picked up by the neuron. Recall that in silence, some cilia micropores are open, and so some neurotransmitter will be released. The auditory system is thought to recognize that this firing is not important, and will not associate it with sound being present. One reason that spontaneous firing of neurons is not related to encoding sound is that the firing pattern is random. (A neuron that fires on average 6 times per second does not fire exactly once per 10 seconds. The interval between spontaneous firings might once be 9 seconds, once 10.8 seconds, etc.) As introduced in the previous chapter, acoustic stimulation will create patterns to the neural firing. Random spontaneous discharge of neurons is different from the patterned firing that occurs when sound is present.

Threshold of Neural Firing Is Related to Spontaneous Discharge Rate

There is an inverse relationship between the spontaneous discharge rate and how easy it is for a neuron to fire faster than its spontaneous rate. A neuron that fires at a fast spontaneous discharge rate will be excited by a less intense stimulus than a neuron with a lower spontaneous firing rate.

As different neuron groups have different thresholds for firing (at a rate that is fast-

er than their spontaneous rates), this may have some relationship to the encoding of intensity. If only the fast spontaneous rate neurons are firing at a rate that exceeds their spontaneous rates, then the sound is near threshold for that individual. The lower spontaneous rate neurons are going to begin to fire (faster than their spontaneous discharge rate) when the signal levels are at most 30 or 40 dB higher. Intensity is not *just* encoded by which neurons are firing, as all neurons can be made to fire above spontaneous rate for moderate intensity sounds. However, which neurons (high, mid, low spontaneous firing rate) are firing might be a cue to intensity discrimination for low-intensity sounds.

About 70% of the neurons would be characterized as having a high spontaneous firing rate (SFR). About 10% have mid SFRs; 20% have low SFRs.

Firing Rate Influenced by Efferent Innervation

Figure 16–6 illustrated the connection of the efferent neuron to the first-order auditory neuron that innervates the inner hair cells. The descending, or efferent, connection to the neuron influences the firing rate. Efferent neuron excitation can cause a sensory neuron to fire slower than it would ordinarily, both while the neuron is responding to a sound and when it is firing only at its spontaneous rate. The efferent nerves that connect to the first-order neurons release an inhibitory neurotransmitter (perhaps GABA, perhaps acetylcholine) that helps to counteract the effect of the excitatory neurotransmitter, slowing the firing rate.

Type II efferent neurons connect to the cell body of the outer hair cells and inhibit the active mechanism. Inhibiting the active mechanism reduces the amount of enhancement of the basilar membrane vibration that occurs. This, in turn, reduces the shearing of the inner hair cell cilia, which of course reduces the firing of the auditory neuron.

Chapter 23 will provide more information on the efferent system.

Pure Tones Frequencies and Intensities That Cause a Neuron to Fire Faster Than Spontaneous Rate

As hair cells are tuned to respond to different frequencies, obviously the neurons connected to the hair cells are also tuned. Just as a hair cell can be stimulated by an intense sound of a lower frequency than its characteristic frequency, a neuron will also fire in response to this intense low-frequency sound.

Before discussing the tuning of the neuron, it is helpful to discuss the **basal spread of excitation**, which is also called the **upward spread of masking.** Let's make the assumption that a certain amplitude of basilar membrane vibration is required for a hair cell to release enough neurotransmitter to create a neural impulse (at a rate above spontaneous firing rate.) In Figure 21–4, this amount of vibration is shown with the thin

lines. Let's examine the different traveling waves that would create enough movement of basilar membrane at one point, marked X, to permit neural firing. Note that as the frequency of the sound is lowered, with the traveling wave peak occurring more and more apically, the intensity required for the traveling wave to stimulate neurons at location X increases.

It is possible for a high frequency to stimulate an area more apical on the basilar membrane than the traveling wave peak location; however, the shape of the traveling wave makes that very difficult. The traveling wave displacement rapidly decreases past the peak of the traveling wave. The areas of the basilar membrane more apical to the traveling wave peak that can be stimulated are restricted to those areas fairly near the peak. Figure 21–5 illustrates.

Another way to describe the basal-ward spread of excitation is to examine which neurons can potentially be stimulated by any given traveling wave. As shown in Figure 21–6, this traveling wave vibrates a broad area of basilar membrane enough to create neural firings. The area of stimulation that is more basal-ward from the wave peak (segment A to B) is much greater than the stimulated area of the basilar membrane that is more apical (segment B to C).

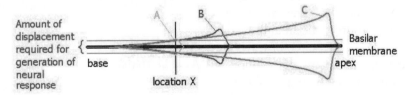

Figure 21–4. Each of the three traveling waves illustrated is just able to create enough basilar membrane motion to stimulate nerve cells at location X. The intensity of wave A, which peaks at location X, is least. As the frequency is lower, as for traveling wave B, the intensity of the signal must increase in order to create enough displacement at location X, which is more basal than the peak of the traveling wave. When the frequency is lower still, as illustrated in C, the intensity of the signal must be greater still.

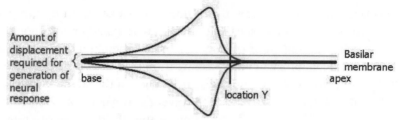

Figure 21–5. Location *Y* is more apical than the traveling wave peak. That is, neurons in this area have lower characteristic frequencies than the frequency causing the traveling wave. It is possible for the higher frequency sound to innervate this lower frequency neuron, but note how intense the sound must be. If the sound is too far above the neuron's characteristic frequency, it will be impossible to create enough displacement of the basilar membrane to stimulate the neurons located at location *Y*.

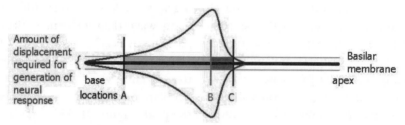

Figure 21–6. A traveling wave for an intense sound is capable of stimulating a broad region of the basilar membrane—from location *A*, where high characteristic-frequency neurons are located, to location *C*, where neurons of a mid-range characteristic frequency are located. Note that a greater area is stimulated from the peak *(B)* toward the base than from location *B* toward the apex. The spread of excitation from a traveling wave is asymmetric; there is a greater basal-ward influence.

Upward Spread of Masking—Masking of One Stimulus by a Second

A single neuron cannot encode two signals simultaneously. Two traveling waves are shown in Figure 21-7. The larger traveling wave (*A*) will drive the neural encoding at location *Z*. The presence of traveling wave (*B*) becomes irrelevant. This sound is not audible; it is **masked** by the presence of sound with the larger traveling wave. This illustrates that an intense sound can mask other signals that are higher in frequency. This is often referred to as **upward spread of masking**, because the frequencies most readily masked by a tone are higher in fre-

quency than the masker. The term **basal-ward spread of masking** may be easier to understand, but this term is not commonly used.

NEURAL TUNING CURVES

How Tuning Curves Are Obtained

Figure 21-8 shows four different traveling waves that cause just enough displacement of basilar membrane at location *X* to create a neural impulse (assuming each were presented, one at a time). Of course, the traveling wave from the 1700-Hz tone which

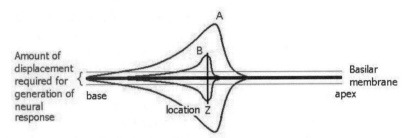

Figure 21–7. The neurons at location *Z* are excited by the sound illustrated with traveling wave *A*. The neuron cannot simultaneously encode information about the presence of the sound creating traveling wave *B*. Therefore, this sound is masked. A traveling wave tends to create more masking for areas more toward the base; that is an intense low-frequency sound will mask weaker high-frequency sounds. This is termed upward spread of masking.

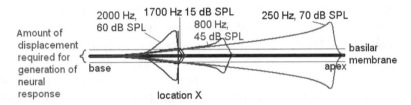

Figure 21–8. In order to stimulate neurons at location *X*, only a 15 dB SPL tone is required when the pure tone is at the characteristic frequency for location *X*, which is 1700 Hz. Because of the basal-ward spread of excitation, 800 Hz is able to stimulate location *X* with only 45 dB SPL of intensity. The more apically peaking 250-Hz, 70 dB SPL traveling wave also can stimulate neurons at location *X*, assuming that this is the only sound in the cochlea at the time. Note how intense the higher frequency pure tone must be to create a firing of neurons at location *X*. The 2000-Hz tone needs to be 60 dB SPL to stimulate the neurons located at the 1700-Hz place on the basilar membrane.

peaks at location *X* requires the least intensity to create a neural impulse. The traveling wave from the sound slightly higher in frequency must be fairly loud to create this response, whereas the 800-Hz traveling wave does not need to be as loud. When the frequency is quite low, 250 Hz, then it needs to be intense to stimulate nerves at location *X*.

If the intensities required to fire the neurons at location *X* of Figure 21–8 are graphed, a pattern such as that in Figure 21–9 emerges. Note that the low frequencies are now on the left, although in the classic figure of the basilar membrane, low frequencies are shown toward the right. The solid line in Figure 21–9 shows the combinations of frequency and intensity that are just loud enough to stimulate a single neuron to fire above spontaneous firing rate. Of course, pure tones louder than these levels will also create a neural impulse. This type of curve is called a **neural tuning curve**. The tip of the curve points toward the neuron's characteristic frequency.

It is helpful next to think about how a physiologist could develop a neural tuning curve. A needle electrode could be placed in a single nerve fiber of an experimental animal. This is called a **single unit recording**. At first, no stimulus would be present-

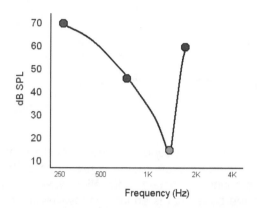

Figure 21–9. Neural tuning curve derived from the hypothetical data in Figure 21–8. The intensities of the different frequencies that allow a neuron at one location on the basilar membrane to fire faster than spontaneous firing rate are illustrated.

ed, and the spontaneous firing activity of the single nerve would be monitored. The electrode output could be sent to an amplifier and speaker so that the experimenter could listen to the firing pattern, with a random pattern, with neural firings occurring several times per second. Instead of listening, a recording of the rate could be made, either viewing the electrical activity on an oscilloscope or by monitoring a tracing that shows the action potentials. To present sounds to an experimental animal, a pure-tone generator would be connected to an amplifier and to a speaker or earphone, which is put at or in the animal's ear. First, a series of very low-intensity pure tones would be produced. The level would start so low that the neural firing rate would not change, no matter what the frequency. The intensity would then gradually be increased until the physiologist detected that, at a certain frequency, the neuron was firing faster than spontaneous firing rate. That frequency and intensity would be noted. That is the neuron's **characteristic frequency**. The signal intensity would be increased slightly, and then,

not just one frequency would create a response—a range of frequencies would cause the firing to be above spontaneous rate. As you have learned, these frequencies would be near the neuron's characteristic frequency. Frequencies that are slightly lower than characteristic frequency would be more likely to create a response than frequencies above characteristic frequency. The physiologist would repeat this process, increasing the stimulus intensity each time. Figure 21–10 illustrates the results that might be obtained. The light horizontal lines indicate that the pure tone at that intensity, across those frequencies, did not create an increase in the neural firing rate. Darker lines indicate that the nerve was stimulated.

Neural tuning curves traditionally are not shown as in Figure 21–10. Rather, the outside edges—the frequency/intensity combinations that allow the neuron to fire above its spontaneous rate—are shown, as illustrated in Figure 21–11. Sometimes the tuning curves are shaded, to represent all the frequency and intensity combinations that could cause the firing of this nerve, but generally this is not done.

The low-frequency side of the tuning curve has a change in the slope once the signal intensity reaches a moderate intensity. The narrower tip portion, below this inflection point on the tuning curve, is called the **tip of the tuning curve**, whereas the broader area in the low frequencies is called its **tail** (Figure 21–12). The tail of the tuning curve reminds us that the traveling wave for most any low frequency can stimulate higher frequency neurons, if the intensity is sufficiently loud.

Figure 21–12 illustrates five tuning curves on one figure. It is common to show a "family" of tuning curves in this manner. Figure 21–12 demonstrates two new points. Note that the lowest intensity that generates responses differs among neurons. Although that can happen if neurons with different

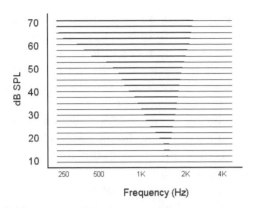

Figure 21–10. The combinations of frequencies and intensities that cause a single nerve to fire above spontaneous firing rate are illustrated with the thicker lines. This process can be used to develop a neural tuning curve.

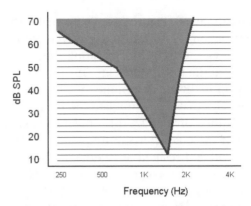

Figure 21–11. Another illustration of the neural tuning curve. The thicker line shows the frequencies and intensities at the threshold of firing of this neuron. The shaded area is typically omitted. Here the shaded area illustrates all the combinations of frequencies and intensities that create a firing of this single nerve at a rate that is faster than the neuron's spontaneous discharge rate.

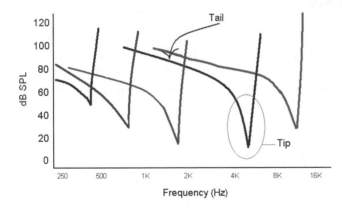

Figure 21–12. A hypothetical family of neural tuning curves from one experimental animal is shown. Each tuning curve represents the response from a different neuron. The tip of a tuning curve points to characteristic frequency for that neuron. The tail region shows the upward (basal-ward) spread of excitation of the neuron (frequencies lower than characteristic frequency can excite a neuron).

spontaneous firing rates are selected, it is also generally true that the lowest thresholds (measured in dB SPL) occur in the mid- to high-frequency range. Greater intensity is required to make low-frequency neurons fire faster than their spontaneous firing rate. Also, the shape of the neural tuning curves is not identical for neurons tuned to low versus high frequencies. When viewed on an octave scale, as in Figure 21-12, the tuning curves are wider for low frequencies.

$Q_{10\ dB}$ Calculations Describe Width of Tuning Curve Tips

The width of a tuning curve provides information about whether or not the neuron is highly selective in terms of the frequencies that innervate it. If a neuron has a sharp tip and narrow tail, there is a limited range of frequencies that stimulate that neuron.

A standard means of describing the frequency specificity of the tip area of a neuron's tuning curve is the $Q_{10\ dB}$ calculated measurement (Figure 21–13). To make this calculation, first find the characteristic frequency—the frequency creating the neural firing at the lowest intensity. Turn the intensity up 10 dB and determine the range of frequencies that now stimulate the nerve. The CF is then divided by this range. For example, if the characteristic frequency is 2000 Hz, with a threshold of 10 dB SPL, then one would see what range of frequencies excites this neuron at 20 dB SPL. If 20 dB SPL pure tones swept from 1850 Hz to 2050 Hz stimulated the nerve (a 200-Hz frequency range), then the $Q_{10\,dB}$ would be 2000/200 or 10.

Low-frequency neurons have smaller $Q_{10\,dB}$, reflecting the less specific tuning of these neurons. The $Q_{10\,dB}$ values for guinea pigs range from about 2 at 500 Hz to about 10 at 10 kHz.

Neural Tuning Curve Summary

Neural tuning curves are important for understanding the function of the ear. They are directly related to the frequency tuning of the cochlea and show that one single nerve will respond best to one frequency (characteristic frequency), but is more easily stimulated by tones of lower than characteristic frequency than by those with frequencies above characteristic frequency. This is directly related to the asymmetry of the traveling wave envelope, which gradually builds to its maximum amplitude, then quickly dies once it passes the point of maximal displacement.

In preparation for later readings, it is helpful to introduce a few more terms. This discussion has focused on single-unit recordings of one nerve's action potential. The response of a group of neurons, or the entire nerve, can also be measured. The **compound action potential** is measured from **whole nerve recordings**.

SUMMARY

The hair cell membranes and nerve cell membranes allow the chemistry inside and outside a cell to differ. The differing electrical charges inside versus outside the cell

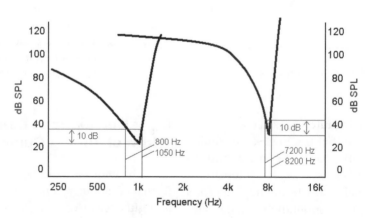

Figure 21–13. The method of calculating the $Q_{10\,dB}$ for tuning curves is illustrated. Threshold at characteristic frequency is noted. The experimenter measures the range of frequencies that excite the neuron when the signal level is 10 dB higher than threshold. The characteristic frequency is divided by this difference number. For example, the 1000-Hz neuron is responding to frequencies from 800 to 1050 Hz, so the $Q_{10\,dB}$ is 1000/250, or 4. The 8000-Hz neuron responds over a range of 1000 Hz, and has a $Q_{10\,dB}$ of 8.

create the potential for electrochemical polarity change within the cell.

The hair cell receptor potentials are the summating potential and the cochlear microphonic. The hair cells are tuned so that the summating potential of the inner hair cell changes when the frequency of the stimulus is near that cell's characteristic frequency. In contrast, cochlear microphonics show the result of the ciliary shearing of the inner and outer hair cells, but do not directly reflect whether the hair cell is releasing neurotransmitter.

Neural action potentials are created when the neuron absorbs sufficient glutamate, released from the bottom of the hair cell. These spikes of activity travel down the axon, and permit the release of neurotransmitter to the second-order neuron.

Auditory neurons are also tuned, as are hair cells. There is a limited range of frequencies that create the neural firing. The neuron's tuning curve shows which frequencies, at what intensity, will create a firing of the single nerve cell at a level above the spontaneous firing rate. The tip of the tuning curve points to the characteristic frequency of the neuron. The tuning curve shape shows the upward spread of excitation—a given neuron can be stimulated by a frequency that is lower than characteristic frequency if the signal intensity is loud enough. It is much harder for the neuron to fire in response to a signal frequency higher than its characteristic frequency.

A neuron that is firing to a low-intensity characteristic frequency signal will change its firing pattern when a loud, lower than characteristic frequency sound is present. In that case, the firing pattern results from the loud low-frequency sound. The signal at characteristic frequency is no longer encoded or heard. This is called the upward spread of masking.

Understanding upward spread of masking is a key physiologic concept. It shows understanding of traveling wave mechanics. It also is useful clinically, as in many situations, loud, low-frequency sound will mask the audibility of quiet high-frequency sounds. Patients with high-frequency hearing loss have upward spread of masking problems, often to an even greater degree than normal hearers. The later chapters on psychoacoustics will discuss that concept.

REFERENCES

Durrant, J. D., & Lovrinic, J. H. (1984). *Bases of hearing science* (2nd ed.). Baltimore: Williams & Wilkins.

Santos-Sacchi, J. (2001). Cochlear physiology. In A. F. Jahn & J. Santos-Sacchi, (Eds.), *Physiology of the ear*, (2nd ed.). San Diego, CA: Singular Thompson Learning.

22

How Frequency and Intensity Information Is Encoded by VIIIth Nerve Fibers

At this point, the reader would probably accept two fundamental points about neural encoding of frequency and intensity. First, you know that the cochlea is tonotopically organized, so it will make sense that different frequency sounds stimulate different regions and cause different neurons to fire. This is referred to as the "**place**" theory of frequency encoding. However, Chapters 20 and 21 discussed that place alone is not enough to encode frequency. A loud, low-frequency pure tone can stimulate a neuron that is at the base of the cochlea.

Second, you understand the change in size of the traveling wave with sound intensity, and how this creates movement on the basilar membrane in a broader area. You also know that more intense sound creates more ciliary shearing, and thus more neurotransmitter release. Let's explore this further. Consider the neurotransmitter released by one inner hair cell, and recall that multiple nerve fibers are connected to that inner hair cell. The greater release of neurotrans-

mitter increases the likelihood that those neurons attached to the single inner hair cell will fire.

You also have seen in Chapter 21 that there is a spread of excitation of energy on the basilar membrane when the signal increases, and that most of that spread is toward the base. So, the louder the signal, the larger the area in which neurons are firing. Those areas toward the cochlea base are more readily activated than areas more toward the low-frequency apex.

As you read this chapter, hold onto these two concepts. Frequency encoding is related to place, although not just place, and intensity encoding is related to the number of individual nerve fibers that are firing. The purpose of this chapter is to expand on how frequency and intensity are encoded, and solve part of the puzzle—how can frequency be encoded if one neuron is capable of responding to a variety of different pitch sounds? The answer will be that the firing *pattern* of the neuron differs depending on the frequency of the stimulus.

RATE OF FIRING OF ONE NEURON INCREASES AS THE STIMULUS FREQUENCY APPROACHES CHARACTERISTIC FREQUENCY

Chapter 21 introduced the neural tuning curve, an outline of the frequencies and intensities that cause a neuron to fire faster than its spontaneous firing rate. As the physiologist is presenting swept pure tones (pure tones that change gradually in frequency) at one intensity, recall that she or he monitors the rate of the neural firing. The tuning curve showed which frequencies are creating a firing at a rate faster than the spontaneous discharge rate, but additional information can be obtained from the experiment. The actual rate of discharge can be measured at different frequencies. For example, Figure 22–1 illustrates the hypothetical neural discharge rates recorded for a neuron that fires spontaneously 20 times per second. As frequency approaches characteristic frequency, the discharge rate increases. It reaches a peak firing rate of 70 per second, then, as frequency exceeds characteristic frequency, the rate of discharge falls rapidly. Expanding on this idea, Figure 22–2 graphs the firing rate increase a

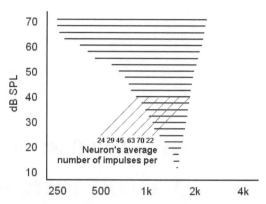

Figure 22–1. Illustration of the type of data that can be recorded while developing a neural tuning curve. The neuron's actual average firing rate is measured as the frequency that is presented is changed. Although spontaneous firing rate of this neuron is 20 firings per second, when the signal reaches approximately 900 Hz, the firing speeds up to an average of 24 firings per second. The neuron's firing rate continues to increase until the stimulus presented is 1700 Hz, at which point the average firing rate of the neuron is 70 per second. Note that the neuron's characteristic frequency is 1700 Hz, and it is at this frequency that the most rapid firing rate occurs. Increasing signal frequency above 1700 Hz causes the rate of neural firing to drop.

second way. The height of the curve illustrates the amount of increase in firing rate.

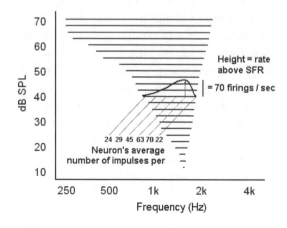

Figure 22–2. The curve height represents the amount of increase in firing rate of the neuron as a tone of a given intensity is presented at different frequencies.

DIFFERENT COMBINATIONS OF FREQUENCY AND INTENSITY CAN CREATE THE SAME OVERALL NUMBER OF NEURAL DISCHARGES PER SECOND

Figure 22-3 illustrates two concepts. First, different combinations of frequency and intensity can elicit the same average firing rate. In Figure 22-3, tones at 55 dB SPL / 750 Hz and at 40 dB SPL/1100 Hz each create the same average firing rate, measured in impulses per second. The second important concept is that, regardless of the signal frequency, increasing that frequency's intensity will increase the firing rate.

The major concept that Figure 22-3 illustrates is that firing rate alone is not enough to encode the frequency/intensity. Different intensity tones can create the same overall firing rate, if the frequencies are different. Moreover, as you know, different frequency sounds can cause firing of one single neuron. So knowing which neuron is firing, and even knowing that neuron's firing rate in spikes per second, would not be enough to know the stimulus's frequency and intensity. However, it remains true that increasing intensity while keeping the frequency the same will increase the neuron's firing rate.

Figure 22-4 has a different vertical axis than used in the prior figures. Rather than the *y*-axis being intensity of the pure tone, it is now the neuron's firing rate. This view shows **frequency response curves.** Keep in mind that both Figures 22-3 and 22-4 are

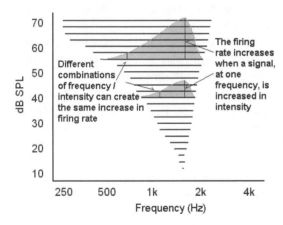

Figure 22–3. Height of the curves indicates the firing rate (as an increase above the neuron's spontaneous discharge rate). Different combinations of pure tone frequency and intensity elicit the same overall firing rate. When intensity increases, as frequency is held constant, the firing rate increases.

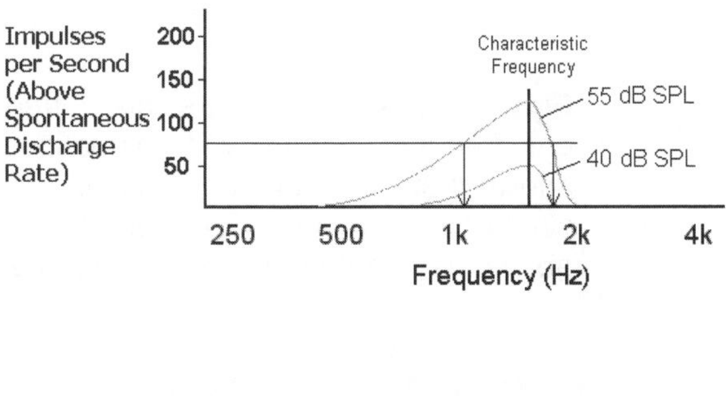

Figure 22–4. Two frequency response curves are shown. This illustrates that when sweeping frequency at one intensity, the neural firing rate increases as characteristic frequency is approached. It also shows that the average firing rate is higher for any signal frequency if the signal intensity increases. The same overall rate, for example, 75 impulses per second, occurred at two different frequencies when the pure tone intensity was 55 dB SPL. Both a frequency just above 1000 Hz and one just below 2000 Hz created this firing rate.

illustrating the response of a single neuron. The firing rate of the neuron increases gradually approaching characteristic frequency, where the rate will be the highest for any given intensity of stimulation, then the rate falls sharply as frequency is increased. Note that the firing rate increases as intensity increases, but that it is possible to obtain a given firing rate, such as 75 impulses per second, with different combinations of frequency/intensity pure tones.

Figure 22–5 provides yet another opportunity to illustrate the point that the firing rate alone is not enough to provide specific information about signal intensity/frequency. It again also illustrates the point that the number of discharges (spikes) per second will increase with signal intensity if you maintain the frequency.

PROBLEMS WITH THE THEORY THAT FREQUENCY IS ENCODED BY RATE OF DISCHARGE

Since the discovery of the traveling wave's gradual increase in amplitude as the wave travels base to apex, it was realized that place alone is not enough to encode frequency. Any one place on the basilar membrane could be stimulated by a variety of different frequencies. Therefore, other theories of how frequency is encoded were developed. An early theory of frequency encoding was that the rate of discharge conveyed

this information. The most simplistic explanation used in this **frequency theory,** also called the **telephone theory,** would be that if the frequency is 100 Hz, then the neuron fires 100 times per second. A 1000-Hz signal would create 1000 firings per second, and so on. However, the refractory period of the neuron prevents this means of encoding. Auditory neurons can't fire faster than perhaps 1000 or 2000 times per second, yet humans can hear sounds as high as 20,000 Hz.

A modification to this theory was the **volley theory**. It proposed that different neurons would take turns firing to the peak of each wave. In a simple explanation of this theory, we could suppose that there were 10 neurons located at the place on the basilar membrane for encoding 10,000 Hz. As each neuron can fire up to 1000 times per second, neuron one would fire first, and then the second cycle of the 10,000 Hz tone would stimulate neuron two, and so on. After neuron 10 took its turn encoding the signal, neuron one would come back into play. Some portions of this theory are true. Different neurons do respond to the peaks of a sound wave, and not all neurons fire in response to each cycle. However, the simplest version of the volley theory has some serious problems. How would a neuron "know" not to fire until the ninth cycle? Why wouldn't they all start firing in response to the first cycle? And more importantly, how would intensity be coded? If there were 10 neurons, each firing to every tenth wave peak, there would be no way to increase the neural firings when the intensity increased.

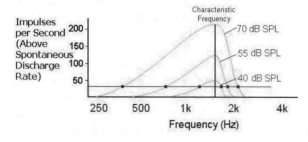

Figure 22–5. There are six different frequency/intensity combinations shown that would create a firing of this single nerve at 30 spikes per second above the spontaneous discharge rate.

PATTERN OF NEURAL DISCHARGE ENCODES FREQUENCY AND INTENSITY

As you know from Chapter 20, there are about 30,000 neurons per ear. At any single place on the basilar membrane, there are a number of neurons that can be stimulated. In the previous chapter, it was mentioned that neurons have different spontaneous firing characteristics—some are spontaneously firing faster, and these neurons respond to lower intensity signals.

Let's propose that at some given location on basilar membrane, nine auditory neurons are connected to a single inner hair cell. That hair cell is tuned to 1000 Hz, and the sound presented to the ear is 1000 Hz. Let's assume that three neurons have low spontaneous firing rates, three have mid, and three have high spontaneous firing rates. In our example, let's further assume that the intensity of the signal is loud enough that even the low spontaneous firing rate neurons are

being excited by the 1000-Hz tone. The low, mid, and high spontaneous discharge rate neurons will be firing with different overall rates. As illustrated in Figure 22-6, those neurons with high discharge rates are firing faster in response to this sound than those with mid or low discharge rates. Note that the spikes tend to occur around the time when the pure tone reaches its peak. In this illustration, one or more of the nine neurons has fired in response to each cycle of the wave. The neurons do not fire in the pattern theorized by the simplistic volley theory. Whether or not a firing occurs around the time of the pure tone peak is determined by whether that cycle of the wave has made the hair cell secrete enough neurotransmitter to excite that neuron.

In reality, not all neurons within a group are equal in their responsivity—for example, not all high spontaneous discharge rate neurons are firing at the exact same rate, which means that one might be more prone to firing in response to stimulation than the next neuron. This is what creates the differenc-

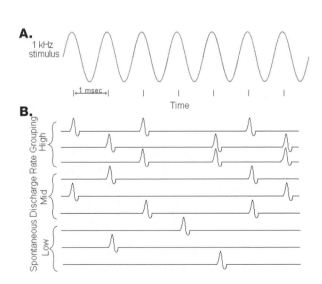

Figure 22–6. A. The 1000-Hz sine wave that is presented to the ear is illustrated. Presume that the signal is stimulating 1000-Hz hair cells and is loud enough to innervate the neurons with 1000-Hz characteristic frequencies. **B**. The discharge pattern across time of nine 1000-Hz characteristic frequency neurons is sketched. The "blips" on the horizontal line represent action potentials. There are three neurons in each spontaneous discharge rate grouping: low, mid, and high. The high spontaneous discharge rate neurons will fire more often in response to the signal. Note that when observing across these nine fibers, one or more neurons is firing to each wave peak. The brain thus can receive a neural signal each time the sine wave reaches 90 degrees of phase.

es in the neural firing between neighboring neurons, even those that fall loosely into a category (low, mid, or high discharge rates).

For this text, we will refer to the type of firing illustrated in Figure 22-6 as firing "in phase" with the signal peaks. That does not imply that the firing occurs to each peak, but when a firing occurs, it is likely to occur at or near the peak of the signal.

What happens if intensity increases? In Figure 22-6, typically three of the nine neurons discharged to each cycle of the pure tone, though for some wave peaks fewer neurons fired in phase with the signal peak. Figure 22-7 shows what might happen to the firing of these same neurons when the pure tone intensity increases. The discharge rate of the individual neurons increases; for each cycle of the wave four or more neurons are activated. Notice now that there is little difference in the firing rates of the low versus high spontaneous rate neurons—both are firing at almost their maximum rate. The careful observer will note that the action potentials in Figure 22-7B are not invariably at the wave peaks. Sufficient neurotransmitter may be present before the sound reaches 90 degrees of phase—before the cilia are fully

deflected toward stria vascularis—allowing for an earlier firing. Sometimes the neuron needs extra time to absorb neurotransmitter and the neuron fires a bit late.

Return to the Digital System Analogy

Chapter 7 discussed digital systems. The neuron is analogous to a one-bit coding system in that each neuron can only say "on" or "off"; either an action potential occurs or it does not. Furthermore, the absolute refractory period of the neuron limits its "sampling rate."

If a neuron can only fire once per millisecond, and there are 100 nerve fibers encoding that place on the basilar membrane, then the maximum number of neural firings the brain can "see" per second is 100,000 (1000 times per second times 100 neurons). These firings will occur not randomly; rather, the firing will be clustered around 1-msec intervals. The neurons will tend to fire in phase with the sine wave reaching 90 degrees of phase. As the acoustic signal strength lessens, the timing of the clusters

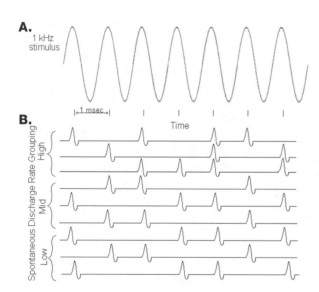

Figure 22–7. A. The stimulus level is higher than Figure 22-6. **B**. The increase in the intensity of the signal causes any given neuron to fire more often, though generally still at or near the peak of the sine wave. Overall, in response to any given cycle of the stimulus, more of these hypothetical nine neurons are firing.

of nerve firings is still once per msec, but at any given time, fewer neurons would be firing. The brain would receive a fewer total number of impulses per second.

WHOLE NERVE POTENTIALS VERSUS SINGLE NERVE POTENTIALS TO SINGLE PURE TONES

Assume that the measuring electrode is not in one single neuron. In this next hypothetical experiment we are not doing **single unit recordings**, but rather **whole nerve potential recordings.** The electrode is placed either near the nerve path, or even on the surface of the skull. When a group of nerves fire simultaneously, the electrochemical activity will diffuse through the brain tissues and will reach the recording electrode. (The activity at that electrode needs to be referenced to [compared to] the electrochemical charge somewhere else, so we need to place a second, reference electrode elsewhere on the surface of the skull or in the central nervous system to make the recordings in this experiment.)

When measuring the whole nerve potential to a soft sound, few neural units are firing and the size of the whole nerve potential is small. However, if many neurons are together firing in response to a loud sound, then the amplitude of this potential, measured in **far field,** is greater. The brain could be thought of as a final stage detector of this **compound action potential**. It is able to abstract the signal frequency from the periodicity of the firing, as well as from knowing, in general, which neurons (by tonotopic organization characteristics) are firing. ("Abstract" means to figure out from the available information. Just as an abstract art painting is not an exact image of the object, but the viewer knows what the image

represents, the brain is going to deduce the original sound from a representation of the sound in the form of the neural code. Thus, we say the brain "abstracts" the information.) The size of the compound action potential (how many neurons are firing to each cycle of the wave) provides information on intensity.

LIMITS ON A NEURON'S FIRING "IN PHASE" WITH SIGNALS

Can *a single neuron* phase-lock to a signal that is not at the neuron's characteristic frequency? Yes, but only within limits. If the signal is up to one-half octave higher in frequency than the neuron's characteristic frequency (the traveling wave peaks more toward the base), phase-locking is possible. Pure tones with traveling waves that peak more apically are better able to recruit neurons into phase-locking. The tone can be 1 octave lower and still the neuron will phase-lock to it (Figure 22–8).

Careful reading is required here. The paragraph above referred to the frequencies to which a *single nerve* will phase-lock. Figure 22–9 reviews this in a *different perspective*—from the view of *which neurons* are phase-locking to a given signal. Those neurons with characteristic frequencies one-half octave lower (located apically from the signal peak) and those with characteristic frequencies 1 octave higher are phase-locking. (Recall that, here, phase-locking does not mean responding to each cycle, but when responding, the neuron fires at or near signal peaks.)

Neurons can be stimulated to fire faster than their spontaneous discharge rate by sounds that are even further away in frequency. However, if the stimuli are more than one-half octave above or 1 octave below the neuron's characteristic frequency, the firing rate is not in synchrony to the

Clinical Correlate: What the Auditory Brainstem Response Measures and How the Auditory Steady-State Response Differs

The reader might hope that the conclusion of this section was that, clinically, we can tell when the auditory system is encoding a sound of 1000 Hz because we can record a single wave that pulses 1000 times per second, and that gets larger when the intensity increases. If you could make a whole nerve recording near a single area of the neuron, this is more or less true. However, the neural signal ascends the auditory system. When recorded from far field, as done in auditory electrophysiologic testing, we can't measure just one nerve. For example, after the VIIIth nerve fires, the second order neurons at cochlear nucleus will fire. The response from one nerve and that from one higher in the auditory system creates a jumble of the response—multiple neural responses overlap in time. When testing clinically, we can use a brief signal and we can observe the neural response over time, as it ascends the auditory pathway, but we can't record information about the firing pattern.

Perhaps it should be mentioned that one technique does allow some information about the firing pattern. Auditory steady-state recordings use pure tones that rapidly change in intensity. In essence, they pulse on and off. The link between the pulsing rate and the firing rate can be measured. However, we aren't measuring the firings at the actual stimulus frequency.

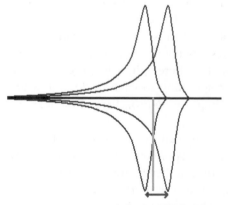

A neuron at this location
can phase-lock to signals
1/2 octave higher to 1 octave lower
in frequency than its CF

Figure 22–8. The vertical line shows the location of a single neuron. Two pure tones that are at the frequency limits for that neuron to be able to fire in response to the pure tone wave peaks (to phase-lock) are shown. Pure tones that peak more apical or more toward the base would either not stimulate the neuron, or would cause it to fire in a random pattern. A given neuron can phase lock when the pure tone frequency is up to one-half octave higher (peaks more basalward) or up to 1 octave lower (peaking more toward the apex.)

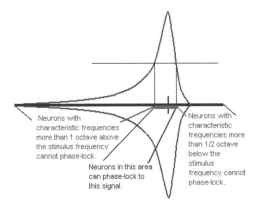

Figure 22–9. An intense sound creates phase-locking of neurons that are close to the peak of the traveling wave. Neurons with characteristic frequencies up to 1 octave higher (located toward the base of the cochlea) and one-half octave lower in their characteristic frequency (located more toward the apex) can phase-lock their responses to wave peaks (fire at integer intervals of the wave period).

stimulus—the firing pattern is random. The firing pattern of these neurons, then, does not aid in encoding frequency; however, the fact that these neurons are firing may indicate to the central nervous system that the signal is intense.

MASKING OF ONE SOUND BY A SECOND SOUND

The process of masking occurs when one sound cannot be encoded by the neurons because a stronger stimulus is triggering the firing of these same neurons. Take the case illustrated in Figure 22–10. If the low-intensity signal, creating the traveling wave that is filled in, were presented alone, in quiet, then the mid-frequency characteristic frequency neurons near the wave peak would phase-lock to encode this low-intensity sound. The simultaneous presence of the louder, lower frequency signal masks the less intense signal. The mid-frequency neurons that were responding to the softer signal are now firing in a random fashion, but at a rate above their normal spontaneous discharge rate. In this case, these mid-frequency neurons would not phase-lock to the louder tone's period, because the loud, low-frequency sound is not near those neurons' characteristic frequencies. The fact that the mid-frequency neurons are made to fire

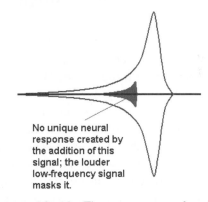

Figure 22–10. The presence of a louder pure tone masks perception of the softer signal when the traveling wave of the louder signal completely envelopes the softer sound's traveling wave. The neurons that would encode the softer signal's presence are "busy" responding to the more intense signal, and do not change their firing patterns in response to the addition of the softer pure tone.

randomly in response to the louder sound means that those neurons cannot phase-lock to the quieter sound (the one at the neuron's characteristic frequency) and therefore the quieter sound is masked. This illustrates upward, or basal-ward, spread of masking. The high frequency tone is masked by the low-frequency tone—or said a bit differently, the masking effect of the low-frequency tone spreads upward to the high frequencies.

Can a high-frequency tone mask a low-frequency sound? Yes, but that's harder to do, given the shape of the traveling wave. Only signals that peak just a bit more apically than the masker tone can be masked (Figure 22–11).

POSTSTIMULUS TIME HISTOGRAMS OBTAINED WHEN STIMULATING THE EAR WITH CLICKS AND THE CONCEPT OF PREFERRED INTERVALS

There is a way to determine a neuron's characteristic frequency without obtaining the neuron's tuning curve. This experiment is not done using pure tones. Instead, clicks are used. Clicks are very brief-duration square waves—that is, very short duration pulses of direct current sent to an earphone. Click signals sound like the snapping of your fingers, or the tapping of a pen on a table. On spectral analysis clicks are shown to contain energy across the frequency spectrum. The traveling wave from a click starts at the base and progresses to the apex. The basilar membrane is deflected up and down along its whole length. Each neuron along the way can be stimulated, if the click is loud enough. If the signal is loud, the basilar membrane will continue to oscillate for a few milliseconds, even though the brief tone pulse has ended -- the principle that a body in motion tends to remain in motion until an external force acts on it applies in this case. The moving basilar membrane will oscillate until the membrane's mass, stiffness, and friction forces damp the vibration. Thus, the neurons beneath the basilar membrane may not fire just once; they may fire a second or third time as well.

The experiment to find the neuron's characteristic frequency using clicks is set up

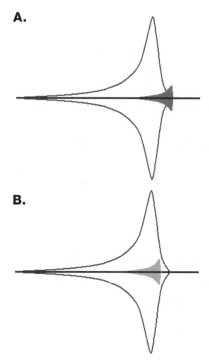

Figure 22–11. A. The shaded pure-tone traveling wave is not within the envelope of the louder, higher frequency sound's traveling wave. Masking does not occur. **B.** Here the lower intensity pure tone is masked. It is possible to mask a tone with one that is higher in frequency, as long as the masking tone is intense and the frequency to be masked is not much lower than that of the stimulus doing the masking.

as follows. A needle electrode is inserted into one single neuron and a click is presented. Sometimes, just one single action potential will be recorded. Sometimes, a second or a third firing occurs (Figure 22–12). Researchers will record the firing of one neuron, not just to one click, but also to many clicks, presented one at a time. They will note how often the firings of the neuron occurred, and the times at which they occurred. The first firing in response to the acoustic click occurs not immediately after presentation, but after a brief amount of time has passed. The latency of the firing (time between stimulus

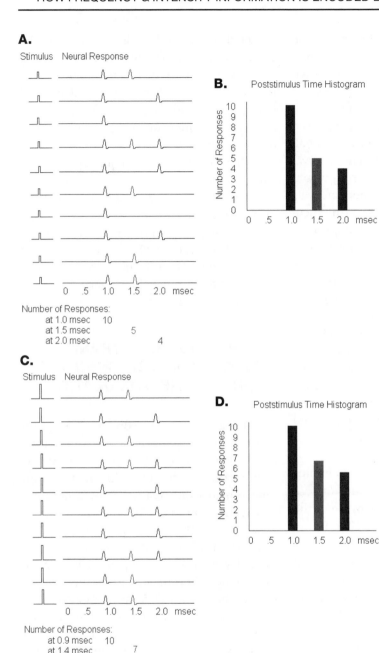

A.

Stimulus   Neural Response

0   .5   1.0   1.5   2.0   msec

Number of Responses:
at 1.0 msec   10
at 1.5 msec   5
at 2.0 msec   4

B. Poststimulus Time Histogram

Number of Responses

0   .5   1.0   1.5   2.0   msec

C.

Stimulus   Neural Response

0   .5   1.0   1.5   2.0   msec

Number of Responses:
at 0.9 msec   10
at 1.4 msec   7
at 1.9 msec   6

D. Poststimulus Time Histogram

Number of Responses

0   .5   1.0   1.5   2.0   msec

Figure 22–12. Construction of a poststimulus time histogram. **A.** A click stimulus is presented 10 times to one neuron, which is monitored using a needle electrode. The time at which the action potentials occur is noted. **B.** The results are tallied and displayed in the form of a histogram. The interval between firings on the poststimulus time histogram is the neuron's preferred interval—for example, the difference between 1.5 msec and 2.0 msec is 0.5 msec. This hypothetical neuron will fire in increments of 0.5 msec when stimulated by a broadband signal, such as the click. **C.** The intensity of the click stimulus has increased. Note that the latency of the initial firing is slightly shorter. The interval between firing times remains increments of 0.5 msec. **D.** The poststimulus histogram shows that there were more neural firings when the intensity increased. Adapted from the work of Gulick, Gescheider, and Frisina (1989).

and the action potential) is dictated by the travel time on the basilar membrane and the time required for the neuron to absorb the neurotransmitter. Thus, high-frequency neurons will fire with a shorter latency than low-frequency neurons.

The second and/or third firing of the neuron does not happen immediately after the first firing—as one would expect given neural refractory periods. Rather, the firing occurs after a pause. Figure 22–12 illustrates this. By examining the time between the intervals at which the neuron has been noted to have fired, we see that neuron's preferred timing pattern. The neuron shown in Figure 22–12 has a firing latency of 1.0 msec. The interval between the initial firing and the next firing is again either 0.5 msec or 1.0 msec (not illustrated, but it could also be 1.5, 2.0, 2.5 msec. . .). The interval between the second and third firing would also be 0.5 or 1.0 msec (or other intervals with 0.5-msec increments). Thus, this neuron prefers to fire at intervals that are multiples of 0.5 msec. We say that its **preferred interval** is therefore 0.5 msec. A sine wave that has a period of 0.5 msec has a frequency of 2000 Hz. The characteristic frequency of this neuron is 2000 Hz. If it were stimulated with a 2000-Hz pure tone, it would fire in response in increments of 0.5 msec (e.g., firing once, then perhaps 1.0 msec after, then again perhaps in 1.5 msec, then 2.5 msec later, 1.0 msec later, etc.—always with pauses that can be divided by 0.5 msec). If a neural tuning curve for this neuron were obtained, the tip would point to 2000 Hz.

Figure 22–12B shows a poststimulus time histogram obtained from the experiment's results. It shows how many times the neuron fired, measured at which time intervals. The timing is relative to the presentation of each click. In this example, each time the click was presented, there was a neural firing at 1.0 msec. Therefore, the poststimulus time histogram bar at 1.0 msec has a height of 10. There were five neural firings that occurred 1.5 msec after the presentation of the signal, and 4 at 2.0 msec after the stimulus, which gives the heights of the other two bars. When examining a poststimulus time histogram, look at the time *between* the bars to determine the preferred interval. The first bar shows the neuron's latency, whereas the spacing between subsequent bars tells the preferred interval. Note in Figures 22-12C and 22-12D that

the click intensity has increased. This decreases the initial latency of the neural firing. The time between the histogram bars remains unchanged: the preferred interval is unchanged. Note that this increase in intensity causes more second and third firings of the neuron.

The characteristic frequency is found using this formula:

1/preferred interval in msec × 1000 msec/1 second = characteristic frequency. In this example, the preferred interval is 0.5 msec. 1/0.5 × 1000 = 2000 Hz. Of course, the period of 2000 Hz is 0.5 msec, so it is equally correct to consider the preferred interval the period of the characteristic frequency.

PERIOD HISTOGRAMS: HISTOGRAMS OBTAINED WITH PURE-TONE STIMULATION

It is also possible to obtain a histogram of neural firing patterns using a pure-tone signal. This type of plot is called a **period histogram.** In this experiment, the pure tone remains on. Again, a single neuron's activity is monitored. As shown in Figure 22–13, rather than tallying the time of the firing from the start of the signal, we tally the delay *between* subsequent firings. Note that the neuron is firing with delays that are integer multiples of 0.5 msec. The time between the histogram bars is 0.5 msec. That provides information on the frequency of the signal creating the neural firing. The period of 0.5 msec is 2000 Hz, which is the stimulus frequency. It is not correct to say that is the neuron's preferred interval, or to say that 2000 Hz is this neuron's characteristic frequency. Remember that a neuron can "phase-lock" to a variety of frequency signals (i.e., the neuron can phase-lock to a signal up to 1 octave lower in frequency or one-half octave higher), so the time be-

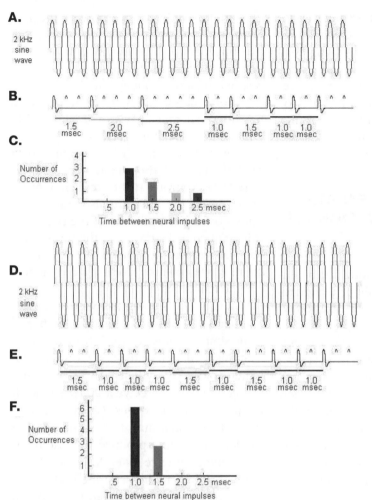

Figure 22–13. Histograms for a single neuron. **A.** The signal is an ongoing 2000-Hz pure tone. **B.** The signal triggers an action potential initially, and then another after a delay of 1.5 msec, then another after another 2-msec pause, and so forth. (The latency of the first firing is not shown.) **C.** The number of times when a given time delay was observed between firings is tallied, creating a histogram. **D.** The signal intensity increases, but frequency remains the same. **E.** The time between firings tends to be shorter. **F.** The histogram reflects the more frequent firings at shorter intervals. The time between bars remains equal to the stimulus frequency period. Adapted from the work of Gulick, Gescheider, and Frisina (1989).

tween the histogram bars tells us the signal period, but not necessarily the neuron's preferred interval. Increasing the signal intensity causes the neuron to fire with less delay (with a shorter latency). The period histogram shows more firing occurrences at the lower delay times.

REVIEW OF THE RESPONSE OF THE VIIITH NERVE TO PURE TONES

In review, the VIIIth nerve fibers will respond to a pure tone after a certain la-

tency, which is greater for lower frequency sounds, due to the traveling wave delay, and which is slightly longer for low-intensity sounds. Each neuron does not fire to the peak of each sound wave, but rather fires to some percentage of the peaks. One or more neurons fires to each sound wave peak, so the period of the signal can be abstracted. Increasing intensity increases the average firing rate of single neural units—they "skip" fewer cycles between firings. Additionally, more neurons will fire as the intensity is increased due to the spread of excitation on the basilar membrane. Because of the shape of the traveling wave, the increased intensity would particularly cause more neurons located toward the base of the cochlea to fire.

The phase-locking of neural firing does not always occur. If the signal is too far different from the neuron's characteristic frequency, either the neuron will not fire, or the firing pattern will be random, rather than firing pattern being at intervals that are multiples of the signal period.

RESPONSE OF THE VIIITH NERVE TO COMPLEX SIGNALS

When two or more frequencies are present in the same ear, either both can be encoded, or one can be partially or completely masked by the second sound. Additional combination tones may also be perceived.

If the signal has multiple frequency components, the traveling wave will peak at multiple different locations. The cochlea acts as a spectral analyzer. Neurons near each peak will encode sound by firing at multiples of the sound wave period. If one examines the firing of all the VIIIth nerve fibers, there would be some nerves that are firing synchronously with the period of each of the sound waves. For example, an ear is stimulated by two equally intense pure tones, one at 500 Hz and one at 2000 Hz. This complex sound wave creates two peaks to the traveling wave—one nearer the base, one nearer the apex. There are neurons at the base firing each 0.5 msec. Not all neurons fire each 0.5 msec, of course; rather, some fire at one 0.5-msec increment, others at the next 0.5-msec increment, and so forth. Additionally, there are neurons nearer the apex firing. Any single neuron located near the 500-Hz wave traveling peak is firing in intervals that are multiples of 2 msec, and one or more of those neurons fires each 2 msec. Therefore the listener perceives both tones.

If one sound is significantly louder than another, and the traveling wave for the loud-er sound completely overpowers the traveling wave from the less intense tone, then masking occurs. The less intense sound is not heard because the neurons are instead responding to the louder sound.

Combination tones, for example the cubic difference tone, may also be audible. The cubic difference tone is calculated by taking the lower frequency (F1) and multiplying by 2, then subtracting the higher frequency tone (F2). Neurons at the frequency of the cubic difference tone are also responding, phase-locking to multiples of the period for this frequency. Likewise, in the healthy ear, hair cells at this location are active, and are creating a backward traveling wave, an otoacoustic emission.

If you are listening to two frequencies, another type of distortion that may be audible is the simple difference tone. For example, if listening to 100 Hz and 120 Hz, presented simultaneously, you will hear those two tones, and additionally perceive a 20-Hz sound. In Chapter 4 on sine waves, Figure 4-12 illustrated how combining two waves that are similar in frequency produces a "periodicity" that is the difference tone. How does the cochlea "resolve" a complex tone such as this one? This complex wave (Figure 4-12B), also shown in Figure 22–14A vibrates the stapes footplate and creates pressure waves in the cochlea. The basilar membrane creates three different traveling waves simultaneously, as illustrated in Figure 22–14B. Neurons at the locations of the peaks of the traveling wave will fire in phase with these different traveling wave peaks (Figures 22–14 C and D). The ear will detect all three tones.

Additional Information Is Obtained from Early and Late Neural Firings

Figure 22-14 and others in this chapter are unrealistic in the degree to which

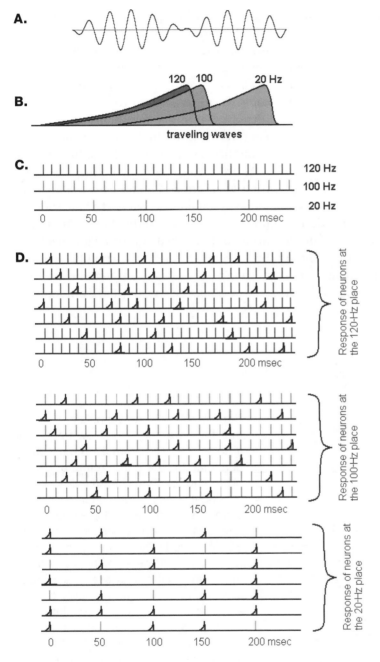

Figure 22–14. The complex sound illustrated in (**A**) is broken down into three different traveling waves, illustrated in (**B**). In (**C**) the period of the three constituent sine waves is illustrated. The traveling wave from the difference tone is 20 Hz and basilar membrane up and down motion at that location has a period of 50 msec. A traveling wave originates from the 100-Hz component; 100 Hz has a period of 10 msec. The 120-Hz component has a period of 8.33 msec. **D.** Assume that 7 neurons at each of the three locations of the traveling wave peaks are monitored for 250 msec. Note that neurons at each location are phase-locking to the driving signal's period. These groups of neurons are phase-locking differently, and are located in different areas within the VIIIth nerve bundle (because of the tonotopic organization of the cochlea.)

the neural discharges phase-lock just to the 90-degree phase portion of the sine wave. In reality, the proportion of the neurons that fire earlier and later than at 90 degrees is proportional to the amplitude of the sine wave at that phase angle. For example, when the sound is at 45 degrees, the sine wave amplitude is 0.707 the size of the sine wave at 90 degrees. The neural firings that occur when the sound is at 45 degrees phase are occurring at 0.707 times the rate that occurs when the pure tone reaches 90 degrees of phase. For example, if 10 neurons fire when the sine wave reaches 90 phase, then there are about seven neurons firing when the neuron reaches 45 degrees of phase. However, the firings only occur for one phase of the wave. The only firings that occur when the sound is at 180 to 360 degrees are just those that would occur spontaneously. This is illustrated in Figure 22–15.

SUMMARY

The neural firing patterns, across a group of neurons, are used to encode frequency and intensity. The pattern of firing mimics the stimulus, allowing the central nervous system to encode frequency. Specifically, for each wave peak, neurons with characteristic frequencies at and near the signal frequency are firing. There are nerves firing to each cycle of the stimulus, although any single neuron is not firing to each wave peak. There will be more neurons firing to each wave peak when the signal intensity increases. Information about whether the neurons firing are high, mid, or low spontaneous firing rate units, and whether the neurons are firing randomly or in phase with the signal, are additional cues available for intensity encoding. That is, if a loud sound is present, not only will there be a high rate of firing for individual neurons with characteristic frequencies near the stimulus frequency, but other neurons, located farther from the traveling wave peak (that cannot phase-

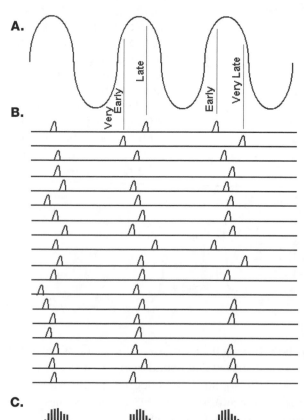

Figure 22–15. A. Stimulus: Assume that this is a very loud, low-frequency tone so that we can make the assumption that the neuron's refractory period is shorter than the stimulus period making it possible for a neuron to fire to each wave peak. B. Multiple neurons at one location on the basilar membrane are observed. The firing times, relative to the peak of the stimulus, are noted. Although most firings are near 90 degrees of phase, some fire early or late, and a few fire very early or very late. C. If this experiment is repeated using many neurons, and the timing of the firings is noted with histograms, it can be seen that the proportion of the firings that are early or late is similar to the relative amplitude of the wave at this phase. Firings do not occur for the rarefaction phase of the wave. The nervous system can use the information on the relative time of firings of the neurons to more precisely determine stimulus characteristics.

lock to the sound), will be firing randomly, providing a cue that the signal is intense.

When clicks are presented to the ear, the neurons respond by each firing at their preferred intervals. Although a click is a short-duration stimulus, neurons frequently fire more than once, and when they do, the repeated firings are at increments of the period of the characteristic frequency. Increasing the intensity of a click signal will result in more neural firings. There will be more firings initially as more neurons are activated, and there will be a higher number of second and subsequent firings of the neurons.

REFERENCE

Gulick, W. L., Gescheider, G. A., & Frisina, R. D. (1989). *Hearing: Physiological acoustics, neural coding and psycahoacoustics*. New York: Oxford University Press.

23

The Efferent Auditory System

To this point, the anatomy and physiology section of this text has focused on how the acoustic signal is converted into mechanical energy, processed by the cochlea, and encoded by the auditory system. In this chapter, the mechanisms by which higher central nervous system structures effect the transmission or encoding of the auditory signal are overviewed. These descending, or **efferent, pathways** serve to reduce the strength of the signal—they "turn down the volume." They may also improve hearing in noise ability. This chapter introduces the efferent pathways from central nervous system to the ear, and the pathway for the acoustic reflex is described.

OLIVOCOCHLEAR BUNDLE

The best known of the descending nervous system pathways is the **olivocochlear bundle** also called **Rasmussen's bundle**. As the name implies, the origin of these nerve fibers is in the area near the superior olive, and these fibers terminate in the cochlea. There are two general sections of the olivocochlear bundle, named for the location of their origination: the medial and lateral efferent systems. Figure 23-1 diagrams the connections for these pathways. The ef-

ferent system releases acetylcholine and other neurotransmitters that have inhibitory effects (e.g., GABA) from its terminal buttons.

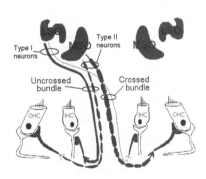

Figure 23–1. Schematic of the efferent system. Type II nerve fibers of the medial system terminate at the outer hair cells (OHCs), where they act to reduce the active mechanism. These fibers are myelinated, which is schematically represented with the lines that look like a string of sausages, which is meant to represent the myelin sheathes found on the individual nerve fibers. The fibers from the lateral superior olive are not myelinated. These fibers send an inhibitory signal to the first-order neurons whose dendrites connect to inner hair cells. Line thicknesses illustrate the relative number of fibers. The crossed pathway is made up mostly of fibers from the medial system; the uncrossed bundle is mostly fibers from the lateral superior olive.

Medial Efferent System

The fibers of the medial efferent system originate in and near the medial superior olive. Recall that medial means toward the center of the body. In addition to the medial superior olive, some of the fibers in this bundle come from other nearby structures; however, for this introduction these other structures will not be listed. The medial efferent system nuclei are at about the level of the fourth ventricle within the brainstem.

In most animals, most of these neurons will decussate, crossing to the contralateral cochlea. (In humans, there is less information available, but some data suggest that only about half of the fibers decussate. This overview will retain the traditional view that even for humans, the plurality of the fibers do decussate.) When medial efferent fibers reach the cochlea, they synapse on the body of the outer hair cells. Stimulation of these nerve fibers appears to decrease the active mechanism. The reduction of the action of the outer hair cells reduces the "boost" that this action normally provides within the cochlea, and as a result, the inner hair cell cilia will not shear as much. This reduces the amount of neurotransmitter released by the inner hair cells, and the VIIIth nerve firing rate is reduced. The medial efferent fibers (both those that cross midline and those that do not decussate) are myelinated, so the nerve conduction rate is relatively fast.

Recall from Chapter 20 that there are two types of neurons in the ascending system. Type I sensory neurons originated from inner hair cells and have myelinated axons. Type II afferent neurons have their dendrites beneath outer hair cells, but their axons are not myelinated. There are also type I and type II efferent nerve fibers. It is relatively easy to remember which are which, as the type I efferent neurons are still associated with inner hair cells and the type II efferent neurons with outer hair cells. The

medial system is composed of type II fibers, which synapse on the outer hair cells. These descending type II fibers differ from the ascending ones not only in the direction of the nerve conduction, but also in myelinization. As noted, the medial efferent nerves (which synapse on the outer hair cells) are myelinated, whereas the ascending type II neurons are not.

Some of the nerve fibers that come from the medial system have a different path—to the outer hair cells on the same side. These are less common than those that cross midline. The discussion below on crossed and uncrossed efferent fibers will cover this issue.

Lateral Efferent System

The fibers coming from the lateral superior olive and nearby structures synapse on the VIIIth nerve cells that receive stimulation from the inner hair cells. These efferent neurons are termed type I neurons, as they are associated with inner hair cells. Note the difference from the type II fibers: Type II efferent neurons synapsed on the outer hair cells; type I efferent fibers synapse on the afferent neuron. These descending pathway neurons are not myelinated. The type I neurons release acetylcholine and other inhibitory neurotransmitters such as GABA, which inhibits the firing of the VIIIth nerve. It therefore takes more excitatory neurotransmitter from the inner hair cell for the afferent neuron to fire.

Interestingly, it seems that inhibitory neurotransmitters are not the only neurotransmitters that the descending nerve fibers can release. Type I efferent neurons have also been linked to some neurotransmitters that are capable of increasing the afferent neuron's response to sound.

Whereas in most animals most of the medial efferent fibers decussate, most of the lateral fibers do not. The majority of the lateral efferent fibers will synapse with the afferent nerve fibers for the cochlea on the ipsilateral side of the body. A minority are "crossed fibers," ones that cross midline and synapse on the contralateral afferent nerve fibers.

Crossed and Uncrossed Efferent Fibers

Some texts and research articles prefer to discuss the olivocochlear bundle as being composed of the **crossed** and **uncrossed** efferent fibers. The crossed fibers originate on one side of the brainstem and then terminate in the contralateral cochlea. The uncrossed fibers remain on the same side of the body. The crossed fibers are mostly those myelinated type II fibers coming from medial superior olive, going to outer hair cells, although a few unmyelinated fibers from lateral superior olive going to the afferent neurons will also cross. The uncrossed fibers are mostly the unmyelinated fibers originating from lateral superior olive that synapse on the first-order neurons, although some uncrossed fibers are the myelinated ones from medial superior olive that go to the outer hair cells.

Effect of Activation of the Efferent System

Medial Efferent System Activation

If the fibers originating from the medial superior olive are activated, the motility of the outer hair cells is reduced. Otoacoustic emissions are lessened. Noise, presented either ipsilaterally or contralaterally, can trigger activation of the descending system. As Figure 23–1 illustrates, the medial pathway is strongest contralaterally. Therefore, putting noise in the contralateral ear is the best way to elicit the suppression effect. Decreasing the active mechanism has a secondary result—the VIIIth nerve evoked potentials will be reduced. The reduced hair cell motility creates less fluid movement in the subtectorial space; the inner hair cell cilia shearing is lessened, and thus it is more difficult to generate an VIIIth nerve potential.

In animal studies, electrical activation of the medial efferent system causes about a 20 dB shift in auditory sensitivity. Human and animal studies of threshold shifts resulting from contralateral noise has similar, though slightly less, effect. Given this, it is somewhat surprising that contralateral noise only creates a slight reduction in the size of the measured otoacoustic emission (OAE). One would typically see less than a 3 dB reduction.

One effect of activation of the medial system appears to be protection of hearing in loud noise situations. Experiments have been conducted to determine if the amount of noise-induced threshold changes in one ear can be lessened by putting noise in the opposite ear. As expected, the contralateral noise reduced the noise damage.

How is it that many students are able to "tune out" background noise when studying? Does visual attention and mental concentration activate the efferent system, reducing hearing sensitivity? This may be true. One study measured a cat's auditory afferent system responsiveness (using electrophysiologic measures.) When the cat was involved in a visual stimulus detection task (that was rewarded with food), the cat had less auditory-evoked electrophysiologic activity, even though the auditory signal in the environment stayed at the same intensity. (The lateral efferent system may play a role in this process as well.)

The medial efferent system may also assist with understanding speech in noise. One theory holds that when the medial system is activated, ongoing noise encoding is reduced. The nerve is better able to encode the speech signal, which changes its frequency and intensity quickly over time. The efferent system does not reduce the speech signal encoding because it is a quickly changing signal. Background noise is often fairly constant, so there is time for the efferent system to reduce the ear's sensitivity to the ongoing noise.

Other studies have shown that the efferent system helps us differentiate between similar frequency sounds. Animal studies show that this ability is reduced when the efferent system is surgically severed. The descending pathways synapse not just within the cochlea, but also at the cochlear nucleus. It may be that the input from the descending system helps to sharpen the ascending neuron's tuning curves, which aids in frequency discrimination. Good frequency discrimination aids in speech-in-noise recognition. Speech sounds with similar spectra will be easier to identify if the auditory system is more sensitive to small differences in pitch.

Lateral Efferent System Activation

It is hard to study the effect of innervating the lateral efferent system because the neurons are not myelinated. They are harder to find, and can't be electrically stimulated as a group. Because of this, the effects of the lateral system are more speculative.

One theory is that activation of the lateral fibers will release inhibitory neurotransmitters and decrease firing rate of the VIIIth nerve. As previously described, the inhibitory neurotransmitter helps counteract the effect of the excitatory neurotransmitter released by the inner hair cells. Activation of the efferent system would raise the threshold for firing of the auditory nerve. It may also make the neuron less frequency selective; the tuning of the neuron may broaden. The Q_{10dB} is smaller as a result. (Recall that the Q_{10dB} is the characteristic frequency di-

vided by the bandwidth, so increasing band width reduces the calculated Q_{10dB}.) Figure 23-2 illustrates this, although the same effect would theoretically occur with medial efferent system activation.

As mentioned, the lateral system is associated mostly with inhibitory neurotransmitters, but there is also evidence that it releases some chemicals that will enhance the auditory system's responsiveness. Given this, the lateral efferent system fibers may sometimes increase, and sometimes decrease, the ability of the afferent type I nerves to respond to sound.

OTHER EFFERENT PATHWAYS

The olivocochlear pathway is the best understood pathway; however, others exist. Fibers descend from the cortex to the olivocochlear bundle, with some fibers synapsing at medial geniculate body, inferior colliculus, and lateral lemniscus. Fibers from inferior colliculus to the medial efferent sys-

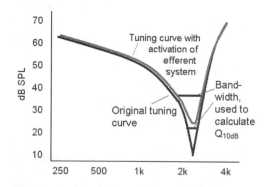

Figure 23–2. The tip of the tuning curve is elevated when the efferent system is activated, indicating that the auditory system has been made less sensitive. The tuning is also broadened; the neuron is not as frequency-specific for sound that is slightly above threshold. Another way to view this situation is that the neuron retains the same ability to transmit louder signals.

tem have been described. The presence of descending fibers originating from the cortex would help explain how attention could affect the efferent system.

THE ACOUSTIC REFLEX

Stapedial Reflex Pathway

The contraction of the stapedial reflex also decreases auditory sensitivity, and is controlled by brainstem structures; it is worthwhile to consider this as part of the way in which the central nervous system controls auditory sensitivity. Chapter 13 discussed the acoustic reflex, primarily as it relates to the conductive mechanism.

When the acoustic reflex is elicited, the normal contraction is bilateral. That is, even if just one ear is stimulated, the reflex will occur in both ears.

If the reflex is stimulated in one ear and measured in the same ear, the reflex is referred to as **ipsilateral. Contralateral** reflexes are measured in the opposite ear. A right contralateral reflex is one where the

loud, reflex-eliciting sound is presented to the right ear, but measurement of the contraction occurs in the left ear.

Figure 23–3 illustrates the reflex pathways. The ipsilateral pathway starts, of course, with the VIIIth nerve. After synapsing at cochlear nucleus, some reflex path fibers go directly to the facial nerve, that is, the motor nucleus for cranial nerve VII. Other fibers first synapse at superior olive, then go to this motor nucleus. The stapedial muscle is innervated by a branch of the VIIth nerve. There is also a possibility of a pathway from superior olive to the motor nucleus for tensor tympani, although most studies indicate that the tensor tympani is not contracted in response to sound.

The contralateral reflex pathway goes from the VIIIth nerve to the ipsilateral cochlear nucleus, then to the contralateral facial nerve nucleus (motor nerve VII), both directly and indirectly by way of the contralateral superior olive. From there, the neural signal is via the VIIth nerve to the stapedial muscle.

Figure 23–3 shows just one ear's pathway. Figure 23–4 illustrates both ears' pathways, but just for the stapedial reflex.

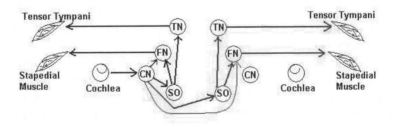

Figure 23–3. The reflex pathways for one ear are illustrated. The ipsilateral stapedial pathway goes from the cochlea to the cochlear nucleus (*CN*), then both directly and indirectly (via superior olive [*SO*]) to the VIIth cranial nerve motor nucleus—the facial nerve nucleus (*FN*). This nerve pathway then goes to the stapedial muscle. There is also a pathway to tensor tympani via its nucleus, which synapses with the trigeminal nerve (*TN*, cranial nerve V). The contralateral pathway decussates after cochlear nucleus. Some fibers synapse on the contralateral superior olive; others go directly to the nucleus for the facial nerve. Again, there is also a pathway for tensor tympani, although there is evidence that in humans there is no acoustic contraction of this muscle.

A.

B.

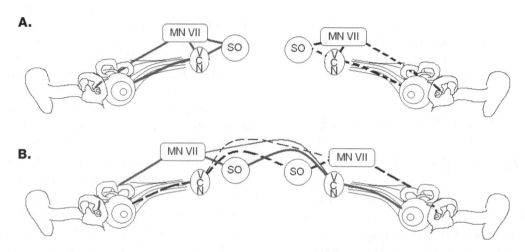

Figure 23–4. The acoustic reflex pathways. The left ear pathway is shown with the dotted lines. **A.** The ipsilateral pathways are schematically represented. The path is from the VIIIth nerve to ventral cochlear nucleus (*VCN*), then to motor nerve VII (*MN VII*) either directly, or after the synapsing at superior olive (*SO*). From there, the VIIth nerve controls contraction of the stapedial muscle. **B.** The contralateral pathway is from ipsilateral *VCN* to contralateral *MN VII* directly, and by way of the contralateral superior olive.

Effect of Stapedial Reflex Contraction

As was discussed in Chapter 13, contraction of the stapedial muscle does not attenuate all sounds equally. Stiffness reduces low-frequency sound transmission, but does not limit the vibration of the ossicles for high frequencies.

Measurement of acoustic reflexes occurs by placing a probe in the external auditory meatus. A low-frequency sound is introduced into the sealed meatus, and the intensity of the sound reflecting off the tympanic membrane is measured. When the stapedial muscle contracts, stiffening the ossicular chain, less sound is transmitted through the middle ear, so more reflects back off the tympanic membrane. The increase in intensity of the low-frequency probe tone in the ear canal provides evidence that the reflex has occurred. Chapter 8 provides additional information about this type of measurement.

There is a **latency** to the contraction of the stapedial muscle. Not only is there trav-

el time through the neural system, it takes some time for the stapedius to contract. The louder the signal, the quicker the contraction. However, the contraction still requires at least 20 msec to occur, meaning that the ear will not be protected from impulse sounds, such as from gun fire.

The acoustic reflex will also **fatigue** or **decay** over time. The rate of the fatigue is greater for high-frequency sounds. For example, a normal hearer may be able to sustain a stapedial muscle contraction for 20 seconds if the signal is low frequency, but for a 4-kHz pure tone, the reflex may not last more than a few seconds. However, when the signal changes frequency or intensity, the reflex is renewed, so in real-life situations, the reflex may provide attenuation of loud sounds for longer periods of time.

Role of Tensor Tympani

Tensor tympani does not contribute to the acoustic reflex in humans. One way that we can verify this clinically is by testing patients with **Bell's palsy**, which affects the VIIth nerve. These patients have no acoustic reflex if the location of the facial nerve problem is central to the branching of the innervation of the stapedial reflex. If tensor tympani (which is innervated by cranial nerve V, the trigeminal nerve) were contributing, then these patients would still have some form of acoustic reflex, which they do not.

Tensor tympani might be contracted during (and just before) vocalization, however. The intensity of one's own voice at the ear is high—just a few inches separate the mouth and ear. Both tensor tympani and stapedius may be contracting in anticipation of speaking, in order to attenuate air-conducted sound transmission.

Acoustic Reflexes Elicited by Nonauditory Stimuli

Sound attenuation will occur not just when loud sounds are present, but in response to other stimuli. A puff of air to the eye or forceful blinking also can elicit the reflex. Try squeezing your eyes shut quickly—perhaps you hear a sound that might be the middle ear muscles in action. Attention (e.g., visual) can affect reflex results; so can body movement. When clinically measuring the acoustic reflex, it's important to keep the patient still and quiet, and it is best not to let patients watch the immittance measuring system.

SUMMARY

The acoustic stapedial reflex pathway has an ipsilateral and a contralateral pathway. Stimulating just one ear creates a reflex in both middle ears, if the reflex pathways are normal. The reflex creates a stiffening of the ossicular chain, causing more sound to bounce off the eardrum. Less sound is transmitted into the cochlea as a result. The reflex does not remain on indefinitely, so it is designed to attenuate brief sounds. However, the reflex would not protect from very brief-duration sounds, because there is a latency between the sound onset and the muscle contraction. Changes in sound intensity and frequency reinvigorate the contraction. The acoustic reflex helps protect the ear from some loud sounds, such as one's own voice.

The tensor tympani muscle does not contract in response to sound in humans. It may be active at other times, such as when speaking.

The best known part of the neural efferent system that affects the cochlea is the olivocochlear bundle, which arises from the superior olive. The efferent system has the ability to limit the neural signals from the ear. The efferent system also has an ipsilateral and contralateral pathway, but the terms most often used are uncrossed and crossed pathways. The uncrossed pathway is comprised mostly of the fibers from the lateral superior olive that synapse on the afferent VIIIth nerve dendrites, reducing their ability to absorb excitatory neurotransmitter from the inner hair cells. The crossed pathway is primarily made up of myelinated nerve fibers from the medial superior olive that synapse on the body of the outer hair cell, functioning to reduce the size of the active mechanism.

Activation of the efferent system not only reduces auditory sensitivity, it also potentially improves hearing in noise.

24

Peripheral Vestibular Anatomy and Physiology

Most of us give little thought to our sense of balance. Having a normal balance system means more than not being dizzy, and our balance systems comprise more than just the vestibular structures in the inner ear. The vestibular sense organs are connected to brainstem structures that reflexively control the movement of the eyes. This permits unblurred vision as we turn our heads. Nerve fibers in the brainstem go to the cerebellum, to the neck, and to motor pathways, all of which control body motions and allow us to remain upright. This chapter describes the peripheral system; Chapter 25 describes the central nervous system and the ways in which the central system integrates information to help us resist the effects of gravity, know where we are in space, and keep us from falling down.

THE VESTIBULAR SYSTEM BONY AND MEMBRANOUS LABYRINTHS

As was discussed in Chapter 16, the same fluids are in both the vestibular system and the cochlea. Perilymph is found between the bony walls of the vestibular system and the membranes; endolymph is within the membranes. A small stalk, **ductus reuniens,** connects the endolymph-filled scala media to the **saccule**, which is connected to the **utricle**. The utricle and saccule are portions of the membranous labyrinth that sense when our bodies are moving in a straight line (e.g., driving in a car, or descending in an elevator.) The **semicircular canals** contain the sense organs that detect rotation, such as the head pivoting on the neck. The three semicircular canals open into the utricle, as shown in Figure 24-1. Each of the semicircular canals has an enlargement, or ampulla, at one end. The sensory cells are in the ampullae. (Ampulla is singular, ampullae is the plural from.)

A tube, called the **cochlear aqueduct,** runs from the scala tympani of the bony labyrinth to the brain above. It appears that the opening to the cerebrospinal fluid (CSF) space of the brain is not patent; CSF is not freely flowing. (The chemistry of CSF and perilymph are a bit different.) There is also a connection, which is called the **endolymphatic duct**, between the saccule and utricle and the **endolymphatic sac**. The endolymphatic sac rests in the dura mater of the brain—the outside of the meninges,

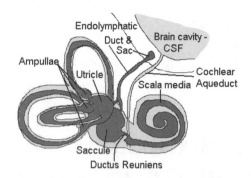

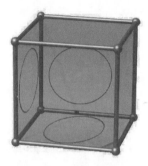

Figure 24–1. The membranous labyrinth includes the scala media of the cochlea, the utricle and saccule in the vestibule, and membranous arcs within the semicircular canals. Perilymph is found outside the membranous labyrinth. There is a stalklike extension of both the endolymph-filled membranous labyrinth and the perilymph-filled scala tympani. The perilymph in scala tympani connects via the cochlear aqueduct to a space in the cranium, filled with cerebrospinal fluid (*CSF*). The membranous labyrinth connects to the endolymphatic duct, which connects to the endolymphatic sac, tucked into the dura mater covering the brain.

Figure 24–2. The three semicircular canals lie perpendicular to each other, just as three sides of a cube are perpendicular to each other.

the covering of the cranium. The presence of these ducts to the brain hints at the inner ear's ability to regulate the pressure of the inner ear fluids. If the system were to create too much endolymph or perilymph, there is some room for expansion. The endolymphatic sac could bulge a bit; the cochlear aqueduct might allow some pressure relief into the CSF-filled brain cavity.

Arrangement of the Semicircular Canals

Each of the three semicircular canals is oriented at right angles to each other. This is easier to envision in the sketch of the circles superimposed on three of the sides of a cube, shown in Figure 24-2.

However, the actual arrangement of the semicircular canals is not as simple as sketched in Figure 24-2; it is more like that in Figure 24-3. The semicircular canals are named for their anatomic location. The **horizontal** or **lateral semicircular canal** is tilted about 30 degrees off horizontal. It is lower in the back than in the front (Figure 24-4A). The canal that is most anterior also is the highest one; thus, this canal is either called the **superior** or **anterior semicircular canal.** The third canal is named either the **inferior** or **posterior semicircular canal.**

Planes of the Canals of the Right and Left Ears Are Aligned

As shown in Figure 24-5, the left posterior canal and the right anterior canal are both angled in the same orientation. The right posterior and left anterior canals also line up. Thus, movement of the head in one direction will cause stimulation in pairs of canals. That holds true for the horizontal canals, too. Moving the head as if shaking "no" causes the pair of the horizontal canals to be stimulated.

Clinical Correlate: Orienting the Horizontal Semicircular Canal

When testing people with dizziness using a test called videonystagmography or electronystagmography, there is a portion of the test that requires that the horizontal semicircular canal be positioned straight up and down. To do this, recline the patient into a supine position, and then elevate his or her head 30 degrees. This will place the semicircular canal in the desired direction (Figure 24–4).

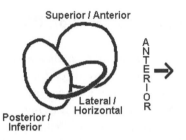

Figure 24–3. The semicircular canals are named by their anatomic arrangement. Each canal may be known by one of two names.

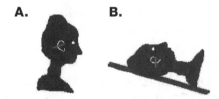

Figure 24–4. Illustration of the orientation of the horizontal semicircular canal in the upright patient (**A**), and when the patient is supine, with her head elevated 30 degrees (**B**). In the latter case, this canal points more or less straight up and down.

ANATOMY AND PHYSIOLOGY OF THE SEMICIRCULAR CANALS

Structures Within the Ampullae of the Semicircular Canals

Recall that the cochlea has a membrane covering the hair cells (reticular lamina) and that the hair cells themselves are bathed in perilymph (or perhaps, cortilymph). The vestibular system's setup is similar. The sensing cells are below a membrane barrier; the sensing cell cilia will project into the potassium-rich endolymph. Collectively, the sensing cells in the ampulla are called the **crista** or **crista ampullaris**. You will sometimes read that the crista is made up of **sensory epithelium.**

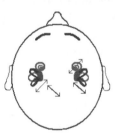

Figure 24–5. The orientation of the right anterior and left posterior, and left anterior and right posterior canals, are in line. Thus, these pairs of canals will be stimulated by the same direction head motion.

The crista contain hair cells. Just like in the cochlea, there are two types of hair cells. They are not arranged in the same way, so the terms outer and inner would not be appropriate, as the two types of cells are mixed together. We call them **type I and type II vestibular hair cells.** The type I cells are more bulb-shaped, similar in shape to the inner hair cells. The type II hair cells are taller and straighter, like the cochlea's outer hair cells. Both types of cells have cilia on them, and when deflected, the cilia will open microchannels, allowing potassium into the cell, depolarizing the hair cells.

In the cochlea, the cilia of the hair cells project into the gelatinous tectorial membrane. In the ampulla of the semicircular canals, the hair cells project into a gelatinous mass called the **cupula.** The cupula hangs from a stalk on the top of the ampulla, as illustrated in Figure 24-6.

The cupula is essentially floating in endolymph, although it is gently attached with a stalk to the roof of the ampulla. This means that it can move somewhat when the fluid moves. A nice analogy for this situation is to consider the twisting of a Hula-Hoop. When the Hula-Hoop spins, the pebbles inside lag behind because of their inertia. If viewed from a camera mounted inside the Hula-Hoop, the pebbles would appear to be moving backward. The moving semicircular canals, which are firmly attached as they are

to the head, lead when the head rotates— the cupulas lag behind.

The cupula can only move so far: it will hit the walls of the ampulla if the movement continues, for example, if you are on a merry-go-round. As you spin and spin on the merry-go-round (at a constant speed), the fluid eventually is going to catch up to the speed of the body and the cupula will float in a relatively neutral position again. When you slow down, the fluid will be moving still as the body decelerates, and the cupula would be forced in the opposite direction.

Angular Head Motion Directions

The semicircular canals are arranged to detect motion in any direction. Sometimes these motion directions are referred to as **yaw, pitch, and roll**. Yawing is moving around a vertical axis. Shaking your head "no" is an example of this motion. A boat at anchor in a shifting wind yaws back and forth. The horizontal semicircular canals would be stimulated with this type of movement. A boat crashing through the waves has its bow (front) tossed upward and downward; it is said to be pitching. Shaking your head "yes" creates the same sort of movement. Looking at Figure 24-5, note that both the anterior and posterior canals would be partially stimulated by this type of motion. Rolling is when a boat tips left to right, as when a wake from a passing boat hits the sides of the boat. Repeatedly tilt your head toward your shoulder—left ear down to the left shoulder, then right ear down toward the right shoulder. Again, the anterior and posterior canals sense this motion.

Stand up. Put your left foot out to the left and forward a bit. Now move your head so that your face points to your foot—in one straight, smooth motion. Which semicircular canals are activated? You've done a bit of a roll, a bit of a pitch, and a bit of yaw—and you've stimulated hair cells in all the ampullae.

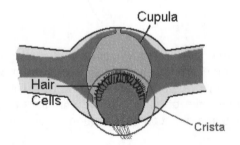

Figure 24–6. Arrangement of structures within the ampulla. The hair cells are in the crista, and are not within the membranous labyrinth, although the hair cell cilia project into it. The cupula is a gelatinous structure into which the cilia embed.

Cilia and Kinocilium in the Ampullae

The cilia on a vestibular hair cell look a bit different from those on an auditory hair cell. First, a kinocilium—a very tall cilium—exists on vestibular hair cells (both type I and type II). Second, the cilia aren't neatly in rows, they form a central mound. The tallest stereocilia are nearest the kinocilium (Figure 24–7).

Just as with auditory hair cells, the adjacent cilia are linked together. Deflecting the tallest cilia therefore moves the entire bundle. And again, as in the auditory system, the movement of the cilia will open and close channels in the cilia. Moving the stereocilia in one direction (toward the kinocilium) will open the channels allowing potassium to enter the cell and excite it. Movement in the opposite direction closes the channel and slows the neural firing rate.

Direction of the Endolymph/Cupula Movement That Is Excitatory

This next section describes how moving the vestibular hair cell cilia changes the nerve's firing rate. As each ampulla opens up into the utricle, it is convenient to use this as an anatomic reference point. We will speak of the movement of the cupula (and hair cell stereocilia) as being **utriculofugal,** meaning away from the utricle, or **utriculopetal,** toward the utricle. "Fugal" comes from a Latin word meaning "to flee," "petal" from the Latin word "to seek."

Deflecting hair cell cilia away from the utricle (utriculofugal movement) stimulates the hair cells inside the posterior and anterior canals. The horizontal semicircular canal structures, in contrast, are stimulated by utriculopetal fluid flow, pushing the cupula toward the utricle.

This means that, depending on the canal, either movement toward or away from the utricle will be excitatory. In all cases, though, movement toward the kinocilium is always excitatory. This means that the tall kinocilium are located toward the utricle in the horizontal semicircular canal. However, in the anterior and posterior canals, the cilia are arranged so that the kinocilium are on the side of the hair cell that is away from the utricle.

Any head motion that creates excitation of one ear's ampulla will cause a corresponding inhibition in firing of the other' ear's complementary ampulla. Figure 24–8 is an illustration of this for the horizontal ca-

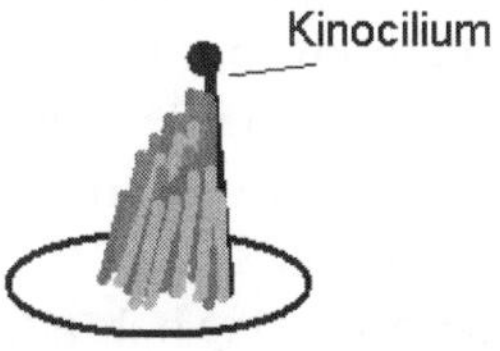

Kinocilium

Figure 24–7. Illustration of the cilia on top of a vestibular hair cell. Hair cells in the vestibular system have a tall kinocilium. The cilia are clustered together and linked together, so that movement on any one part moves the entire bundle.

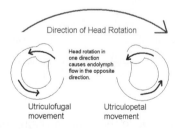

Direction of Head Rotation

Head rotation in one direction causes endolymph flow in the opposite direction.

Utriculofugal movement   Utriculopetal movement

Figure 24–8. The horizontal semicircular canals viewed from above. Rotating the head clockwise creates counterclockwise fluid motion. In one ear, this deflects the cupula utriculopetally (toward the utricle); the other ear's cupula's deflection is utriculofugal.

nals. As discussed earlier, the two ears' anterior/posterior canals work in pairs. Remember that the anterior and posterior canals are stimulated by utriculofugal flow. Figure 24-9 illustrates that a head motion that creates inhibition of firing of the left ear anterior canal also results in excitation of the right posterior canal.

THE UTRICLE AND SACCULE

Inside the vestibule of the inner ear are the **utricle** and **saccule**. The utricle is located closer to the semicircular canals. Each structure has a membranous portion and a bony portion.

The sensory structures are the maculae—there is a **macula** of the utricle and a macula of the saccule. The utricle is oriented mostly horizontal, whereas the saccule is essentially vertical. Both the utricle and saccule have some curvature to them; they are not perfectly horizontal or vertical, which allows different sections to be stimulated by slightly different motions. Both of these organs are said to respond to gravity and linear acceleration, rather than rotating head movements. As discussed in greater detail below, these structures respond to gravity because they contain crystals that have mass. The structures will also respond to straight-line motion, which is called linear acceleration, because when we move in a horizontal or vertical plane, the rate of movement changes over time, which is the definition of acceleration.

Hair Cells of the Utricle and Saccule

The hair cells in the utricle and saccule are similar in make-up to those in the ampulla—they have kinocilium; there are a mix of type I and type II cells. The cilia project upward into a gelatinous layer. However, in the utricle and saccule, above the gelatinous part is another layer with otoconia in it. **Otoconia** is the Latin word for "ear stones." These calcium carbonate crystals are in the **otoconial layer** of the **otoconial membrane**.

The calcium crystals are heavier than the endolymph, so the force of gravity is always acting on the cilia. Movement will create additional forces (Figure 24-10). For example, if you are moving forward or backward (or left or right), the heavy otoconia in the horizontally arranged utricle will lag behind due to inertia. Coming to a sudden stop (deceleration) causes the utricular otoconia to continue moving forward due to their inertia, which deflects the cilia. Dropping suddenly, as in an elevator or on a roller coaster, moves the body, but the otoconia of the saccule lag behind, deflecting the cilia upward. Conversely, if you are going up in an elevator, the saccule's macula is on the rise, the calcium crystals lag behind, and the cilia deflect downward. Head tilt will also affect the motion of the cilia. Looking down at the floor causes the horizontal utricle to slope, and the cilia will bend as a result.

The cilia on the hair cells of the maculae are arranged in many different orienta-

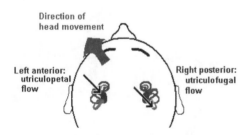

Direction of head movement

Left anterior: utriculopetal flow

Right posterior: utriculofugal flow

Figure 24–9. In this head motion, the fluid in the left anterior canal would move toward the utricle. The right posterior canal, which is in the same plane, would have utriculofugal fluid motion. The left anterior canal would send an inhibitory signal; the right posterior would send an excitatory signal.

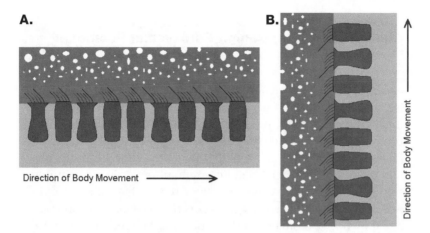

Figure 24–10. Hair cells of the macula have cilia that project upward into a gelatinous layer that has calcium particles called otoconia. Movement of the body in one direction causes the cilia of the utricle and saccule to move in the opposite direction. Different parts of the macula have the kinocilium arranged in different orientations, so some portion of the cells will send an inhibitory signal whereas other parts will send an excitatory signal. **A.** The horizontally oriented utricle is moved to the right, causing the cilia to deflect toward the left. **B.** The vertically oriented saccule moves upward (e.g., when you rise from a seated position) causing the cilia to deflect downward.

tions. For each type of head tilt or up/down, forward/back, right/left motion, different areas within the macula are sending excitatory and inhibitory signals.

VESTIBULAR BRANCH OF THE VIIITH NERVE

Each vestibular nerve has two sections, as illustrated in Figure 24-11. The **superior branch of the vestibular nerve** has dendrites in the horizontal canal crista, the superior crista, the utricle, and part of the saccule's macula. The **inferior section** is innervated by the remainder of the saccule and the posterior semicircular canal. The vestibular branch joins with the auditory branch and courses through the internal auditory meatus. The cell bodies for the vestibular branch are called **Scarpa's ganglia**— there are ganglia for the inferior and for the

superior branches. The ganglia are in the internal auditory meatus.

SUMMARY

The vestibular peripheral system has both a membranous and bony portion, with endolymph and perilymph, respectively. The endolymph within the semicircular canals moves with head rotation, which deflects the cilia that project into the cupula, the gelatinous floating structure above the hair cells.

For the horizontal canals, fluid motion toward the utricle (utriculopetal flow) is excitatory, but for the other two canals, utriculofugal flow increases the firing rate of the nerve. The semicircular canals work in pairs. If one ear's horizontal canal is stimulated, the other ear's canal creates an inhibitory response. The left anterior and right posteri-

Clinical Correlate: Benign Paroxysmal Positional Vertigo

Some patients experience a condition called **benign** (meaning not a progressive or malignant disorder) **paroxysmal** (having sudden attacks) **positional vertigo**. (The condition is pronounced "buh-nine pair-oxs-ĭz-mul ver-tĭ-go." Fortunately, audiologists usually just call it BPPV.) Rotation of the head in a certain direction triggers a brief, intense bout of vertigo (a spinning sensation). For example, a patient may report that rolling over in bed or bending the head down triggers the vertigo. This condition occurs when otoconia from the utricle migrate into one or more of the semicircular canals. The posterior canal is particularly vulnerable, as it is lower than the utricle.

The otolithic debris may be free-floating within a semicircular canal, or it may adhere to the cupula. If the debris is free-floating (termed canalolithiasis), then head movement causes the otoconia to hit the cupula as the head rotates, which causes an intense sensation of spinning. If the debris adheres to the cupula (cupulolithiasis), the cupula is heavier than it should be and responds to gravity, again causing exaggerated response to movement.

These patients' dizziness can be treated using specific head repositioning maneuvers that help the otoconia to migrate out of the semicircular canal and back into the utricle. Many of these patients have immediate relief from a treatment that can be completed in about 15 minutes.

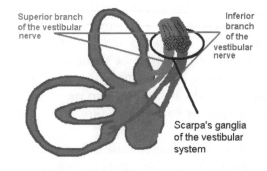

Superior branch of the vestibular nerve

Inferior branch of the vestibular nerve

Scarpa's ganglia of the vestibular system

Figure 24–11. The vestibular portion of the VIIIth nerve has two branches. The superior branch comes from the horizontal and superior semicircular canal cristae and the utricle and part of the saccule. The inferior branch arises from the posterior semicircular canal crista and the saccule.

or canals, and right anterior and left posterior canals, are arranged in the same orientation, so these also work in pairs—when one is creating an excitatory signal the other of the pair creates an inhibitory signal.

Semicircular canals detect head rotation, whereas the utricle and saccule detect straight-line motion, and are affected by gravity. The cilia of the maculae of the utricle and saccule project into a gelatinous

Clinical Correlate: Vestibular Assessment of Each Branch of the Vestibular Portion of the VIIIth Nerve

Electronystagmography and videonystagmography are clinical tests to assess the vestibular system. These tests are discussed in the next chapter. A part of the test battery called "caloric testing" stimulates the horizontal semicircular canal. The superior branch of the vestibular section of the VIIIth nerve is therefore assessed.

Sending a loud sound into the ear creates a large pressure wave in the vestibule and stimulates the saccule. A nerve signal is transmitted via the inferior section of the vestibular nerve, which creates a reflex that will cause the sternocleidomastoid muscle in the neck to contract in response. We can measure to see if stimulation of the saccule created this muscle contraction. Measuring this **vestibular evoked myogenic potential (VEMP)** allows us to assess the health of the inferior branch of the vestibular nerve and the health of a macula, to complement our examination via caloric testing.

layer that has calcium crystals, which will respond to gravity as they have mass. Movement in a straight line causes the cilia to deflect because the heavy, crystal-laden membrane lags behind due to inertia. Even when the body is not moving, gravity affects these structures. Cells in the macula of the utricle and saccule are arranged in various directions. Movement that stimulates some cells will cause inhibition of others.

There are two branches of the vestibular portion of the VIIIth nerve. The inferior branch connects to the saccule and the inferior semicircular canal; the superior branch connects to the other two semicircular canals, to the utricle, and to part of the saccule. The vestibular branch joins the auditory branch in the internal auditory meatus.

REFERENCE

Baloh, R. W., & Hurubi, V. (1990). *Clinical neurophysiology of the vestibular system*, (2nd ed.). Philadelphia: F. A. Davis.

25

Central Vestibular Anatomy and Physiology

As the introduction to Chapter 24 described, we maintain balance using more than just our peripheral vestibular systems, and there is more to having a working balance system than just not being dizzy. The balance system keeps you from falling as your body moves—especially when you are no longer positioned right over your center of gravity. It also lets you know if you are moving, and if so, how fast and in what direction. It coordinates your eye movement with your body motion, so that you can focus even as you walk or turn.

The balance system involves more than just the semicircular canals and utricle and saccule; it is multisensory. We use **proprioceptive input**—we can feel movement; we know if our feet are solidly on the ground, or if our body is pressed against the car seat as the car accelerates. We make instantaneous muscle movement corrections to keep balanced, so our **motor systems** are involved as well. We use **visual input**—we can see where we are and whether or not we are moving. If you have ever hit your car brakes when stopped at a stoplight because the car next to you was creeping forward, you have evidence of the influence of the visual system on the perception of move-

ment. Of course, vestibular input is another sensory input. All forms of information are integrated so that you know your position in space, and can keep from falling. If one sense starts to fail, the patient can be trained to make better use of the information from the remaining senses in order to improve balanced and avoid falling.

This chapter overviews the central nervous system connections that allow for coordination of eye and body movement, and integration of other sensory information. It also provides an overview of some vestibular testing clinical correlates.

FUNCTIONS OF THE BALANCE SYSTEM

This section overviews some of the functions of the balance system. First, the obvious one. We need to receive information cortically so that we understand our body's position. (If you don't know where you are, you don't know what volitional movement to make next.) Next, the text describes why it is so important to have the ability to have unblurred vision as the body moves, and how horizontal eye motions are coordinated as the head turns. Lastly, we need reflexive mechanisms that will coordinate our muscle movement so we don't lose balance and fall. These are termed the reflexes for postural control, and this section describes these reflexes in more detail.

Awareness of Head Position

The peripheral vestibular structures are similar to the peripheral auditory structures: both have the same fluids, hair cells, cilia, and ciliary shearing. However, there are few corollaries in the central nervous system. Because balance is inherently multisensory, there is connection between vestibular inputs, visual inputs, proprioceptive inputs, and motor inputs at all areas of the central nervous system. Just as there is no one single major path for vestibular information to ascend to the brain, there is no "primary vestibular cortex" region.

Within the brainstem, nuclei receive input from multiple senses. That is, one structure can receive somatosensory, visual, and/or vestibular information. There can then be efferent signals sent from that nucleus to motor pathways. Our brainstem structures can receive information back from peripheral motor systems. Some of this is covered in the sections below on the reflex pathways involved in maintaining vision as one moves, and in the section on the reflexes of postural control.

Balance information is sent from midbrain to multiple regions of the cortex, and sensory and motor information is interconnected. These amorphous, diffuse pathways are difficult to study. It is generally accepted that there are four major areas of the brain involved in balance. As balance involves making motor movements, the major motor areas of the frontal lobe are involved. Specifically, precentral cortex and its connections to the pyramidal system are implicated

in making the voluntary motor movements for balance. Visual information must be processed, which involves the occipital lobe, with connections back to the frontal cortex to control eye movement. Deep brain, basal ganglia processing also helps to coordinate motor movements, and the limbic system is involved in processing the emotional aspects of the need to keep from falling. Lastly, the cerebellum has a role in control of posture, and in coordination of the sensory and motor information.

As this overview indicates, recognizing one's head/body position uses multiple areas of the brain. Because of this, there are a variety of ways in which persons with lesions and brain injuries (including brain circulation insufficiencies, such as strokes and transient ischemia) can experience balance problems. Also, drugs that affect the central nervous system can affect a patient's balance.

The Vestibular-Ocular Reflex

Movie fans who remember the *Blair Witch Project* will recall the bouncing video images of the running videographer. If you take a video with a camera firmly mounted to your head, you would have this sort of blurred image. So why is it that when you walk or run, your vision is clear? The answer is the **vestibular-ocular reflex (VOR)**, which coordinates your head and eye movements, so that your eyes remain focused on one point, even as your body moves.

The classic way of describing the vestibular-ocular reflex is to detail how moving the head in the horizontal plane affects the movement of your eyes. You typically won't read about the pathways between the eyes and the ear for vertical head rotation. Does this mean that your eyes will stay focused when you shake your head "no," but not if you shake your head "yes"? Of course not. But, there are good reasons that we describe the horizontal system but give only passing mention to the ways in which the eyes stay focused as you nod your head, or do the head roll described in the previous chapter. First, an understanding of the principle of how horizontal head movement relates to horizontal eye movement will give you the basic idea, and you will be able to generalize to the concepts to other head/eye motions. There is another reason for audiologist's perseverance on horizontal eye motion. One of our clinical tests of balance stimulates the horizontal semicircular canal, mimicking the effect of moving the head in the horizontal plane. As we stimulate this pathway in our clinical tests, we have to be well versed in the anatomy of the pathway.

Ewald's First Law

In the late 1800s, Ewald studied the vestibular system and recognized that if you rotate your head in one direction (e.g., to the left), the fluid in the semicircular canals moves in the opposite direction (e.g., to the right). As described in Chapter 24, the fluid lag due to inertia creates the out-of-synch motion of head and fluid within the semicircular canals.

Ewald's first law is that head motion in one direction will create endolymph motion in the opposite direction, which causes the eyes to move in the direction of the endolymph. Although this sounds quite complex, it really isn't. Imagine a camera mounted on your head, facing your eyes. Look at something straight in front of you. Rotate your head to the left slowly as you keep your eyes fixed on that original point. The camera would show that the eyes are moving to the right (Figure 25–1). Ewald showed us that there is reflexive coordination of this head/eye movement.

Muscles Controlling Eye Movements

Each eye has three pairs of muscles. Superior rectus and inferior rectus move the

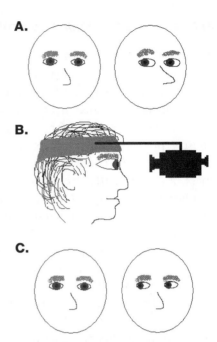

Figure 25–1. A. This cartoon illustrates that when a person turns his or her head, it is normal for the eyes to remain fixed on a point in the visual field. **B.** Consider the view from a video camera mounted to a person's head, so that the eye movements can be recorded as the person rotates his head. **C.** From this view point, the eyes can be seen as deviating in the direction opposite from the head turn.

eye up and down. These two muscles work in concert—one relaxes and one contracts. For example, if you contract the superior rectus muscles and relax the inferior rectus muscles, your eyes will deflect upward. For horizontal eye movement, the muscles are medial and lateral rectus. There are two more muscles which are not located directly opposite from each other. They are superior oblique and inferior oblique. As illustrated in Figure 25–2, superior oblique (when contracted) rotates the eye in one direction, inferior oblique provides the opposite direction rotation for a single eye. Contraction/relaxation of combinations of the eye muscles allows us to deviate our eyes in all directions.

Neural Pathways for Ocular Control

Moving your eyes is, of course, under neural control. The three cranial nerves involved are III (oculomotor), IV (trochlear), and VI (abducens). Cranial nerve VI connects to the lateral rectus; contraction of this muscle pulls the eye away from midline. Cranial nerve IV controls the superior oblique. Cranial nerve III has connections to all the other ocular muscles. Cranial nerve II (optic nerve) conveys the visual information to the central nervous system.

Upholding that long-standing tradition of describing the horizontal eye movements and ignoring the control of other eye movements, we will focus (no pun intended) on the central control of the medial and lateral rectus. Figure 25-3 illustrates the pathways that can either excite (contract) the medial

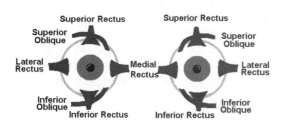

Figure 25–2. Schematic of the muscles of the eye.

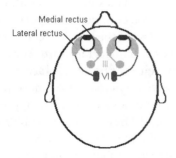

Figure 25–3. Cranial nerve III innervates medial rectus. Cranial nerve VI innervates lateral rectus, which pulls the eyes away from midline. The signal sent to the nerve may be to contract, or to relax, the muscle.

and lateral muscles or inhibit (relax) these muscles.

Pathways from Vestibular Nucleus to the Nerves Controlling Eye Movement

The nerves that originate at the horizontal semicircular canals synapse at vestibular nucleus. The nerves then synapse at motor nuclei VI and III, then traverse to the eyes, causing contraction/relaxation of these ocular muscles. Figure 25–4 shows the schematic.

Neural Control of Eye Deflection During Head Turn

Recall from Chapter 24 that utriculopetal endolymph flow (toward the utricle) creates an excitatory signal from the horizontal semicircular canal, and utriculofugal motion would slow the neural firing rate. As was shown in Figure 24–8, movement of the endolymph from head rotation in one direction will excite one semicircular canal and inhibit the nerve firing for the other ear's canal. That is, one ear sends an excitatory signal, one sends an inhibitory signal. In order to move the eyes in the opposite direc-

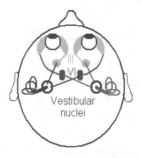

Figure 25–4. nput from the horizontal semicircular canal is received in the vestibular nucleus. There is a connection from the vestibular nucleus to the contralateral VIIth nucleus and then to lateral rectus, and from vestibular nucleus to the ipsilateral IIIrd nucleus and then to medial rectus.

tion from the head movement (same direction as the endolymph flow), the signal from the excited semicircular canal will cause the contralateral lateral rectus and the ipsilateral medial rectus to contract. Simultaneously, the inhibitory signal from the other ear tells the same-sided eye's medial rectus to relax, and the other eye's lateral rectus to relax. Thus, each eye has one muscle relaxed and one muscle contracted, and the eye moves in the opposite direction from the head turn. Figure 25–5 illustrates this.

Limited Range of Eye Deflection

The eyes can only move so far to the side. Once they have reached their limit, if the body is still rotating, the eyes cannot keep the im-

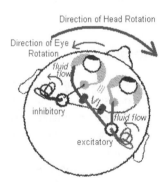

Figure 25–5. Moving the head to the right causes the endolymph in the right horizontal semicircular canal to move left. This movement is utriculopetal for the right ear, so the right horizontal canal sends an excitatory neural signal (*illustrated with thicker lines*) to right eye medial rectus and the left eye lateral rectus causing muscle contraction. Simultaneously, the left semicircular canal has utriculofugal flow, so an inhibitory signal (*thin lines*) is sent to the right eye lateral rectus and left eye medial rectus, causing these muscles to relax. The eyes deviate to the left, the same direction as the endolymph flowed, which is opposite the direction of the head turn.

age in focus. The central nervous system will cause the eyes to rapidly move back toward center line, establishing a new focus point. A rapid eye movement in one direction such as this is called a **saccade.** Saccadic movements are controlled by (mediated by) the central nervous system. Of course, the same sets of eye muscles are involved in saccadic movement as are involved in the slower deflection that is controlled by the vestibular system.

Nystagmus: Repeated Slow Drift, Rapid Saccadic Return Motion

If the body continues to rotate after the eyes have returned to the center position, there will be a repeat of the slow eye movement in the direction opposite the body movement. The speed of the slow part of the eye movement should match the speed of the head rotation quite closely. If you are spinning left at 30 degrees per second, the eye movement should be right at 30 degrees per second. The return to midline gaze is much faster movement in the opposite direction (toward the head turn).

The repeated slow movement of the eyes in one direction and fast saccadic movement back to midline is called **nystagmus.** Nystagmus occurs normally with head rotation. You can also elicit nystagmus visually by watching something moving in front of you. For example, if you are in the car stopped at a railroad crossing, if you are watching the moving train, your eyes will follow one train car for a while, then snap back to center and pick up a new target to track. Nystagmus elicited by the visual system is called **optokinetic nystagmus**.

Nystagmus is called "left beating" if the saccadic portion, called the **fast phase,** is to the left. The **slow phase** is the part of the eye movement that is under vestibular control if you are turning. To reiterate, fast phase motion is controlled centrally rather than by the ears.

It will be important to remember that the direction of the nystagmus beat is in the same direction as the head turn. If the head turns to the right, the eyes drift left, then beat back to the right: the nystagmus is "right beating."

Introduction to Ewald's Second Law

The nystagmus that comes from turning your head is created by the excitatory signal from one canal and an inhibitory signal to be sent from the opposite ear. That doesn't mean that the importance of the excitatory and inhibitory signals are equal. The excitatory signal has greater importance to the central nervous system than does the inhibitory signal. This is **Ewald's second law**: excitation is stronger than inhibition. This merits elaboration. Suppose a patient with a weak right horizontal semicircular canal turned to her right. As described above, endolymph flows left; this excites the right vestibular nerve and inhibits the left nerve's firing. If the right canal has a weak receptor, it cannot properly excite the contraction of the right medial rectus and left lateral rectus in order to make the eyes deviate to the left. However, there would still be an inhibitory signal from the left ear to the left medial rectus and right lateral rectus, so the patient will have some eye motion. Perhaps, when moving her head to the right at 30 degrees per second, the eye movement might be left at 10 degrees per second. This gross difference would prevent visual fixation while turning to the right, and the patient is going to avoid turning her head toward the ear with the problem, which we speak of as "toward the lesioned ear." When turning the head away from the lesioned ear, left in our example, the normal left ear sends an excitatory signal. The loss of the inhibition signal from the right ear may alter the speed of the VOR slightly, but the mismatch between head and eye speed is less, so this motion is tolerated better by the patient.

Summary of the VOR and Introduction to VNG Testing

The vestibular-ocular reflex (VOR) creates a slow-phase reflexive eye movement in the opposite direction from the head movement, followed by a fast return of the eyes to midline. The nystagmus created by continued head movement beats in the direction of the head movement, as nystagmus is named for its fast phase. The VOR helps us to maintain our vision when we turn our heads. The VOR causes nystagmus. Nystagmus can also be present in other conditions, and is often found in patients with dizziness even when the patient is not moving. Audiologists measure the nystagmus that may be present spontaneously, or that is present when stimulating the ear during the procedures called videonystagmography and electronystagmography. This clinical measurement is discussed later in the chapter.

Velocity Storage

In Chapter 24, it was mentioned that if a person continues to spin round and round at a constant speed, eventually the speed of the endolymph would catch up with the speed of the semicircular canals, and there would no longer be a vestibulo-ocular reflex. This occurs after just a brief amount of time; however, the VOR lasts longer than the time it takes the endolymph to move with the canals. The endolymph will move at the same speed as the canals after about 5 seconds, but the VOR remains for about 20 seconds. This observation lead to the understanding of a **velocity storage mechanism.**

Interneurons create the velocity storage. One single vestibular neuron synapses with several nerves. One of these nerves sends the signal directly to the ocular system. However, another nerve first synapses with an intermediary nerve (or interneuron), then sends the single to the ocular system. This creates a delay—the signal is

Clinical Correlate: Unilateral Peripheral Lesions Cause Nystagmus That Beats Toward the Unaffected Ear

Just as in the auditory system, the vestibular nerves are firing spontaneously even when not stimulated. When turning, the neural firing rate increases in one ear, and decreases in the other ear: There is a difference in the firing rates between ears. If a patient suddenly loses vestibular input from one semicircular canal, there is an imbalance—there is more of a signal coming from the unaffected ear. The weak or dead ear sends less (or no) signal. The imbalance means that the brainstem receives a stronger signal from the good ear. Normally, when the central nervous system receives a stronger signal from one ear, it means that the head is rotating toward that ear (and the endolymph is moving in the opposite direction).

The patient with a weak or dead unilateral peripheral vestibular has a "stronger from the good ear" signal and has the sensation of the head moving toward the good ear. So, this patient will have a slow drift eye movement away from the good ear, and then a beat toward the good ear. Recall that nystagmus is named for the fast phase, and the fast phase will be toward the good ear. Your patient with a unilateral vestibular lesion can be expected to have **spontaneous nystagmus** (nystagmus that is present without head turn or movement in the visual field) that beats toward the unaffected ear. Need help remembering the rule? "Good fast, bad slow" might help. The fast phase of the nystagmus is toward the good (unimpaired) ear; the slow phase is toward the bad (lesioned) ear.

It bears mentioning that the person with a stable vestibular lesion won't have the spontaneous nystagmus forever. The central nervous system will adapt to the unequal inputs and learn that this is the normal condition. Patients who remain on medication that suppresses the central nervous system have relief from the initial dizziness, but these patients' central nervous systems won't learn to compensate.

still being sent, even after the neural event has occurred. When several interneurons come between the first afferent neuron and the ocular nerve, then the degree of delay can be further increased. This is the mechanism that allows the VOR to continue longer than the time during which the endolymph is lagging behind the canal.

Reflexes of the Balance System for Postural Control

We have reviewed two of the three functions of the balance system so far. The balance system sends a signal to the brain to allow us to know our head position, so we can decide on subsequent head motions. The vestibular-ocular reflex allowed unblurred vision during the time when the head moves. The final function of the balance system to be overviewed is how the balance system has reflexes for postural control that allow us to reflexively adjust our body positions to avoid falling. This final function is permitted through integration of the various senses: proprioception, vision, and vestibular systems all work together. The input from the proprioceptive system that tells us about our body position goes to vision centers (cervico-ocular reflex) and to the muscles of the body (cervicospinal and cervicocollic reflexes). There are also reflexive pathways from the vestibular system to the muscles of the body (vestibulospinal reflex) as well as the already discussed vestibulo-ocular reflex. In sum, we have an amazing feedback loop between the different senses.

Vestibulospinal Reflex

The muscles of the body termed "antigravity muscles" are the ones that keep us upright, so that we don't collapse from the forces of gravity. As the utricle and saccule are our gravity receptors, it is no surprise that they are involved in the **vestibulospinal** reflex pathway. The nerves conveying the signal from these receptors synapse in the lateral vestibular nucleus, then descend to the muscles of the hands and legs. When we sense our body tilting, we reflexively compensate with body movements that will keep us from falling.

Cervico-ocular Reflex

As the name implies, the cervical area of the neck and the eyes are reflexively coordinated. Input from the neck about head position influences the **cervico-ocular reflex**. Thus, shaking your head versus having your body rotate creates different signals. When the VOR is weak, the patient can learn to rely more on the cervico-ocular reflex: Input from the neck can help to compensate for loss of vestibular input, particularly for patients who have bilateral vestibular lesions. The cervico-ocular reflex also helps to lets us know when the body is *not* moving. For example, when watching a train move, the eyes have optokinetic nystagmus (visual field movement-induced nystagmus.) The cervical receptors are not signaling movement, (and the proprioceptive system agrees,) which provides the body with information that the visual field, not the body, is moving.

Cervicospinal and Cervicocollic reflexes

The **cervicospinal** and **cervicocollic** reflexes provide coordination between movements of the neck and movements of the body. There are reflexes that don't involve the eyes or ears. Head/neck movement can be reflexively coordinated with body movements, and vice versa.

Vestibulocervical and Vestibulocollic reflexes

The **vestibulocervical** reflex helps to stabilize the head as the torso and head move at different rates. The vestibular input tells of total head rotation; input from the cervical proprioception centers gives input on head relative to trunk rotation. The **vestibulocollic reflex** allows for vestibular input to create reflexive motion of the shoulders and upper back. Both of these reflexes come from input from the utricles and saccules.

Summary of the Functions of Balance and Clinical Implications

As you have read, balance does not involve just the ears, but is multisensory. Obviously, problems with the vestibular peripheral system, the semicircular canals, the utricle and saccule, and/or the vestibular branch of the VIIIth nerve, can cause balance problems. As you may expect given the information about how the different nervous system inputs interconnect, and how there are many different reflex pathways involved in balance, disorders affecting any of a number of neurologic sites or muscle groups can affect balance. Problems with proprioception also affect balance, including a condition called peripheral neuropathy. This is the loss of sensation in the periphery (e.g.,

feet) that is relatively common in elderly patients with cardiac problems that have led to disease of the small blood vessels. The poor blood flow has damaged the sensory receptors. For patients with neuropathy, the proprioceptive input is weakened and is a less effective signal for the balance system.

Because balance involves multiple inputs, there are mechanisms for compensation when one system is weak or absent. A blind person maintains balance by relying on the vestibular and proprioceptive systems. A person with peripheral vestibular lesions can learn to make better use of the visual and proprioceptive inputs. The patient with neuropathy can learn to better use vision and input from the vestibular system. This is the basis for **vestibular rehabilitation** training, provided by physical therapists. The area of deficit is identified, and strategies are taught to either strengthen a weak system, or provide compensatory input and tune existing reflexes.

Clinical Correlate: Overview of Balance Assessment

Overview of Posturography

A form of balance assessment that goes beyond evaluating the peripheral vestibular input is **dynamic posturography**. In this testing, the patient is put in ever more challenging situations, where one of the three balance senses is in conflict with the others, or is prevented from assisting the patient. The patient is assessed in each of these situations to determine what situations will create risk of falls, and to evaluate the strengths and weaknesses of the balance system.

Dynamic platform posturography places the patient on a platform that can move. The patient is in a safety harness so that he or she cannot fall. The sensor on the floor measures the patient's relative stability—does he or she sway or would the patient fall if not harnessed? In front of the patient is a screen that wraps around the sides of the patient, so the screen is seen even in peripheral vision. The platform that the patient stands on can move under computer control (Figure 25–6). The patient is placed in a variety of situations. First, the patient just stands with eyes open. Next, the patient closes his or her eyes. The effect of removing vision (any decrease in stability) is measured. In the third condition, the visual field moves. If a patient is heavily reliant on vision, as happens when proprioception and/or vestibular inputs are compromised, this will cause the patient to sway or fall. In the fourth condition, the platform moves, but the visual field in front stays constant. This assesses the patient's reaction to conflict between vision and vestibular/proprioceptive input. Next, the patient is asked to close his or her eyes, and again the platform moves. A good vestibular system is required to keep from falling in this condition. Lastly, the platform moves and so does the visual field—but in different ways. This is the most challenging condition, as the inputs from the vision and vestibular/proprioception centers differ. Posturography can help to establish a treatment program, and can give information on risk of fall.

Overview of Video- and Electronystagmography

As you have learned, the eyes are reflexively controlled by the vestibular system, and good central nervous system function is required for eye movement. When a patient is "dizzy" we want to know why, and we want to objectively document the problem. Video- and electronystagmography give us the tools to evaluate the patient, and to help distinguish between problems coming from the vestibular periphery versus the central nervous system. This testing relies on measurement of the movement of the eyes.

Videonystagmography (VNG) records eye movements using infrared cameras. The eye movements are displayed and recorded by a computer system. The camera system is mounted on goggles, and the goggles can be closed to exclude light and examine the patient's eye movements when the patient is no longer able to visually fixate (Figure 25–7). **Electronystagmography** (ENG) is the older form of testing. Electrodes are placed near the eyes to measure the eye movements. The front and back of the eyeballs have different electrochemical charges, so that moving the eyes toward or away from an electrode can be detected. The eye motion is shown graphically. Modern systems use computers to analyze and display the results.

ENG/VNG testing uses a "battery" or group of tests. Some of the tests assess the ocular system, without vestibular input. Other tests put the patient into different positions to determine if movement or body positioning provokes the nystagmus. The last test in the ENG/VNG battery is caloric testing, which stimulates the horizontal semicircular canals, one at a time.

The tests of the ocular system and its central nervous system connections are saccadic testing, smooth pursuit testing, and optokinetic testing. In these tests, the patient is seated in front of a bar that has a row of red light-emitting diodes (LEDs) on it. LEDs light up, and the patient watches the movement of these little light dots. In **saccadic testing,** the dots jump from location to location. The patient's ability to follow the rapidly moving image is assessed. Inability to quickly and accurately follow the target would indicate a central problem. **Smooth pursuit tracking** is sometimes called pendular tracking, because in the earliest days of testing, the audiologist had the patient watch the back and forth movement of a pendulum. When the light bar is used, the lighted dot smoothly moves left and back to the right, over and over, at varying speeds. This tests the ability of the central nervous system to make controlled eye movements. During **optokinetic testing,** the lights on the bar continue to travel right to left—"falling off" the end of the bar. The patient is asked to watch the dots, or perhaps to try to count them. This creates visual nystagmus. When the dots are moving to the right, it will be left-beating nystagmus. The direction the dots move is then reversed, and the ability of the patient to track these dots is assessed, in both directions of travel, and usually at more than one rate. If the central nervous system is intact, there will be "well-formed" nystagmus.

Gaze tests examine whether nystagmus is present without head movement. The patient looks straight ahead, and up, down, left, and right. The audiologist is looking for spontaneous nystagmus. Spontaneous nystagmus from peripheral lesions (and some central lesion) is worse when looking in the direction of the fast phase, which is known as **Alexander's law**. Recall that spontaneous nystagmus from horizontal canal problems beats toward the unaffected ear. The patient with a right lesion has left-beating nystagmus. Gazing left makes the nystagmus even worse.

Positioning and positional tests determine if we can evoke nystagmus by placing the patient in different head and body positions, such as lying down, rolling on one side, or turning the head. The **Dix-Hallpike test** is a specific positioning test that is used to examine patients for **benign paroxysmal posi-**

tional vertigo (BPPV). The patient's head is turned to the side, and the patient is rapidly moved down to a lying position, with his or her head off the edge of the examination table, so that it is hanging slightly. If this triggers a **tortional** nystagmus (where there is a rotary eye movement) that has a brief latency, subsides quickly, and is less severe when the movement is repeated, then the patient has posterior canal BPPV. As discussed in the previous chapter, this can be treated with specific head movement to remove the otoconial debris.

Caloric testing stimulates the horizontal semicircular canals using thermal stimulation. The stimulus can be air or water, which the audiologist introduces into the ear canal. The audiologist will alternately use cold and warm stimulation. To understand how caloric testing works, you need to remember that the horizontal semicircular canal bulges out into the middle ear space (Figure 12–2).

When the audiologist puts the cold/warm air or water into the ear canal, this is called performing an "irrigation" of the ear, a term that was introduced in the earlier days of testing, when the stimulus was traditionally water, rather than heated/cooled air. The caloric irrigation heats or cools the middle ear space, as the tympanic membrane is not a good insulator. This will in turn heat/cool the fluid in the horizontal semicircular canals. The patient is supine, with his or her head elevated 30 degrees. As was illustrated in Figure 24-4, this places the horizontal canal into a vertical position. When the fluid in the semicircular canals is heated, the fluid rises. Cool irrigations cause the fluid to fall. Movement of the endolymph will move the cupula and create nystagmus. The audiologist will assess whether the irrigations caused equal degrees of nystagmus in each ear. A weak peripheral system causes little or no nystagmus in the affected ear. Although "peripheral" tends to mean the conductive system and the cochlea when describing the auditory system, the "peripheral vestibular system" includes the VIIIth nerve as well as the end organs. A person with an VIIIth nerve tumor or with damaged sensory receptors will also have reduced response to caloric stimulation.

SUMMARY

The vestibular peripheral system has reflexive connections to the eyes, and the vestibular ocular reflex (VOR) permits us to keep our eyes focused, and our vision clear, as the head turns. There are also reflexive connections between the vestibular periphery and the muscles of the head, neck, and trunk, that help keep us from falling as we

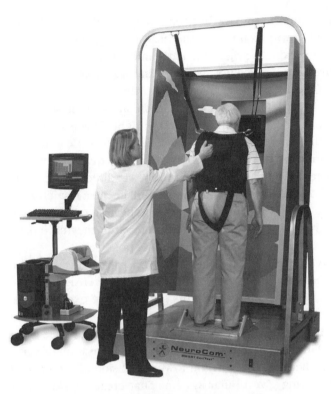

Figure 25-6. A dynamic platform posturography system. Photo courtesy of NeuroCom International, Inc., with permission.

A.

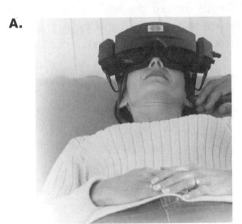

Figure 25-7. A. The patient is shown wearing the goggles. **B.** The infrared cameras provide a picture of the eyes, and the computer will record the eye movements. Photo courtesy of Maico Diagnostics, Eden Prairie, MN, with permission.

B.

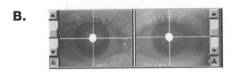

change positions away from our center of gravity. Visual input and proprioceptive input are also integrated into what we think of as the balance system.

Audiologists assess patients with balance problems, primarily with VNG testing. Some tests assess the central nervous system by evaluating the accuracy of eye movement. Other tests in the battery determine if body position creates nystagmus, the slow movement of the eyes in one direction and fast movement in the opposite direction, that signals a vestibular problem. Caloric testing stimulates the horizontal semicircular canal, which is innervated by the superior branch of the vestibular nerve. Chapter 24 mentioned VEMP testing—evaluation of the vestibular evoked myogenic potential, which evaluates the inferior branch of the vestibular portion of the VIIIth nerve.

Patients with a weak or dead peripheral vestibular system often have the sensation of rotation—vertigo—which the VNG testing evaluates. Familiarity with the anatomy and physiology of the vestibular system underlies the interpretation of the clinical tests, and merits a brief review. Moving the head in one direction (e.g., left) causes the fluid in the semicircular canals to lag behind the head movement; it is as if the fluid were moving right, in this example. Movement of the endolymph toward the utricle creates an increase in the neural firing rate of the nerves arising from the horizontal semicircular canal. In this example of the head turning left, fluid moving right, the left semicircular canal sends an excitatory signal. That signal goes from the vestibular nucleus to the VIth and IIIrd cranial nerve nuclei, then on to the muscles that move the eyes to the right. This is called the vestibular-ocular reflex or VOR. Head motion in one direction causes an equal velocity eye movement in the opposite direction. The central nervous system will create a fast leftward moving motion (or left-beating nystagmus) to move the eyes to center after they have drifted as far to the right as possible.

Weakness in one ear means that the normal ear is sending a stronger signal to the brainstem. This imbalance of excitation/inhibition from the two ears is like the signal sent when the head rotates toward the good ear, so the patient has the sensation of vertigo, a turning toward the side of the normal vestibular system. That creates a slow drift of the eyes toward the bad ear side, and a fast return to the good ear side—nystagmus that beats toward the good ear.

SECTION FOUR

Basic Psychoacoustics

26

Introduction to Psychoacoustics

This chapter provides an overview of psychoacoustics, the study of perception of sound. Psychoacoustics is a branch of psychophysics, which is the study of all sensory perception.

To be semantically correct, when speaking of the signal's physical characteristics, use terms such as "intensity" and "frequency." Perceptual judgments are of "loudness" and "pitch." Psychoacoustics is the study of the link between the physical characteristics of sound, and the perceptual dimensions.

There are three basic ways that pure tones can be manipulated. Frequency and intensity can be changed. The temporal (timing/duration) characteristics can be altered. The earliest studies of psychoacoustics sought to understand how human perception was affected when sound frequency, intensity, and duration were manipulated. The fundamental questions asked were—what are the limits of hearing: when does sound become audible, how does loudness perception change with intensity increase, and how does frequency relate to pitch perception? Does signal duration alter those perceptions?

Although psychoacoustic phenomena are interesting in and of themselves, psychoacoustics has some practical implications as well. Knowing the lowest intensity that normal hearing people can detect is critical if we are to define hearing loss. Understanding psychoacoustics aids in our understanding of anatomy and physiology as well. The study of threshold of hearing and loudness perception helps us understand the active mechanism of the cochlea, discussed in Chapters 18 and 19. Pitch perception allows us to gain insight into what frequencies are detected at what place in the cochlea, because the place theory assumes that each time we can detect a change in pitch, we have increased some distance on the basilar membrane. It allows us to "map" the basilar membrane, that is, to understand its **tonotopic organization** (the relationship of the location on a structure and the pitch encoded at that location.)

Duration studies give us some insight into neural encoding. Enough neurotransmitter has to be released to create a signal. A brief, louder signal can release enough neurotransmitter to permit hearing, or a less intense but longer signal will also create the same intensity perception. Perhaps that is related to there being a similar total amount of neurotransmitter release. It takes a certain duration for the sound to not just be heard, but be perceived as a tone, because to know the sound's period, the neurons need to fire more than once in order for some neurons in the nerve bundle to fire to each wave peak.

How hearing differs monaurally (sound presented to a single ear) and binaurally (sound presented to both ears) is another interesting area. Understanding binaural advantage gives insight into how the central nervous system functions—the neural pathways decussate (cross the midline of the brain) and interact, and therefore binaural sound stimulation improves most forms of perception. Understanding binaural advantage helps the audiologist appreciate the impact of unilateral hearing loss, and it provides the audiologist with ability to understand when and why binaural amplification will be beneficial.

Another basic psychoacoustical study area is masking—how the presence of one sound (the **masker**) alters or eliminates the perception of a second sound (the **probe**). Study of masking helps us understand the function of the cochlea and the traveling wave, discussed in Chapter 18, and along with pitch perception studies, provides information on the tonotopic organization of the cochlea.

This chapter highlights a few of the most important and/or most interesting psychoacoustical findings. It provides an overview of what will be covered in the rest of this text.

THRESHOLD FOR PURE TONES DEPENDS ON FREQUENCY

One of the earliest psychoacoustics questions, dating back to the 1930s, was "How loud does a tone need to be in order to be detected by a normally hearing person?" Figure 26-1 shows the results of the merging of two studies that examined how well people hear when sound is presented via a sound-field speaker. This figure reveals the intensity of the signal in the room at each frequency when the average normally hearing person first detects the pure tone (warbled, to avoid standing waves). Figure 26-1 shows that the best hearing is for mid- to

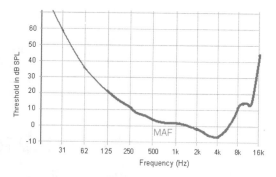

Figure 26–1. Minimal audible field (MAF) is the lowest intensity required for the average normally hearing person to detect a sound presented in sound field, that is, through loudspeakers. Note that threshold is highest in the low and high frequencies.

high-frequency sounds. In psychoacoustics, we often look to the data to provide support for what we know about auditory anatomy. We know that the pinna and external auditory meatus increases the intensity of sound in this frequency range (see Figure 13-1) and that the middle ear also has high-frequency resonances. However, the resonance data don't completely explain the threshold curve. It appears that the inner ear also has some differences in ability to detect sound at different frequencies.

TWO EARS ARE BETTER THAN ONE

Listening with two ears improves hearing sensitivity, assuming each ear is equal in hearing ability. The magnitude of the binaural advantage is about 3 dB for threshold-level sounds. The advantage can be an increase in perceived intensity that is as much as 6 dB at higher intensities. This shows that the brainstem is integrating the information provided by the two ears. Other abilities, such as detecting changes in the signal pitch or loudness, are also generally better with two ears.

UNDER IDEAL CIRCUMSTANCES, A PERSON CAN DETECT A 1 DB INTENSITY CHANGE

Humans are able to detect very small changes in intensity. About 1 dB is enough of a change to be detectable, if conditions are just right. It's easier to detect changes in louder pure tones. Very low-intensity tones, that is, those below about 20 dB SPL, need a larger intensity change for us to recognize a loudness increase.

IN GENERAL, A 10 DB INCREASE IN INTENSITY IS ABOUT A DOUBLING OF LOUDNESS

Those who tackled Chapter 2 know the "joys" of working in the decibel system. The actual physical units of sound, either measured in μPa or watts per cm², have to be converted to decibels. There is a good reason though. The ear responds to these logarithmic increases in loudness. One of the earliest studies of loudness found that increasing sound about 10 dB created a perceived doubling of loudness. The methodology used does influence this result, and others would argue that 10 dB is not the best number to use; however, what is clear is that we perceive loudness changes in fairly equal intervals on the decibel scale.

LOUDNESS GROWS A BIT DIFFERENTLY IN THE LOW FREQUENCIES: AN INTRODUCTION TO PHON CURVES

An exception to the idea that some increase, like 10 dB, is a doubling of loudness occurs for the low frequencies. In the lowest frequency range, our ability to hear sound is not as sensitive. However, when we increase the loudness to something that is very loud, we find that almost equal sound pressure levels are perceived as "very loud." Figure 26–2 illustrates, but requires the introduction of the term "**phon**," a unit of equal loudness. All sounds that are 10 phons are equal in loudness to a 10 dB SPL, 1000-Hz pure tone. The number of phons is always the dB SPL of the 1000-Hz tone at that loudness, or of any sound that is equally loud. Notice that as frequency decreases, more intensity is required for the low-frequency sound to be equal in loudness to the 1000-Hz sound. This is expected, because the threshold

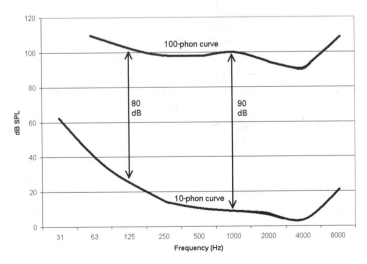

Figure 26–2. Phon curves show what sounds are equally loud. Two phon curves are shown: 10 and 100. The curves are named after the SPL of the sound at 1000 Hz, which is the reference. Every combination of frequency and intensity on the curve is equally loud. Note that the 10-phon curve is curvier than the 100-phon curve. The spacing between the two changes, particularly for the lowest frequencies.

changes with frequency and more intensity is required to detect low-frequency sounds. However, note the shape of the 100-phon curve, which shows which frequency/intensity pure tones are equal to the loudness of a 100 dB SPL, 1000-Hz tone. There is less variation, though the effect of the ear resonances in the high-frequency range is still obvious. Focus on the closing space between these two phon curves in the lower frequencies. Loudness is growing more quickly as shown in that it only takes an increase of 80 dB of a 125-Hz tone to be 90 phons. It took a 90 dB increase for the 1000-Hz tone to be 90 phons.

PITCH

When Is a Pure Tone Tonal?

Let's turn to the topic of the perceptions associated with changing frequency. The most fundamental question is "What frequencies can we hear?" We can hear from 1 Hz to about 20,000 Hz, though the upper limit of hearing decreases as we age. By the "ripe old age" of about 18, hearing in the highest frequency range is on the decline. As Figure 26–1 illustrated, it takes more intensity to hear in the extreme high and low frequencies. In addition to not being very sensitive to low-frequency sounds, there is a limit on the quality of the perception. The lower the frequency, below about 50 Hz, the less tonal it is. Below about 20 Hz it isn't really perceived as tonal at all. "**Infrasound**" may be perceived as a rumble or a thrusting sound. It is also known to invoke a "spooky" feeling. If you had loudspeakers capable of producing these very low frequencies, which if loud enough can also be felt as vibrations in the chest cavity, it would make an interesting addition to a haunted house.

Detecting Change in Pitch

Of course, frequency is determined by the period of the sound. When we are asking the question "What is the smallest change in frequency that is detectably different" we are presenting sounds that vary in their periods. Think back for a moment to how the nervous system encodes frequency/period. Although not every neuron located near the peak of the traveling wave will fire to each cycle of the sound wave, neural firings are triggered in some neurons by each successive cycle of the wave, which codes the period of the sound wave. Investigating the "just noticeable difference for frequency" reveals how accurately the ear can make these neural encodings. The ear is able to detect a change in period as small as 1/1000 of a millisecond (0.001 msec) for mid- to high-frequency sounds. That is the difference in the period of 4000 Hz (0.25 msec) and 4016 Hz (0.249 msec), for example. You won't be able to detect a smaller frequency difference; for example, 4000 and 4005 Hz would have the same pitch. However, if you were listening to a low frequency, for example 250 Hz, you could distinguish a 1-Hz change under ideal listening conditions. That's because the period of 250 Hz is longer: 4 msec. The period of 251 Hz is 0.02 msec shorter (2/100 msec), so detecting that change is easier. When examining the ability to detect change in frequency, measured in number of Hz, our ability to discriminate frequency change is best in the low frequencies. From the way this is worded, you might guess that there is another way to view things. We could also think about what percent change in the signal frequency is detectable, in which case, as Chapter 31 elaborates on, you would conclude that we are better able to detect mid-frequency signal changes.

The ability to detect change in pitch was of interest to early cochlear physiologists because it was assumed that the same distance on basilar membrane must be involved in this ability. When it was found that a greater number of Hz are found in a high-frequency just noticeable difference for pitch, then it was concluded that the base of the cochlea has greater "frequency density." A given distance (in mm) on basilar membrane spans a larger number of frequencies.

Doubling Frequency Creates a Musical Sameness, but Not a Doubling of Pitch

The musical scale is based on an octave scale: for example, C2 is twice as high a frequency as C1. The ear does respond to these doublings of frequency with a "sameness" sort of scaling; however, if we ask a person to listen to a sound, and then adjust a second tone to be twice as high in pitch, the listener doesn't double the frequency. Typically, the frequency change is less than a doubling. The **mel** scale was created to describe the perceptual scale of pitch change. It is described in Chapter 31.

MASKING

Masking occurs when one sound reduces or eliminates the audibility of another sound. Most, but not all, of masking occurs within the cochlea and can be explained by the traveling waves of the sounds. In order to mask a sound, "cover up" or "swamp" its traveling wave with the traveling wave from another sound. For example, a 1000-Hz pure tone creates a gradually rising traveling wave that peaks near the middle of basilar membrane. As we know from von Bekesy's work, the traveling wave dies out very rapidly after it peaks. The mass of the area of basilar membrane above the **characteristic frequency** area, that area that encodes that given frequency, keeps basilar membrane from moving in response to the tone. As shown in Figure 26–3, another sound put into the same ear, such as a slightly more intense narrowband noise centered at 1000 Hz, can mask the audibility of the 1000-Hz pure tone.

Upward Spread of Masking

Figure 26–4 illustrates what is termed **upward spread of masking**. The 1000-Hz pure tone can mask signals with higher (upward) frequencies more readily than those with lower frequencies, which peak toward the apex. Said another way, low frequencies can mask high frequencies much more readily than a high frequency can mask a low frequency.

The phenomenon of upward spread of masking has implications in speech understanding in background noise. Many types of background noise are predominantly low frequency. Traffic noise, the sounds of a dishwasher, and lawnmower are low pitch, and the sound of many people talking contains mostly the more intense vowel energy,

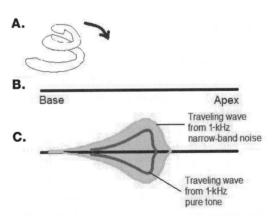

Figure 26–3. A. Basilar membrane coils base to apex, but is often drawn schematically as a straight line (**B**). **C.** The envelope of the traveling wave for a 1-kHz pure tone is completely within the envelope of the 1-kHz narrow-band noise that is slightly more intense. The narrow-band noise masks the pure tone.

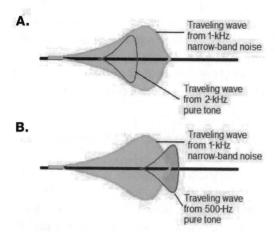

A.

Traveling wave from 1-kHz narrow-band noise

Traveling wave from 2-kHz pure tone

B.

Traveling wave from 1-kHz narrow-band noise

Traveling wave from 500-Hz pure tone

Figure 26–4. A. The 1000-Hz narrow-band noise is able to mask a less intense pure tone that is higher in frequency, shown here as 2000 Hz. **B.** Because of the shape of the traveling wave, the 1000-Hz narrow-band noise does not mask the 500-Hz traveling wave, which peaks more apically.

which is low frequency. The low-frequency content of the background noise can interfere with hearing for lower intensity high-frequency sounds, such as consonants.

Critical Bands

For any given masking signal, there is a range of nearby frequencies that are easily masked. This frequency range is called the **critical band**.

Critical bands relate not only to masking, but also to loudness perception. The neurons within a critical band are situated close together, of course, and they are capable of being stimulated by sounds within that frequency region. For example, a critical band ranges from 900 to 1060 Hz. A 950-Hz pure tone would stimulate the 900-Hz characteristic frequency neuron, and also the 1060-Hz characteristic frequency neuron. Let's suppose that instead of hearing just a 950-Hz tone, simultaneously a 900-Hz and a 1060-Hz pure tone are also presented.

All those pure tones are stimulating neurons within the same area (the same critical band.) Those three tones won't be perceived as being as loud as if the tones were not all in the same critical band. For example, if the experimental subject is listening to 500-Hz, 1000-Hz, and 2000-Hz tones presented simultaneously instead of 900, 950, and 1050-Hz, that will be perceived as louder, because, in total, more neurons are being stimulated.

TEMPORAL PROCESSING

Sounds Are Louder and of More Distinct Pitch if at Least One-Quarter Millisecond Duration

If a group of neurons were to fire just once, the central nervous system has limited information available. Because neurons are tonotopically organized, so that different neurons are associated with different places on basilar membrane, it is possible that some information about the frequency of the stimulus would be provided. However, the central nervous system uses the time between neural impulses (coming from different nerves, some responding to one peak of a sound wave cycle, others responding to subsequent peaks) to encode frequency. Because of this, it makes sense that the listener won't be sure of the pitch of the sound unless the sound has been on for at least a few cycles of the sound wave. To fully develop the sensation of pitch, the sound needs to be of 200 to 250-msec duration.

Also, perception of loudness is increased if the brief signal remains on for a greater duration. When a sound is shorter than 200 to 250 msec, it is not perceived as being as loud. The neural system seems to sum up the firing of neurons over time to create part of the perception of loudness.

Temporal Order Detection

If two sounds are presented very close together in time, the listener will not perceive them as two sounds. A generalization is that it takes about 1 to 2-msec difference in the onset times to know that there were two sounds. It takes a greater separation between the onsets to recognize which one started first—about 20 msec.

Gap Detection

A common way to evaluate the ear's ability to recognize timing is to put a brief pause, or a "gap," in a noise signal. If the gap is too small, it is not detected. Under ideal circumstances, a gap of 1 to 2 msec can be detected.

Temporal processing is of interest because part of how speech is detected is by processing time information. Some speech sounds change frequency and intensity rapidly, and require good time-processing ability.

SUMMARY AND IMPLICATIONS FOR SPEECH PERCEPTION

Understanding the limits of human perception is of interest, as that relates to our ability to understand speech. We know that the ear is most sensitive to mid- to high-frequency sounds, which helps in detecting consonant sounds, that are predominantly high-frequency sounds. We know that loud low-frequency sounds are able to mask the perception of the consonants that are so important to speech understanding. We know that if a speech sound is very brief, it will be perceived as less intense. The class of phonemes called stop consonants are shorter duration, and thus expected to sound less loud than equal intensity sounds of greater duration.

The remainder of this text provides a more thorough introduction to psychoacoustics. The final chapter introduces some of the ways in which cochlear hearing loss changes how the ear processes sound, and describes how this may affect the understanding of speech.

27

Classical Psychoacoustical Methodologies

Before describing the limits of human perception, a foundation in how psychoacoustics experiments are and were conducted is helpful. This chapter discusses the classical methodologies, and introduces some of the newer procedures. The following chapter provides more information on signal detection theory and some of the modern adaptive methods.

CLASSIC PSYCHOACOUSTIC METHODS

How we ask questions influences the answer. Just as a course examination can have multiple choice and essay questions, psychoacoustic experiments can use different methods to study the same perceptual phenomenon. Generally, similar results are provided, and the methods differ in efficiency and with the purpose of the experiment.

As audiologists are interested in assessing hearing threshold, that example will be used in this chapter. The ways in which changing the method alters threshold, and clinical implications, are discussed.

Method of Limits

The **method of limits** is familiar to the audiologist, as a form of this method is used clinically in establishing "the limits" of the patient's hearing thresholds. Clinically, the frequency of tone is set, then the intensity is adjusted by the audiologist or experimenter, and the patient or subject responds, one hopes, as instructed. These responses are noted and used to define threshold, the lowest intensity that the patient responds to at least 50% of the time.

Effect of Instruction

How you instruct the research subject or patient affects the threshold obtained. (Rather than always saying subject or patient, this chapter will use the term subject, but keep in mind that what is true about subjects is true of patients.) Threshold will be lower (better) if the subject is told to respond whenever he or she "thinks the sound may be present." When the subject is encouraged to guess, the subject more often correctly identifies low-intensity signals; however, the patient also will make more mistakes—responding when there is no sound present.

Correctly responding to an audible tone is called a **hit**. Failing to respond to an audible signal is a **miss**, or **false negative.** The baseball-esque terminology ends there; the next two terms are false positive and correct rejection. **False positive** or **false alarm** is when the subject responds when no signal was present. A **correct rejection** is when the subject does not respond, and no signal was present. So, using these terms, we say that instructions that encourage guessing will increase the number of hits, decreasing the misses. It will also increase the number of false positives and decrease the correct rejection rate.

False positive responses can be difficult to differentiate from true positive responses in clinical testing and during manually controlled method-of-limits experimental testing. It can even be a problem when a computer is controlling the presentation and recording of responses.

Instructing the subject to be sure that the tone is present before responding would increase correct rejections, but at the expense of increased misses. Threshold is also increased.

Because of the problems with false positive responses, psychoacousticians typically use experimental methods other than the method of limits. However, this method is time efficient, and it is sufficiently accurate for clinical purposes, where it is acceptable to measure a threshold that is 5 dB different from the patient's true threshold of hearing.

Response Latency and False Positive Responses

A skilled experimenter or clinician (or a good computer program used to collect experimental data) uses the **latency** of the subject's response (the time interval between the start of the signal and the subject's response) as a clue to determining if a response is likely a false positive. When the signal is well above threshold, there is a short time between stimulus onset and subject response. Near threshold, the subject may pause to question whether that was or was not a signal, and the subject may wait until the signal goes off, using the return to quiet as another cue, increasing the response latency. The subject's latency is fairly stable, though different subjects have different response times. The more cautious, and generally the more elderly, tend to have longer response latencies. Carefully observe the subject's response latency. When the time between stimulus and response is uncharacteristically long or short, then the response is more likely to be a false positive.

Effect of Using Increasing Versus Decreasing Intensity Runs

A **run** is a series of stimulus presentations. An **ascending method of limits** run is when the experimenter starts presenting signals at a low-intensity level and records the lowest intensity that elicits a response. A **descending method of limits** run starts at an audible level and goes down.

Subjects tend to have better (lower) thresholds when tested using descending runs. This probably occurs because the subject is more willing to guess. It is easier to track the sound as it decreases in level, and attention is focused on the progressively quieter signal. The size of the difference is not large: it is on average about 2 dB. Clinically, as we test in 5 dB steps, threshold should be the same or 5 dB worse if retested using an ascending procedure.

Experiments can present both ascending and descending runs, and use the average threshold from several ascending and descending runs to obtain threshold. Equal numbers of ascending and descending runs would need to be used, or else threshold would be biased.

Clinical Correlate: How Instruction Affects Patients' Responses

Clinical audiologists differ somewhat in their preferred patient instructions. Some will instruct the patient to respond "even if you think you hear the tone"; others provide no indication that guessing is acceptable saying "press the button if you hear the tone." A middle ground is "press the button even if it is very soft." As younger patients are more likely to guess, this text's first author does not ask patients under the age of 50 or 60 to guess, as some interpret that instruction quite literally, and the audiologist then has to tactfully ask that "now, rather than guessing as I initially asked you to do, please be more certain before pressing the response button." However, with older patients, who often seem not to be inclined to err, it is safer to ask them to guess because they seldom have high false-positive rates.

The classical article on hearing testing, Carhart and Jerger's (1959) description of the **Hughson-Westlake procedure**, used the following instructions, which do not encourage guessing. "The purpose of this test is to see how well you can hear some faint tones. Each tone will be quite short. Some will be easy to hear. Others will be quite faint. Whenever you hear one of these tones, no matter how faint it is, raise your finger. As soon as the tone goes off, lower your finger."

Clinical Correlate: Nonorganic Loss Detection Using Lack of False Positive Responses and Latency Inconsistencies.

A person who is malingering (faking a hearing loss, and is said to have a **nonorganic hearing loss**) is unlikely to give false positive responses. Why would a person who knows that a tone is present and is waiting until it is some predetermined loudness think it normal to respond when *no* tone was present? Clinically, an audiologist is suspicious of the patient who never has a false positive response, as most patients will give at least a few false positive responses when trying to detect soft sounds. Additionally, the latency of the responses of a patient with nonorganic loss can vary dramatically. As the threshold to be simulated approaches, the latency may increase more than usually noted as the patient ponders whether or not to respond to that signal level. This prolonged latency may occur, not just within 5 dB of threshold, but within 10 or 15 dB of threshold. Astute observation of false positives and latencies provides the audiologist with a means of detecting malingering.

Audiologists use a combined ascending/descending approach in clinical threshold testing using the **Hughson-Westlake procedure**; the descending runs are in larger steps (the signal decreases 10 dB with each patient response). The use of descending runs helps the patient focus on the progressively softer sound. The actual threshold measurement is made recording the responses to the ascending runs, which are in 5 dB **steps**.

Method of Adjustment

When the subject is allowed to adjust the stimulus him or herself, a **method of adjustments** is being used. Typically, the intensity increases smoothly, rather than going up so many dB each step, and the signal stays on even if it is not audible to the subject. In regard to threshold testing, the subject could adjust the signal by manipulating a knob, moving it left and right until threshold is reached. The experimenter could then read the level, which the subject would not be able to see. The knob would be reset, and the procedure could be repeated. (Experiments typically require making measurements several times to establish the reliability of the responses.)

However, a more typical way to obtain a method of adjustment threshold is to instruct the subject to press a button while the signal is heard, which causes the signal to gradually become less intense, and release the button when it is not heard, which makes the signal level gradually increase. A graph of the results is shown in Figure 27–1.

The method of limits used clinically in this manner is called **Bekesy audiometry**. It

Clinical Correlate: Ascending Testing in Nonorganic Loss

Although normal hearers and those with conductive or sensorineural pathology have little difference between the ascending and descending thresholds, those with nonorganic loss frequently have large differences between the ascending and descending thresholds. When tested with descending runs, the nonorganic patient uses the loudness of the more intense presentations as a guide to when to respond, and tends to give even more elevated thresholds. If the runs ascend only, lower thresholds are often obtained. The malingerer seems to choose a quieter level to respond to when the sounds "emerge" out of quiet. Audiologists generally retest at least one frequency to see if the patient is consistent. It can be helpful to conduct the threshold retesting, not with the Hughson-Westlake technique, but with an ascending-only approach. If retesting hearing to establish validity of the thresholds is done using an ascending threshold search method, the typical patient will respond at the original threshold level or 5 dB *higher*; the nonorganic loss patient will probably have a threshold more than 5 dB *lower*.

was popular in the 1950s through the 1970's and is still sometimes used in the Veterans Administration. Threshold is considered the midpoint between the **reversal points** (the points where the subject starts to press the button, causing the signal to decrease in intensity, and where the subject stops pressing the button, which causes the signal level to gradually increase).

Similarity of Results of Method of Adjustment and Method of Limits

There is very little difference between the results that would be obtained with a Bekesy method of adjustments, a **Simple Up-Down (SUD)** method of limits, and the clinical Hughson-Westlake method of limits (Figure 27–2). In a SUD method, each time the subject provides a positive response, the signal level is decreased. Each time the subject does not respond, the intensity is increased. In SUD, the step size for increasing and decreasing the intensity is the same (here, 5 dB).

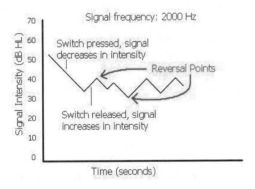

Figure 27–1. When the subject presses the button, indicating the sound is heard, the sound gradually decreases intensity. Releasing the button increases intensity. A graph of the results such as this is used when clinically conducting fixed-frequency Bekesy audiometry.

Method of Constant Stimuli

For clinical purposes, threshold is defined as the lowest level at which the subject hears the signal at least 50% of the time. Although the methods of adjustment and limits can easily define threshold, they do not help us see how the percentage of "hits" changes as signal level changes. If one wants to know how signal intensity affects the subject's response rate, the **method of constant stimuli** can be used. A (constant) number of stimuli per intensity will be presented, and the subject's response (or failure to respond) will be recorded. For example, a 1000-Hz tone may be presented 5 times each at the intensities of 2, 4, 6, 8, 10, 12, and 14 dB SPL. The order of the stimuli presentations is randomized. The results are tallied (Table 27–1) and plotted, as in Figure 27–3. Threshold is considered the intensity at which the curve passes the 50% point, and threshold need not be at one of the intensities actually presented.

Number of Trials and Step Size

The larger the number of trials used in the method of constant stimuli, the less likely one is to be influenced by experimental error. The step size, and the choice of those steps, also affects accuracy. Table 27–2 and Figure 27–4 show data from the same hypothetical subject, obtained by testing in 1 dB steps, and in 8 dB steps.

The obvious drawback to increasing the number of step sizes and trials is that it increases the testing time. Boredom and fatigue from extra trials may reduce accuracy.

Newer Methods

Adaptive Up-Down Methods

The method of constant stimuli allows one to know not just threshold, but the intensity at which the patient achieved 25%

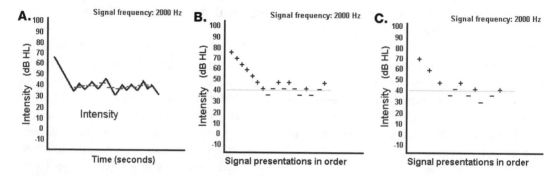

Figure 27–2. Illustration that all methods provide essentially the same threshold estimate, in this case 40 dB HL. Plus symbols indicate that the subject has responded indicating the tone has been heard; negative signs indicate the subject did not hear the tone. **A.** Bekesy method of adjustment. Threshold is considered the average of the points midway between the reversal points. **B.** Results from an experiment using the Simple Up-Down method. The average of the midpoint of the reversal points is also used to determine threshold **C.** Clinical Hughson-Westlake procedure. The intensity decreases are in 10 dB steps, the increases are in 5 dB steps. Threshold is the lowest level that elicits a response in at least 2 of 3 reversals.

Table 27–1. Hypothetical Responses of a Research Subject to Presentations of a Pure Tone at Different Intensity Levels During a Method of Constant Stimuli Experiment. Results are plotted in Figure 27–3.

Signal Level (dB SPL)						
2	4	6	8	10	12	14
Responses						
0/5	1/5	2/5	4/5	5/5	5/5	5/5

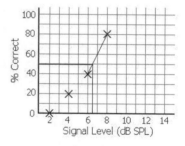

Figure 27–3. The method of constant stimuli presents predefined signals to the patients, with stimuli at each level presented several times. The percent correct data are plotted. Threshold is interpolated from the data available. Here, the 50% point is reached at 6.5 dB SPL.

detection, 33% detection, 67% detection, and so forth. If the experimenter wanted to know the level at which a given detection rate is achieved, there is an option beyond using the method of constant stimuli. An adaptive up-down method can be used. Adaptive up-down methods present several stimuli at the same intensity. The decision to turn the intensity up or down is made based on whether or not the subject reached a certain performance level. For example, in a very simple paradigm, if we wish to know when the subject responds 67% of the time (2/3 times), then we would decrease the in-

tensity when the subject responds 2/3 or 3/3 times correctly, and increase the intensity if there is 0 or 1 of 3 trials correctly identified.

There are many adaptive procedures, and ways to minimize the bias that would come if the subject figures out that the intensity is remaining the same in three trials. This will be discussed further in the next chapter.

Table 27–2. Two More Set of Experimental Results, Using Different Numbers of Steps in the Experiment. Both results are plotted in Figure 27–4.

Signal Level (dB SPL)									
3	4	5	6	7	8	9	10	11	12
Responses									
1/20	3/20	4/20	7/20	11/20	16/20	19/20	20/20	20/20	20/20
Signal Level (dB SPL)									
4									12
Responses									
3/20									20/20

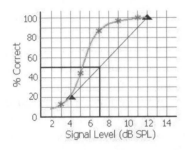

Figure 27–4. When testing in 1 dB steps, the threshold is established at 6.5 dB SPL. The curve is not accurately plotted when 8 dB steps are used, and threshold is estimated as 8 dB SPL.

Introduction to Forced-Choice Methods

Here is an example of the instructions an experimenter may give if using a forced-choice method to measure hearing detection threshold. "A light will go on. There may or may not be a sound present when the light goes on. Tell me 'yes' if you think there was a sound and 'no' if you think there was no sound." That is an example of **a two-alternative** (the only alternatives are to say "yes" or "no") **forced-choice (2AFC) procedure**. It has the advantage of allowing the experimenter to accurately count the false positive responses; however, it doesn't control

for the subject's guessing behavior. One subject may not give a positive response unless she is sure of the signal presence, whereas another subject may tend to respond more readily, being more willing to guess.

The experimenter tells the subject "The white light will go on, and then the green light will go on. The sound will be present either when the white light is on or the green light is on. Tell me which interval, white or green light, had the sound in it." This is a **two-interval, two-alternative forced-choice** (2I-2AFC) **procedure**. The procedure can be modified for 3, 4, or as many alternative periods as desired, and the subject would more likely be viewing a computer screen graphic than simply viewing lights.

The classical method of presenting the signal, and determining if the subject responded with the appropriate latency, is a fairly crude method from a psychoacoustics standpoint. It gives no information on whether threshold was lowered by the subject's tendency to guess, or elevated by reluctance to guess. Forced-choice methods can control for guessing by requiring all subjects to guess (e.g., using a two-interval, two-alternative forced-choice procedure.)

Threshold Is Generally Not 50% Correct Identification in a Forced-Choice Procedure

If a subject is participating in a two-interval, two-alternative forced-choice threshold assessment, and the signal is below threshold, how often will the subject correctly identify the interval with the signal? As the subject must guess between two intervals, you would expect by chance that the subject will select the correct interval half the time. If the task were a three-alternative forced-choice procedure, then the subject would guess correctly one-third of the time.

When using forced-choice procedures, threshold is defined as the halfway point between chance and certainty. That is, the 75% correct identification point is threshold in a two-alternative forced-choice procedure, and it is 67% correct for a three-alternative forced-choice procedure

INTRODUCTION TO SIGNAL DETECTION THEORY

Sometimes, understanding perception across different individuals is complicated by their willingness to guess. For example, a psychoacoustician may want to know how large a frequency change is detected in hearing-impaired and normal-hearing people. The normal hearers tend to be young and willing to guess; the hearing-impaired are more elderly and may be less likely to guess. The two- (or more) alternative forced-choice procedure could be used to control for tendency to guess. A more complicated procedure using signal detection theory gives the scientist even more information, while controlling for willingness to guess.

First, some background on the name "signal detection theory." We theorize that when listening, there is always some back-ground noise present. That noise could be the subject's breathing, the slight noise he or she makes when responding, or ambient noise. (And in many experiments, the subject's task is to listen while noise is experimentally added.) The subject's task is really then to detect the signal in the background noise, whether it is ambient or experimentally manipulated noise.

In signal detection theory experiments, the subject's willingness to guess is manipulated. Consider how you would behave if you were a subject in this experiment. You are told "When the computer reads 'vote' click either "yes" to indicate there was a tone present, or "no" if there was not. If you are correct, you will receive a dime. If you are incorrect, your account will lose a nickel. You can see your running tally of your bonus money on the top right of the computer screen." Of course, to maximize your income, if you even think you heard the tone, you would answer "yes." That is, you would have a high percentage of hits, but many false positives as well.

How would your behavior change if the experimental rules change to gaining a dime for each correct response, but losing a dime if you are wrong? Your hit rate might fall, but you false positives will fall too. Furthermore, if you were to gain only a nickel for being right, and lose a dime for being wrong, you would be even less inclined to respond unless you were sure the signal was present—you would have a very low false alarm rate, but a lowered hit rate.

Signal detection theory uses these sorts of rewards in order to alter the subject's willingness to guess. During these experiments, the signal level is changing too, and for each signal level, the hits, misses, false positives, and correct rejections are tallied. From this data, the psychoacoustician obtains more information than "threshold." He or she arrives at a mathematical calculation of the magnitude of how much greater the subject's perception of the signal is than the "noise." This number is called **d'**, which is pronounced "d prime." Understanding what d' really means is challenging, and a topic covered in the next chapter. At a simplistic level, the d' number relates to the percentage of hits to false positive responses.

Signal detection theory experiments are not required to control willingness to guess. Using a forced-choice procedure has that advantage, and is the reason most of the studies of auditory perception use a form of a forced-choice procedure (with or without signal detection theory elements).

SCALING PROCEDURES

The methods described to this point are applicable to tests of threshold and tests that seek to determine what change in frequency or intensity is just noticeably different. However, they are not applicable (without modification) if we want to experiment on how humans scale or rate perceptions. For example, if one wants to know what intensity is twice as loud as a given sound, how would that information be obtained?

Magnitude Estimation

The **magnitude estimation technique** asks the subject to assign a number to a stimulus. For example, the subject could be asked to listen to various intensity sounds, and give a number to each to represent its loudness. Similarly, this technique can be used to scale for pitch. In some cases, the experimenter might "anchor" the subject by giving the subject a number to use for the mid-range stimulus. That reference stimulus might be termed a modulus or a standard.

Magnitude Production

The subject is given control of the stimulus in a **magnitude production meth-**

Clinical Correlate: Scaling Procedures Used Clinically

If you were to ask a clinical patient to listen to discourse recorded in noise, and asked the subject to estimate the percentage of words heard, that would also be an example of a magnitude estimation task. It is not a terribly reliable estimate, but it is a technique that has been used.

If you obtain the patient's uncomfortable listening level by using a scale from 1 to 7, where you tell the patient that 7 means a sound that is so loud that she would never choose to listen to it, no matter what mood she was in, 4 means it is comfortable, and 1 means it is just barely audible, then you have used a magnitude estimation task. You would not say that a modulus or standard was given. Those who have had a course in statistical methods might recognize this as the use of a "semantic differential" scaling method.

od; that is, it is a form of a method of adjustments task. The subject might be told to adjust the stimulus until the subject thinks it reaches a predefined criterion (e.g., adjust the loudness of this until you think it is "50." Now, make that tone a "25" in loudness.")

Fractionation

The method of fractionation has the subject make the stimulus some fraction of its original quality. For example, the subject may be asked to make the sound half as loud, or half the pitch. The instructions could work in the opposite direction—you could have the subject make the pitch twice as high, for example.

Cross-Modality Matching

Sometimes, the experimenter will use a visual image to help the subject in making the judgment about the stimulus. The subject might be asked to mark off the length of a line on a piece of paper to represent the loudness of the stimulus. The experimenter then records the length of the lines. This is an example of cross-modality matching.

SUMMARY

Psychoacoustic methods vary from the simple and easy to use in the clinic to the complicated methods that require considerable time, may require computer control of the stimulus, but also provide greater information. The right method is a function of the information needed, and the time available. The next chapter delves further into methodologies, but that chapter is not required reading in order to understand Chapters 29 to 38.

REFERENCE

Carhart, R., & Jerger, J. F. (1959). Preferred method for clinical determination of pure-tone thresholds. *Journal of Speech and Hearing Research, 24*, 330–345.

28

Signal Detection Theory and Advanced Adaptive Approaches

One of the most important advances in psychophysical methodology was the routine use of forced-choice paradigms. By requiring all the subjects to make a choice between alternatives, the problem we have clinically of patient reluctance or willingness to guess is eliminated. Another important development was signal detection theory, which provided even more insight into the magnitude of the subject's perception judgments. As the previous chapter started to describe, an additional advance in psychophysical methods was to allow the researcher to experiment more efficiently when finding threshold—or determining any other percent correct identification point (such as 66% or 71% correct detection).

This chapter introduces signal detection theory and some of the terminology and concepts behind the modern methods. It is beyond the scope of the chapter to fully describe all the methods and their advantages and limitations, but the chapter should provide the foundation needed for the reader to read scholarly articles with at least a basic understanding of the techniques used.

Additionally, the chapter will consider some of the issues involved in applying psychophysical techniques to testing for in-

dividual patient preference for hearing aid characteristics. As will be shown, currently there are no practical, scientifically valid procedures for systematically altering the characteristics of a patient's hearing aid to establish the "best" hearing aid settings.

A review of some of the terms from the previous chapter is in order before beginning the discussion of signal detection theory. The patient will be given a *forced-choice* task, that is, required to make a guess after being presented with two or more alternatives. A two-alternative forced-choice procedure could be a task with presentation of one stimulus, which is judged as present or absent. This is called a yes/no method, or a single-interval two-alternative forced-choice procedure. You could also have a two-alternative forced choice procedure where two intervals could be presented, with one containing the stimulus. In this case, the subject indicates the interval containing the stimulus. If the subject correctly identifies a stimulus interval, (or stimulus in a yes/no paradigm) that is a "**hit**." Failing to detect the signal when it is present is a "**miss**" or "false negative," and the percentage of hits and misses tallies to 100%. In a yes/no paradigm, if the signal is not presented, the subject may indicate that it is not present (make a "**correct rejection**") or may incorrectly indicate that the signal is present (have a "**false positive response**"). These two also tally to 100%.

SIGNAL DETECTION THEORY

Understanding "Magnitude of the Sensory Event"

Signal detection theory terms can be challenging. The first to tackle is the concept of the "magnitude of the sensory event" or the synonymous "magnitude of sensory activation." In psychoacoustics, the idea is that the subject is always being stimulated—there is always some sound present. The perception of that sound, whether it is background noise alone, or the signal in the background noise, is conceptually the "magnitude of the sensory event." If there is an audible experimental signal present, a greater magnitude sensory event is perceived.

A key point in signal detection theory is that—even without a signal present—the magnitude of the sensory event is not always constant. Common sense tells us that sometimes the subject will be seated very quietly, sometimes he or she might be breathing or moving, and that activity changes the magnitude of the sensory event at that moment.

Signal detection theory says that the sensory event from noise alone varies around some average level—sometimes it is more than the average level, sometimes it is less. Furthermore, the theory holds that the noise level is most often near the average, and seldom far quieter or far louder. The theory postulates that the magnitude of the sensory event across time has a bell-shaped (Gaussian) distribution. See Figure 28–1.

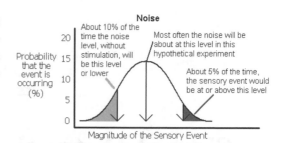

Figure 28–1. Theoretically, the background noise will most often be near some average magnitude. The noise levels may be higher or lower at any given time, creating a higher or lower magnitude sensory event. The percentage of time that the noise levels are higher or lower than average is assumed to have a bell-curve shaped distribution. As shown here, about 15% of the time the magnitude of the perception of the background noise, the "sensory event," will be exactly at average. Less often, it will be higher or lower.

Signal Plus Noise Perception

If the experimenter presents an audible signal, one that is clearly above the background noise, if the research subject perceived just that signal (and not the background noise with it), then hypothetically, that signal alone would be of some relatively high perceptual magnitude, as suggested by Figure 28-2.

However, the perception during the experiment is never just of the signal alone. There is always background noise with it. Most experiments present signals that are very faint, and therefore the magnitude of the sensory events aren't much larger than the sensory events from the noise. Therefore, when we think about the subject's perception when the signal is present, in signal detection theory, we consider that the patient perceives the signal and the noise, not the signal alone. Because the background noise levels vary, the signal and noise levels combined will vary. The theory assumes that the distribution of the signal plus noise sensory event has a Gaussian distribution, as illustrated in Figure 28–3.

If the signal were as shown in Figure 28–3, and the subject knew that the test involved only that signal level, the subject would have an easy time determining if the presentation was of "signal plus noise" or if

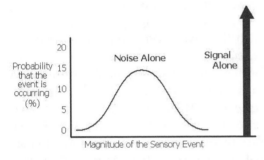

Figure 28–2. Whereas the background noise varies, creating sensory events with magnitudes that fluctuate over time, one might think that the signal alone would theoretically always create a sensory event of some magnitude. The "up" arrow on the signal alone graphic is meant to illustrate that 100% of the time; the signal alone would yield that magnitude of sensory event.

the magnitude of the sensory event came just from background noise. The subject would probably put his or her decision-making point, or "criterion point," at the location of the dashed line. If the "sensory event" is larger in size than that indicated by the dashed line, the subject would decide that the signal is present. The experimental task is an easy one, and the subject would correctly decide whether the signal was present or absent with perfect accuracy.

Criterion Points for Decision-Making and How Hit and Correct Rejection Percentages Reveal Spacing Between the Noise and Signal-Plus-Noise Distributions

Of course, we are seldom interested in knowing about perception of clearly audible signals—we generally study perception when the signal is just barely detectable. For the rest of this example, let's assume that the subject is given a single presentation, and is forced to decide if the signal was or was

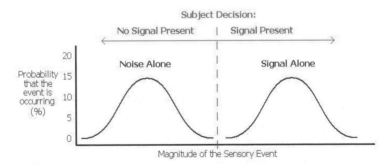

Figure 28–3. The magnitude of the sensory event of the signal, presented in the background noise, varies over time. Again, it averages at some magnitude, but can by chance, at any given moment, be more or less, because the background noise could be higher or lower than average. The noise and the signal both contribute to the magnitude of the signal-plus-noise sensory event. The dashed vertical line represents the subject's theoretical decision on when to consider a sensory event as having been noise alone (if the sensory event magnitude is below, that is to the left of, the dashed line) or signal plus noise (the sensory event is above that level).

not present (if it was noise alone, or signal-plus-noise that created the sensory event). Furthermore, let's reduce the signal intensity, so that sometimes the noise-alone level is higher than the signal-plus-noise level, as shown in Figure 28-4.

In Figure 28-4 let's imagine that the subject is asked four times if there is or is not a signal present. The subject has placed his or her decision point at the location of the dashed line. This subject has decided to respond that a signal is present if the sensory magnitude is to the right (higher than) that noted by the dashed line. In the first interval, no signal is present, and the noise just happens to be lower than average. This is noted by "*a*" in the figure. As the magnitude of the sensory event is low, the subject decides that there was no stimulus present. With presentation "*b*," the signal was present, but the sensory event from the signal plus the low ambient noise was not large enough that the subject would consider it a signal. As the magnitude of the event is to the left of the dashed line, the subject guesses that the signal is not present. The subject

has a "miss": the signal was present but the subject's decision was that it was not. With presentation "*c*," the subject has a false positive response. The sensory event magnitude from noise alone was large, and is to the right of the dashed line. The subject guessed incorrectly that the signal was present. Presentation "*d*" is correctly identified as signal present. It represents a hit.

As shown in Figure 28-5, this subject, with this given criterion point for deciding whether to say the signal was or was not present, if tested repeatedly, would have many hits and a large percentage of correct rejections. Misses are more frequent than false positives. Remember that signal detection theory assumes that the noise and signal-plus-noise distributions are bell-shaped.

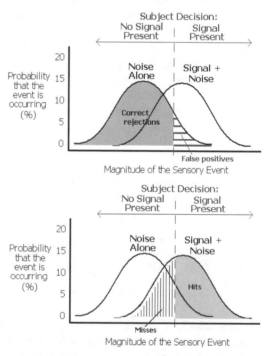

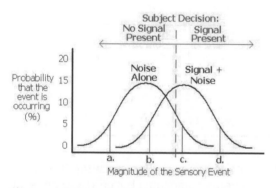

Figure 28–4. Illustration of four presentations made to the subject: two when the stimulus was present, and two control presentations when no stimulus is given. The subject is asked to respond in a one-interval, two-alternative forced-choice experiment. See text for discussion.

Figure 28–5. When the separation between the noise and signal plus noise is a certain distance, and when the subject uses some set criterion point, the subject will have a certain percentage of correct rejections, misses, false positives, and hits.

If we are given the subject's percentage of hits and false positives, we can calculate the misses and correct rejections (because hits plus misses equals 100% and false positives plus correct rejections equals 100%). With help from the appropriate tables to look things up, we could construct a picture such as this one, just knowing the hit and false positive rate. We would be able to know how far apart the distributions are from each other, and where that decision point is. The difficulty is that we do not have a numeric scale for the magnitude of the sensory event. However, we could describe the distances between the noise and signal-plus-noise distributions another way. We could describe it by the relative number of standard deviations apart. Recall that a bell curve has 68% of the events within ±1 standard deviation from the mean, and 95% within ±2 standard deviations. This knowledge lets us derive a standard deviation scale (Figure 28-6).

The standard deviation units act as our "ruler" or scale for the size of the separation between the signal-plus-noise and noise distributions. The signal detection theory would use this scale to describe the noise and signal-plus-noise distribution separation (Figure 28-7). The scale unit is now "d'" units, where each unit is the size of one standard deviation of the distribution. (d' is pro-

nounced as "d prime".) In Figure 28-7, the d' is 2.0, that is, the N and S + N distributions are as far apart as two standard deviations of the noise (or signal plus noise) distribution.

Altering Subject Criteria in Signal Detection Theory and Receiver Operating Curves

Signal detection theory tells us that knowing the subject's percentage of hits, misses, false positives, and false alarms is enough to calculate the d' value. If you wish, you can alter the hits/false alarm rate to make a second estimate of d' and to develop what is called a **receiver operating curve**. If you want to do this, you would alter the subject's decision-making points. As described in Chapter 27, this could be done by altering the monetary rewards for correct decision-making. Alternatively, you could just instruct the subject differently, such as "please be very sure the signal is present before you judge that it is present," or "even if you think there is the slightest chance that the signal is present, please respond that it is." Having two or more sets of the subject's false alarms and hits allows two or more additional calculations of the d'. This would validate the spacing of the two distributions; it

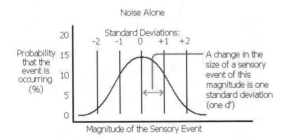

Figure 28–6. As there is no numeric scale for the perception of the magnitude of the sensory event, the only way to measure the horizontal axis is in standard deviation units. One standard deviation unit is called a d' of 1.0.

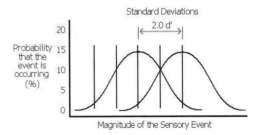

Figure 28–7. The standard deviation scale is used to measure the separation of the noise (N) and signal plus noise (S + N) distributions, and the term d' is given to the size of the distance between the distributions.

would serve as a double check of the experimental results.

If this is done, then a **receiver operating curve** (ROC) can be developed. This is a plot of the same subject's hits versus false alarm rates. Figure 28–8 shows a ROC. The point on the ROC that is closest to the top left is the ideal point on the curve. At that point, there is the best tradeoff of high hits but low false alarms. For a two-alternative forced-choice procedure, at that ideal point on the curve, the hit rate will be 76% when the d' value is 1.0.

The Magic of d'

You can use a variety of different tasks in signal detection theory. In the example above, a two-alternative forced choice was used ("Is the signal present or not?"). In this case, or in one where you ask, "Was the signal in interval one or two," the mathematicians tell us that the ideal hit rate will be 76% when the separation is one d'. That is, the inflection point on the ROC, the point on the curve that is closest to the upper left corner, will be at 76%. (If you use other procedures, for example, a three-alternative forced-choice paradigm, the hit rate wouldn't be 76% for a d' of 1.0. That is only true for the 2AFC procedure. Tables are available to either convert from hit/false alarm to d' or from d' to the ideal hit/correct rejection rate.)

The d' scale is as close as we can come to a universal scale of human perception. You and I may differ in what we consider "comfortably loud," but we don't differ in

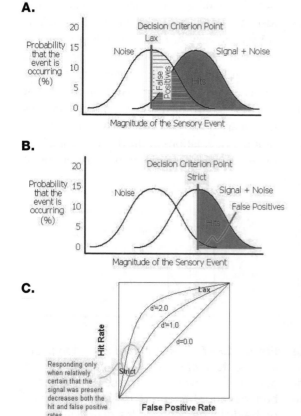

A.

B.

C.

Figure 28–8. When the same subject's decision-making criteria change, the false positive and hit rates change. **A.** With a lax criteria, the subject has a high hit rate, but also a high false-positive rate. **B.** A strict criteria reduces false positives, but the hit rate falls as well. **C.** A plot of the hit/false positive values creates a receiver operating curve. For a given value of d', all the hit/false alarm rates will fall on the same curve. For this reason, it is not necessary to manipulate the subject's decision-making rules in order to find the d' value.

our perception of what a d' is for a given signal. For example, if a hearing-impaired patient and a normal hearer are each tested for threshold at 1000 Hz, when each is presented with the level that gives them a d' of 1.0, then each is experiencing the same intensity. The measure is a measure of perception; it is not influenced by the subject's willingness to guess or other psychological factors.

ADAPTIVE METHODS TO DETERMINE THE SIGNAL LEVEL THAT IS CORRECTLY DETECTED A GIVEN PERCENTAGE OF THE TIME

It was mentioned above that when the d' is 1.0, the hit rate is 76% for the theoretical ideal subject in a 2AFC task. If we aren't interested in finding the d' value for a certain signal level, we may instead be interest-

Clinical Correlate: Clinical Tests Have d' Values

In psychoacoustic experimentation, the subject has many presentations and makes decisions on signal presence or absence, and we record the results as hits, misses, false alarms, and correct rejections. In evaluating clinical test efficacy, for example, which infant hearing screening method works best, data are collected from different patients. If the hearing screening says the baby has a hearing loss, and the baby is hearing-impaired, that result is a hit. False alarms (false positives) are screenings failed by normal-hearing babies. False negatives (misses) are those babies not picked up by the screening. Correct rejections are the children who pass the screening and are not impaired. If data are collected on hundreds of children, a table of hits, misses, and so forth can be obtained. The same tables used in psychoacoustics to compute a d' can be used to give a d' number to the infant hearing screening test.

We can also use d' values to compare different clinical test procedures. For example, we could examine several infant hearing screening programs that use different procedures and note the hits and misses for each of them. If one method has a d' of 3.0, and the second method has a d' of 3.5, the second method better separates the hits and correct rejections (the correct screening passes), and/or better minimizes the false positives and misses. One way to evaluate a test's effectiveness is to describe its d' value. This has been done for tests of retrocochlear pathology, and for means of detecting middle ear effusion (fluid behind the eardrum) when screening children.

ed in knowing what signal level gives a d' of 1.0. That is, we may want to have a forced-choice procedure that tells us what signal level the subject correctly detects 76% of the time. We could later analyze the hit versus false positive rate to ascertain if our subject was reasonably close to being the ideal decision-maker. Therefore, it is helpful to have experiments that can find this 76% correct level. The 76% point is close to the 75% point that is the difference between chance guessing (50% correct) and certainty (100%) correct, which is the threshold point in a two-alternative forced-choice procedure. In Chapter 27, it was mentioned that to find the 66% hit rate, the signal level can be changed adaptively. The signal level would increase whenever the patient misses more than one of three trials, and decreased when the subject correctly identifies the signal in two of three or three of three trials. To find a 75% correct rate, the criterion would be three of four trials correct to increase the signal level.

Block Up-Down and Transformed Up-Down Procedures

The **block up-down two-interval forced-choice (BUDTIF) procedure** can be used to find the 75% correct point. As the name implies, the task is a two-interval forced-choice, and rather than deciding on the next signal level based on one single stimulus, a series (block) of stimuli are used before deciding. If you wished to find the 75% correct identification point, you would decrease the signal intensity unless three of four or four of four trials were correctly identified.

A similar concept is the **transformed up-down procedure**. The transformed up-down procedure uses different numbers of trials to determine when to turn the signal up versus down, and for that reason is more complex than the block up-down pro-

cedure. To obtain the 71% correct response rate, the signal level is decreased if the subject responds correctly to both of two trials, and increased if there is a miss on either one (or both) of the two trials. (For expediency, if the subject misses the first of two presentations, the level would be increased; there is no need to present a second trial.) If a different level of correct identification is desired, the presentation rules differ. In contrast, **simple up-down procedures** change the signal level after each presentation, that is, down for a correct identification and up for an incorrect response.

Interleaving Runs

Often, a psychoacoustic experiment will determine more than one criterion level of performance. For example, the experimenter using a two-alternative forced-choice procedure might wish to know when the 71% and 84% correct rates are achieved.

The experimenter could use a method of constant stimuli, or the experimenter could use two separate adaptive procedure tests with two separate sets of rules. The 71% correct level is achieved by decreasing the intensity only when two sequential presentations are correct, as described above. The 84% correct transformed up-down procedure calls for signal levels to be decreased only when four presentations in a row are correct; otherwise, the signal level is increased.

Especially in the latter case, the subject might develop a bias. If the tone is heard once, and the subject learns from experience that four presentations will occur in a row, the subject will probably tend to respond to the next presentation the same way as the last. To avoid this problem, the different trials are interleaved. That is, the first presentation to establish the 71% criterion is made. The next stimulus the patient hears is the first presentation to establish the 84% correct point. The third presentation is the next signal in establishing the 71% correct identification point, the fourth presentation is back to the testing to find the 84% point, and so forth. By interleaving the trials for different runs, the subject does not have the ability to predict the next stimulus intensity.

Parameter Estimation by Sequential Testing

Adaptive procedures are frequently used to establish an individual's threshold level of perception (whether for hearing detection threshold, or threshold of detection of a difference in pitch or intensity). In order to be efficient, one may wish to vary the step size as threshold is approached. (Start by using big step sizes of stimulus change to "get in the ballpark," then when honing in on threshold, drop to small, precise stimulus magnitude changes.) The **parameter estimation by sequential testing** (PEST) paradigm is a systematic method of reducing the step size. There are different variations. A common procedure is that the step size is cut in half with each "reversal in direction," that is, changing from a judgment that the signal is present to absent, or from absent to present. Figure 28–9 shows an example.

GRIDGEMAN'S PARADOX

Gridgeman's paradox is an example of "method matters." Assume you were the participant in these two experiments. In each, you are using a three-alternative forced-choice procedure, and in each, one of the three presentations will be louder than the other two. In the first experiment, called a triangle experiment, you are asked to select the one of three intervals that sounds

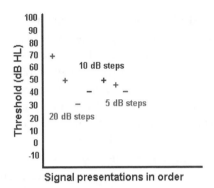

Figure 28–9. Example of a parameter estimation by sequential testing paradigm. Initially, 20-dB step decreases in intensity are used. Once the subject misses a response, it is assumed that threshold is within 20 dB, and it is prudent to start to use a smaller step size. The step size is cut in half, and the ascending run uses 10 dB steps. When the subject hears the signal, the intensity decreases, and the step size is cut in half again. The experimenter sets the minimum step size that will be used in the final threshold determination, and would have rules for how many reversals are needed using this smallest step size before threshold is established.

different. In the second experiment, a standard three-alternative-forced choice procedure, you are asked to select the one that is *louder.* You would think that the results would be the same; however, telling the subject the attribute that is changing (loudness) makes the task easier. If you scored 66% correct identification (threshold level performance) on the triangle method, that same intensity stimulus would be correctly identified about 92% of the time when you are instructed to focus on loudness!

PREFERENCE TESTING IN HEARING AID CUSTOMIZATION

Pure psychoacoustic research seldom involves preference testing. An exception is in the study of what sounds are irritating. However, the audiologist has interest in this area, as it would be ideal if there were reliable, accurate, and robust psychophysical procedures that would allow us to customize the way a hearing aid amplifies sound so that the hearing aid performance characteristics could be tailored to that particular patient's preferences. There is substantial literature in the area of perceptual preference testing. Applications extend to blending the best scotch and marketing a tasty chocolate chip cookie.

If you were to sell a new brand of chocolate chip cookie, what would its texture be? Soft or crunchy or somewhere in between? How big should the chocolate chips be? How many chips should it have? Should there be nuts too; if so, what size and how many? How sweet should it be, how much salt should it have? There are at least as many factors to identifying the most popular chocolate chip cookie recipe as there are factors for adjusting a hearing aid. How much base should the hearing aid have for low-intensity sounds, for mid-intensity sounds, and for high-intensity sounds? How about the mid-range and treble? How much should the aid suppress low-intensity background noise? How much should it filter out steady-state noise such as from air conditioners? How fast should it turn the volume down when the intensity goes way up? How quickly should it return to providing full amplification when the environment grows quiet again?

Unfortunately, there are valid reasons why it is much harder to have a patient customize his or her hearing aid using perceptual testing than it is to create a cookie that will be popular. The fundamental difference is that the cookie marketer will create the cookie that is acceptable to the average consumer. The marketer doesn't have to customize the cookie to your individual tastes. The hearing aid that is enjoyed by the average hearing-impaired patient would only be good if your pa-

tient is average. However, some of the same procedures used to taste test cookies might be applicable to patient hearing aid customization. In any case, the cautions on the limits of application are important to understand.

Paired-Comparisons

Several hearing aid manufacturers allow you to present the patient with two ways that the digital hearing aid could sound, one right after the other. Because the human memory span is short, software that allows rapid comparison of one aid simulation to another is very valuable.

However, before asking the patient to make the comparison, it is advisable to first ask if the patient notices a *difference* between the two simulations, and if so, how large the difference is. If you don't ask the patient, he or she will probably assume that there should be a difference, and provide you with an answer.

Second, it may be advisable to ask the patient if one or the other presentation is louder overall than the other is, and adjust the loudness to be equal. If you are trying to find the best quality or tonality of the hearing aid, you do not want the patient to make only judgments of loudness preference. Although you could ask the patient to focus only on tonal quality rather than loudness, the patient probably will not be able to do that.

Remember the role of chance. If you present the exact same hearing aid simulations to the patient in several trials, although not letting the patient know that you are repeating the preference testing, you may find that the preference is stable, or you may find the patient to be unreliable in his or her judgments. Remember the idea of interleaving trials; it would not be prudent to repeatedly present simulation A versus simulation B, B versus A, A versus B, all in a row. It would be better to evaluate a few pairs in an interleaving fashion.

SUMMARY

Modern psychoacoustic testing typically uses forced-choice procedures. Adaptive procedures may be used. They vary the signal level to find a given percent correct detection rate. Threshold (the midpoint between chance and certainty) is often the target of investigation, whether it is for absolute sensitivity, for detection of a signal in noise, or for the just noticeable change in pitch or intensity.

Results may be reported using terminology from signal detection theory. You may read about experiments that report results in d' values and ones that may seek to find the 76% correct detection level using a two-interval forced-choice procedure. The goal of this chapter was to introduce some of the modern psychoacoustics terminology, so that those who read the literature have familiarity with the more common terms. It also cautioned against using poorly controlled clinical tests of patient preference for the way a hearing aid sounds.

29

Threshold of Hearing Loudness Perception, and Loudness Adaptation

Normal hearing humans can detect sounds in the range of 20 to 20,000 Hz. As will be discussed in an upcoming chapter, we can actually detect even lower frequency tones, but don't perceive them as tonal. However, just because we can perceive tones in this wide range of frequencies doesn't mean we hear them all equally. In general, the most sensitive hearing is in the mid-frequency range.

The curve of hearing threshold across frequency, measured in dB SPL, changes depending on how it is measured. Do we measure in sound field (called **minimal audible field**) where both ears are able to participate, or is the testing conducted monaurally, under earphones, as in a **minimal audible pressure** test? The sound field thresholds show better sensitivity. One major explanation for this is that binaural hearing is more sensitive than monaural hearing.

This chapter discusses not only the absolute threshold of hearing, but also our ability to detect changes in intensity. It will be shown that the larger the physical pressure or intensity present (measured in μPa or watts/m^2, not in dB), the larger the

change in pressure or intensity needed to perceive a change in loudness. This is the basis of Weber's law which states that the size of the just noticeably different change in pressure divided by the pressure of the original sound is always a constant fraction. Weber studied a variety of sensory perceptions, and this law holds reasonably well for audition. We say the results are "a near miss to Weber's law."

It is also interesting to examine loudness and loudness scaling issues. Just as the ear is not equally sensitive to all frequencies, a given moderately intense pure tone (held at the same SPL as frequency varies) is not perceived as equally loud across the frequencies. When comparing the loudness of a sound of one frequency to a different frequency sound, the **phon scale** is used. The phon scale tells us what different sound pressure levels are needed across frequencies for the perception of equal loudness.

To compare the loudness of one intensity sound to a sound perceived as more intense, the scale is the **sone**. Doubling the sone scale value equates to about a 10 dB increase in intensity. Stated another way, increase the tone 10 dB and you have essentially doubled the loudness. This is an example of the beauty of the decibel scale. Across a wide range of intensities, a 10 dB change is an equal change in perception. This is a reminder to us then that a 10 dB hearing threshold change is not necessarily a small amount. The audiologist will recognize that this is particularly true with conductive loss (loss from outer and middle ear pathology). (Inner ear hearing loss affects loudness perception differently.)

Loudness is not constant over time. If sounds are of very brief duration (less than 1/5th second long), the sound seems quieter than longer duration sounds. However, many signals, if present for prolonged periods, will fade in loudness and may become inaudible. This is termed **loudness adaptation** or **tone decay.**

ABSOLUTE THRESHOLD OF HEARING

"Threshold" refers to the minimum level of a stimulus that can be detected (**absolute threshold**), or the minimum change in a stimulus that can be detected (**difference threshold**). In this first section, we discuss absolute threshold.

Threshold is actually a statistical term. As discussed in Chapter 27, if establishing threshold in the clinic using the method of limits or adjustment, threshold is defined as the lowest intensity that can be detected in at least 50% of trials. (When a two-alternative forced-choice procedure is used, threshold would be the 75% correct detection point.)

Minimal Audible Pressure and Field

One of the earliest experiments in psychoacoustics sought to define the average

normal hearing threshold. There are different ways to measure hearing threshold, with the signal either presented via earphones or via speakers. As shown in Figure 29–1, the results differ. Figure 29–1 illustrates **minimal audible field (MAF)**, which is the lowest intensity present in a sound room at the group's average threshold. MAF is measured in dB SPL. Measures of MAF are made by finding the lowest level of the tone that the listeners can detect when in the sound field. (Of course, the experiments are done by testing one person at a time.) MAF testing is accomplished using a loudspeaker, usually placed one meter in front of the listener, to produce the tone. Once the threshold of the listener has been determined, the listener is removed from the sound field and a microphone is placed where the listener's head had been. The level of the stimulus that produced a threshold response is

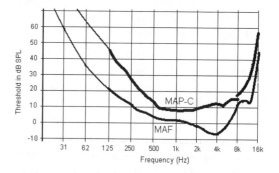

Figure 29–1. Minimal audible field (MAF) is the lowest intensity detected by average normal hearers listening binaurally in a sound field. The minimal audible pressure as measured in a coupler (MAP-C) curve reveals average hearing for monaurally presented sounds. The thicker lines come from data from the American National Standards Institute, an organization that sets reference standards for calibration of audiometers. The MAP-C curve shows a disconnect in the line because a different earphone and coupler was used for testing above 8000 Hz. The thinner lines are data from other experiments.

then determined using a sound level meter. Because the measurements are made without the listener being present, the measurement does not account for any changes in the sound pressure that would occur because of the presence of the listener. If the listener's body absorbs sound, blocks some of the sound, or resonates, these factors are not accounted for in the measurement of MAF SPL. MAF experiments allow the subject to use both ears, and the speaker would typically face directly at the subject (at zero degrees azimuth).

Minimal audible pressure (MAP) is the sound pressure level of the tone measured at the eardrum of the listener while listening under earphones. A true MAP measurement is made by placing a miniature microphone in the ear canal. It is more convenient to measure the level of the sound when the earphone is removed from the ear and is placed into a measuring cavity called a coupler or "**artificial ear.**" These measurements are termed **MAP-C,** for **minimal audible pressure in a coupler**. MAP measures would account for the individual resonances of the listener. MAP-C measurements, made by placing a microphone within the artificial ear, do not reveal information about the resonance of any one subject's ear. The artificial ear is designed to resemble the resonance of the average human ear; however, the coupler typically used in these measurements and used in calibrating audiometers is not a perfect match to the average ear. (Measurements made with a **Zwislocki coupler** would better approximate the average human ear.)

Figure 29–1 illustrates the average MAP-C curve in contrast to the MAF curve. Note that the size of the difference between the curves changes at different frequencies, but the MAF thresholds are always more sensitive. One reason for the poorer hearing when listening through earphones is that as the subject moves during the experiment,

the earphones can rub and make some noise, interfering with the hearing threshold. Measurement differences also affect the results because the MAP measurements already account for the resonance of the ear, either directly if it's a true MAP measure, or indirectly for MAP-C data because the coupler tries to act like the average ear by having its own resonances. MAP shows higher thresholds because the sound that is measured has been enhanced by the resonances of the ear canal and pinna, or by the coupler. The SPL is greater near the eardrum than it is outside the head, and it is greater inside a measuring coupler than it would be outside the coupler. Figure 29–2 elaborates.

Binaural and Equated Binaural Thresholds

Another significant reason for the difference between MAF and MAP is that MAP measures are made monaurally; MAF allows binaural hearing. A general rule of thumb is that **binaural thresholds,** thresholds obtained when both ears are tested, are 2 dB better than monaural thresholds. This wouldn't always be exactly true. If a listener has exactly equal hearing in each ear, when that listener is permitted to listen with both ears, absolute threshold is 3 dB better than when listening with one ear only. **Equated binaural hearing** is also 3 dB more sensitive. An example is the easiest way to explain this concept. Let's assume our listener has a 1000-Hz threshold of 7 dB in the right ear and 5 dB in the left ear. The experimenter can set the tones to 4 dB in the right ear and 2 dB in the left ear (3 dB below threshold in each ear) and the listener will be able to detect them if they are presented simultaneously to the two ears. This better hearing binaurally holds for all frequencies. The 3 dB advantage makes sense, because two ears are working together, and 10 log 2 is

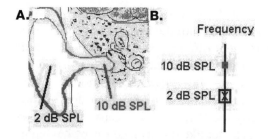

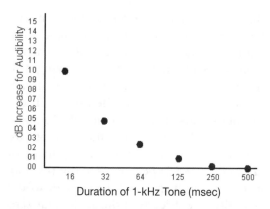

Figure 29–2. As sound enters the ear canal it is enhanced due to the ear's resonances. That is, a threshold at a particular frequency might measure 2 dB SPL at the entrance of the ear, but if enhanced 8 dB by the resonances of the ear at that frequency, it would read 10 dB SPL near the tympanic membrane. If measuring threshold at the eardrum, the level required for hearing is measured as higher. This partially explains the difference between the minimal audible pressure (MAP) and minimal audible field threshold difference. MAP levels are enhanced by the ear canal resonances and read at a higher level. In contrast, MAF measurements are the SPL measured in the area where the listener had been situated. Because MAF measurements are made in sound field without the subject present, they do not take into account the enhancement that will occur as the sound enters the ear. MAP-C measures are similar to MAP measures because the coupler also has resonances that increase the sound pressure levels.

equal to 3 dB. However, most people do not have exactly equal thresholds in each ear; therefore, the actual average advantage is only about 2 dB.

Effect of Stimulus Duration on Absolute Threshold

Thresholds for pure tones are also affected by the duration of the tones, a concept known as **temporal integration**. Figure 29–3 illustrates that as the tones decrease in duration below about 200 msec, thresh-

Figure 29–3. More intensity is required to detect shorter duration tones.

old increases. Figure 29–3 shows data from Watson and Grengel's 1969 experiment, for a 1-kHz tone. Note that threshold is about 10 dB poorer when the duration is reduced from 500 msec to 16 msec. The change just begins to be noted at 250 msec. It is sometimes said that cutting duration to one-tenth of what it was originally elevates threshold by about 10 dB, as long as the tone is below about 200 msec in duration. Another generalization is that doubling duration lowers threshold by 3 dB (until duration reaches 200 msec).

There is a physiologic reason that we would expect that shortening a tone's duration elevates threshold. Each time a cycle of a sound wave is present, the cilia of the hair cells shear back and forth. This creates a release of neurotransmitter at the base of the hair cell. If there are more cycles of the sine wave, there are more releases of "doses" of neurotransmitter. It seems then that "injecting" more neurotransmitter into the synaptic cleft with more back and forth cycles of ciliary shearing improves the chances of the auditory nerve firing. However, this advantage is only effective in that first 200 to 250 msec. Keeping the stimulus on longer might cause the nerve to fire again, but if the nerve has not fired in the first 200 msec of the tone being present, it's unlikely that the nerve will fire at all.

Clinical audiometric thresholds are typically not going to be affected by duration effects. Even an electronically pulsed tone from an audiometer will have pulse durations longer than one-fifth of a second.

Effect of Stimulus Repetition Rate

Not all sounds used to evaluate auditory function are pure tones. Brief segments of pure tones (tone pips) or pulses of energy (clicks) can also be used in certain applications. In these cases, the signal is presented many times each second. How often the signal is presented per second, called the signal **repetition rate**, affects the hearing threshold for these brief signals.

Audiologists use brief-duration stimuli when conducting electrophysiologic measures (measuring the nerve potentials created by sound). If the brief-duration stimuli are presented more times per second, the energy summates—the sound is perceived as louder and the threshold of hearing is lower. Figure 29–4 illustrates a sound that is presented at two different repetition rates.

DIFFERENCE THRESHOLD FOR INTENSITY: DL_I

The term **limen** is a synonym for threshold, and **difference thresholds** are frequently referred to as **difference limens**. Another term that means the same thing as a difference limen is **just noticeable difference (jnd)**. The **difference limen for intensity (DL_I)** is the smallest intensity change that the observer can detect 50% of the time. (Of course, the 50% criterion assumes a method of limits or method of adjustment threshold. Chapter 27 discussed

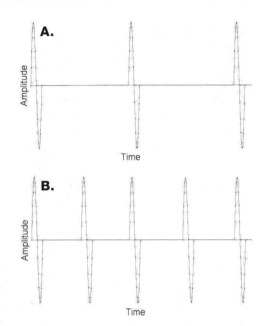

Figure 29–4. The signal has a higher repetition rate in (**B**) and it would be perceived as louder.

how threshold may be another percent correct if determined with other methods.) As with absolute thresholds, intensity of the sound and the method of measurement affect the size of the DL_I. There is some disagreement about whether the stimulus frequency affects the size of the just noticeable difference. When older experimental methods were used, the frequency affected the results, but more recent studies do not show that result.

The objective in establishing a DL_I is to determine the size of the increment of intensity that must be added to (or subtracted from) a reference intensity in order for the observer to just detect a difference in intensity. Weber hypothesized that for all of our senses, we detect a *relative* or proportional or percent change. For example, you might be able to detect the difference between the weight of four pennies versus five pennies. That is, you can tell 4 + 1 pennies versus 4, which would be a ratio of 1/4. Similarly, you might be able to tell the difference between 4 ounces and 5 ounces, or 4 pounds and 5 pounds. You would not notice the added weight of a penny if you were holding a four-pound weight in your hand. That's **Weber's law**. Your ability to detect a change is proportional to the size of the original stimulus. For those who like graphs, Figure 29-5A illustrates. (And in case you are curious, the Weber fraction for weight is not 1/4 under controlled experimental conditions, but about .03. You can tell 1.03 lbs versus 1 lb.)

For sound, to find a Weber fraction we examine the ratio of how much sound power we need to add to the power of the original sound for the change to be noticeable. We would refer to the original power using the letter I. The difference limen increment is typically noted using the Greek letter delta (Δ), meaning difference. It is the amount added that is just noticeably different. When discussing sound power (intensity) we would term this ΔI. If Weber's law is correct, then the fraction ΔI/I would always be the same ratio, as illustrated by the horizontal line in Figure 29-5. The size of ΔI in-

creases as the reference intensity increases, but the ratio of the two stays the same.

We are not used to thinking of sound in absolute power units, but rather in decibels. What decibel increase is needed to detect a change? If Weber's law holds, that too should stay constant. If examining the dB increase that is noticeably different, we would examine the ratio of the just noticeably different power (ΔI + I) versus the power of the sound we heard as the comparison (I), and put that into the decibel form. To calculate the dB increase that is just noticeable, the formula is 10 log (ΔI + I) / I. That decibel number would stay the same if Weber's law holds.

Is the Weber fraction constant for sound intensity change? Do we have a single dB increase that is detectable, no matter how loud the original sound? It depends on the signal (Figure 29-6). For wide-band noise we have a "near miss" to Weber's law. The greatest departure is below 20 dB sensation level (decibels above threshold). At these very low intensities, it takes a greater change in sound level to detect a loudness difference. However, for pure tones, the DL_I continues to improve as sound intensity increases.

Psychoacoustics often helps us further understand auditory physiology, and this de-

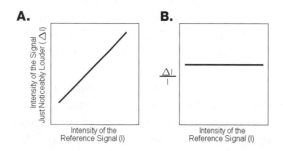

A. Intensity of the Signal Just Noticeably Louder (ΔI) / Intensity of the Reference Signal (I)

B. $\frac{\Delta I}{I}$ / Intensity of the Reference Signal (I)

Figure 29–5. Illustration of Weber's law. **A.** If Weber's law holds for audition, then the magnitude of the increase in intensity that can be detected grows along with the intensity of the sound that it is compared with. **B.** If that is true, then the ratio of the increase in sound (ΔI) to the original sound (I) would stay the same no matter the intensity of the original (reference) sound.

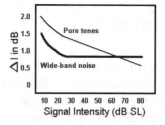

2.0
1.5   Pure tones
ΔI in dB   1.0
0.5   Wide-band noise
0

10 20 30 40 50 60 70 80
Signal Intensity (dB SL)

Figure 29–6. When the experimental signals are pure tones, the difference limen for intensity, expressed in dB, is less for the higher intensities, showing a deviation from Weber's law. When the signal is broadband, then Weber's law does hold, and the line is horizontal, at least above about 20 dB SL.

crease in the difference limen for increased pure tone intensity is one of those cases. In Chapter 18, the traveling wave envelopes for low- and high-intensity pure tones were discussed. We noted that as the pure tone's intensity increased, basilar membrane vibration spread toward the base of the cochlea. The shape of the envelope changes with intensity, as illustrated in Figure 29-7. In the top of Figure 29-7, a low-intensity signal is increased to a level that is theoretically just audibly different. Those neurons near the traveling wave peak that were firing to the lower intensity now change their firing rate to encode the increase in intensity. In addition, a few more neurons located toward the base of the cochlea fire. In the lower part of the figure the pure tones are now more intense. Again, the firing rates for the neurons near the traveling wave peak would change, but that same amount of increase in intensity causes a greater number of neurons near the base to begin to fire, so that is a more easily heard signal. The increase in intensity of the high-intensity pure tone doesn't need to be as great because of the spreading out of the traveling wave.

A broadband noise would occupy the entire basilar membrane regardless of its intensity. Turning up the broadband noise doesn't cause new neurons to fire, so we don't see this extra sensitivity for detecting louder sounds.

Spectral Profile Analysis

Spectral profile analysis also evaluates ability to detect change in intensity, but in this test, it is a change in intensity of one of several tones presented simultaneously. Let's examine a sample of how to conduct a spectral profile analysis experiment. The patient is asked to detect an intensity difference of one of a series of tones. That is, several tones are presented simultaneously, and one of the tones has a higher (or lower) intensity. For example, the 250, 500, 1000, 2000, and 4000-Hz tones might be presented to the subject, and one tone, perhaps 1000 Hz, is adjusted until the patient can detect that the intensity has changed. The subject might be given three sets of tones and asked to select the one that has one tone that is louder than the others. To make this a test of ability to detect the *relative* difference in intensity across the different frequency sounds, the different trials have different overall intensities, as illustrated in Figure 29–8. The subject is given feedback during the experiment on whether the correct spectral profile was selected, which helps the subject learn to evaluate the relative change in the intensities across frequency, rather than focusing on overall loudness. The results are again a reasonable fit to We-

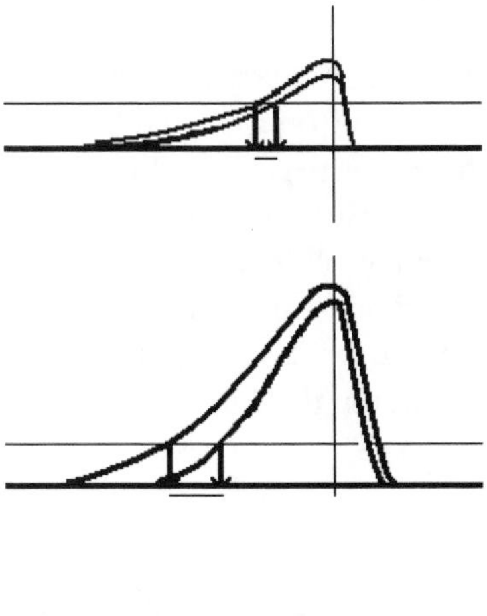

Figure 29–7. One-half of traveling waves is illustrated, with the thick horizontal line representing the basilar membrane. The movement of basilar membrane must be greater than shown by the thin line for neurons to fire. An increase in the intensity of a low-level pure tone (*top of figure*) creates a smaller amount of spread of excitation than when a loud intensity pure tone is increased in intensity (*bottom*). Therefore, it is easier to detect increases in intensity of pure tones that are of high intensity as the ear can use this additional cue to loudness.

Clinical Correlate: Short-Increment Sensitivity Index

Most cochlear loss damages the outer hair cells before inner hair cells are lost. Damage to the outer hair cells means that the active mechanism (Chapter 18) is lost, and basilar membrane vibration for soft sounds is no longer enough to shear the inner hair cell cilia. However, if the sound is loud enough, even without the active mechanism enhancing basilar membrane vibration there is enough movement to shear the inner hair cell cilia. Therefore, when sounds are loud, if there are inner hair cells present, they will be stimulated and the sound will be perceived as loud. This phenomenon is called recruitment. Soft sounds are inaudible, but loud sounds are perceived as loud. The increased spread of excitation described above when a loud sound gets a little louder would still occur with cochlear loss, and we would expect that the person with cochlear loss would have the same difference limen for intensity for loud sounds as would a normal hearer listening to a loud sound.

As an example, let's assume a patient has a 50 dB HL threshold at 1000 Hz. If presented with a 70 dB HL sound, even though this is only 20 dB above threshold (20 dB SL), that 70 dB HL sound is perceived as moderate in intensity. The patient's perception may not be much different from a normal hearer's perception of a 70 dB HL pure tone. A normal hearer's just noticeable difference in intensity for a 20 dB SL sound would be about 1.5 dB, but the normal hearer's just noticeable difference for intensity at 70 dB HL would be below 1 dB. The hearing-impaired person doesn't perceive the 20 dB SL sound as quiet, but as more like what a normal hearer would perceive as 70 dB SL. The hearing-impaired person's difference limen would be below 1 dB.

Dr. James Jerger developed the Short Increment Sensitivity Index (SISI) test in the late 1950s. It is a clinical test to determine if the patient's just noticeable difference for intensity is above or below 1 dB. A pure tone is presented at 20 dB SL (20 above threshold). Every once in a while the tone intensity increases by a decibel. The patient is instructed to push a button to signal if the incremental increase is detected. Those with cochlear loss and recruitment can detect that increase; those with conductive loss (outer/middle ear pathology) or retrocochlear involvement (VIIIth nerve/brainstem pathology) cannot. The principle behind the SISI is still valid, but there are more sensitive tests for diagnosing the site of lesion, so the SISI is seldom used today.

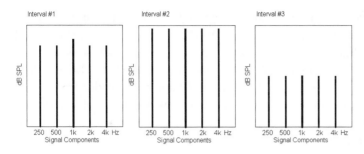

Figure 29–8. Example of a possible spectral profile experiment. The subject is instructed to select the interval that has the different pitch profile while disregarding overall intensity of the signal. Here, the first interval has the spectral profile difference at 1000 Hz.

ber's law—for mid-range intensities, the ΔI, expressed in dB, or as $\Delta I / I$, stay the same.

Green (1988) is the psychoacoustician typically thought of when discussing profile analysis, as he literally wrote the book on the topic. His general findings are that a 1 to 2 dB difference in a single component can be detected, and that intensity difference detection ability holds across a wide range of intensities. Again, as the dB difference is already a ratio, saying that we detect the same dB size increase at different spectral profile intensities means we have a fit to Weber's law.

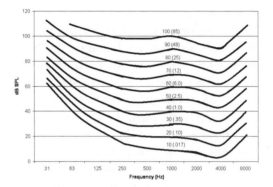

Figure 29–9. Smoothed phon curves that show the SPL required across frequencies for the sound to be of equal intensity. All sounds along a phon curve are perceived as equally loud. The loudness level in phons is noted above the curve. The loudness in sones is in parentheses using data from Stevens and Davis (1938). The phon curves are modifications of Robinson and Dadson's (1956) data.

LOUDNESS PERCEPTION

As intensity increases, the perception of loudness changes. The sound can range in perceived loudness from just detectable to painfully loud, and numbers can be attached to the loudness perception. That is, subjects can describe the loudness on a numeric or quantative scale. Although loudness increases as intensity increases, the relationship of intensity to loudness is not linear. That is, doubling the intensity does not double the loudness.

Loudness Level

By definition, when one refers to the **loudness level** of a sound, one is comparing

the loudness of that sound to the loudness of a 1000-Hz tone. Loudness level is measured in units called **phons**. By definition, the loudness level of a sound in phons is equal to the dB SPL of a 1000-Hz tone judged equally loud. Thus, 20 phons is the loudness of a 1000-Hz tone at 20 dB SPL and the loudness of any other frequency sound that is perceived as equally loud. We defined 40 phons as the loudness of 1000 Hz at 40 dB SPL, 80 phons as the loudness of 1000 Hz at 80 dB SPL, and so forth. Figure 29–9 shows a smoothed family of equal loudness curves. These curves can also be thought of as phon curves with each curve representing the phon level at which the curve crosses the 1000-Hz line. For example, all tones on the 60-phon curve sound equal in loudness to a 1000-Hz tone of 60 dB SPL. Phon curves show how different frequencies relate to the loudness of each other, but phon curves do not show how different phon levels relate to each other. That is, 10 phons sounds are *not* twice as loud as 5 phons sounds, and so forth.

Notice that for low intensity sounds, the dB SPL level difference between the 63-Hz and 1000-Hz 10-phon signals is quite large—the signal must be about 40 dB SPL at 63 Hz and 10 dB SPL at 1000 Hz, a difference of 30 dB. Next, examine the 100-phon curve. A 108 dB SPL 63-Hz tone is equal in perceived loudness to a 100 dB 1000-Hz tone, only a 8 dB difference. This shows that the ear is differently sensitive to intense and quiet sounds of varying frequencies.

Decibel Scales Revisited

Chapter 2 described the physical intensity of sound, and how the pressure or power of the sound can be compared to a standard pressure and turned into a decibel SPL or IL

value. Chapter 3 discussed the dB HL scale—where 0 dB HL is the lowest intensity heard by the normal hearer. Decibels sensation level, dB SL, means the intensity above another threshold. Chapter 8 introduced dB A, B, and C. We can now add to the discussion of these last three types of decibel scales. dB A, B, and C are each derived from the dB SPL measurement system—they are measures of the physical intensity of the sound. The dB A scale was originally designed to provide a measure of intensity that resembled the ear's sensitivity to soft sounds, specifically those at 40 phons. It devalued the decibel value of the low and high frequencies, so that the intensity of sounds in the low-intensity range would be read on a scale not far different from the 40-phon scale (Figure 29–10). The dB B and C scales do not filter out the low and high frequencies as dramatically, and correspond approximately to the 70- and 100-phon curves. Although the original purpose of these scales was to provide some scale that might mimic perceived loudness, this is seldom the reason they are used. The dB A scale happens to reasonably approximate how damaging different frequencies are to the ear. Intense mid- to high-frequency sounds, those not filtered out on the A curve, damage the ear more readily than

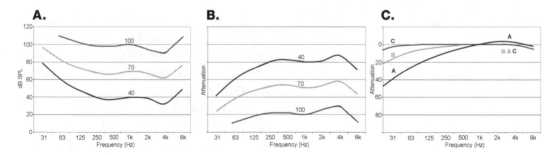

Figure 29–10. A. Phon curves showing the 40, 70, and 100-phon equal loudness contours. **B.** The phon curves have been inverted. Note that the shape of the 100-phon curve is flatter than that of the 40-phon curve. **C.** The dB A, B, and C curves attenuate low-frequency sounds, somewhat like the way the phon curves show less sensitivity to the low frequencies.

low-frequency sounds. Measures of sound to estimate the potential for it to damage the ear typically use the dB A scale.

Loudness Scaling

Loudness level in phons refers to sounds that are equally loud. Understanding the phon scale helps us see how loudness perception changes across frequencies, but it does not give insight into how increasing intensity at one frequency causes a change in the perception of loudness. The **sone** scale gives us information on this aspect of loudness.

Loudness scaling requires us to have one signal that is considered the standard or reference to which others will be compared. S. S. Stevens chose the 40 dB SPL, 1000-Hz tone as this reference, and called it 1 **sone**. Any other 40-phon sound would be as loud, so it would also be 1 sone. A sound that is twice as loud is 2 sones, and a perceived intensity half as loud as a 1-sone sound is 0.5 sones in loudness. (Note that this is loudness, not "loudness level.") The doubling scale continues—a sound twice the loudness of 2 sones is 4 sones. Figure 29-9 shows the sone values next to the phon levels.

Generally, increasing intensity 10 dB doubles the sone value. If you put the value of sones on a logarithmic scale, as shown in Figure 29-11, the data fit in basically a straight line down to about 20 phons.

When a graph, such as Figure 29-11B shows a straight line on a logarithmic scale, then the mathematical equation for the line would have an exponent in it. **Stevens' law** for intensity has just that. The formula he derived for loudness (L) is $L = k \times I^e$ where k is a constant, which changes with frequency. I is the physical intensity measured in µPa or dynes/cm^2. Stevens' original work says that the exponent e is about 0.6, which works out to loudness doubling every 10 dB. This will be discussed further in the next chapter.

It's worth mentioning that other researchers have gotten other estimates of loudness growth. Some find that a 6 dB change is a doubling of loudness for their subjects. Others have noted that using two ears rather than one doubles loudness, which should be about a 3 dB perceptual change. The variety of results may relate to the inherent difficulty we have with the task. We are not inherently used to scaling loudness numerically (Moore, 2004).

A.

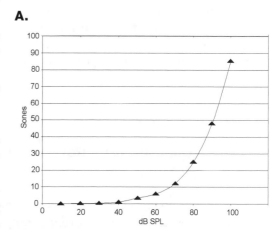

B.

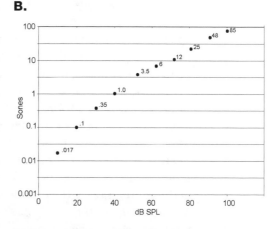

Figure 29–11. The relationship between sones and dB SPL at 1000 Hz looks exponential if viewed with sones on the linear scale; however, the data fit an almost straight line when plotted on a logarithmic scale. Data from Stevens and Davis (1938).

LOUDNESS ADAPTATION

If a sound remains on for a long period of time, that is, a minute or more, and stays the same intensity and frequency, it may begin to be perceived as less intense. This is termed **loudness adaptation** or **auditory adaptation**. A similar term is **tone decay**, which specifically refers to a signal that was at first audible, fading away to inaudibility.

Normal hearers have greater adaptation to low-intensity sounds and to high-frequency sounds. Normal hearers differ considerably in the amount of adaptation they experience. Adaptation can be measured by loudness matching, where the constant tone is presented to just one ear, and the subject matches the loudness of a pulsing on and off sound in the other ear. The loudness match is made just as the sound starts and after some period of listening to the constant tone. Adaptation can also be demonstrated using loudness scaling procedures.

A similar phenomenon is called tone decay. A tone is presented, and the subject indicates when it becomes inaudible. The time required for the tone to fade to inaudibility can be measured, or one can measure how much tone decay (in dB) occurs in a given period of time. To measure it this second way, the tone intensity is increased (without turning the tone off) each time the tone fades to inaudibility.

Clinical Correlate: Tone Decay and Reflex Decay Testing

Although some tone decay is typical, especially for high-frequency sounds, normally functioning ears should not have significant tone decay for mid- or low-frequency sounds. Those who have damage to their retrocochlear systems may experience more adaptation and tone decay. When a tone first initiates, the damaged nerve can initially respond, but the nerve is too weak to continue to fire over a long period of time.

Clinical tests of tone decay determine if the patient is able to hear a sustained tone. Acoustic reflex decay testing is even more sensitive, if the person has an acoustic reflex. (Reflexes are often absent with retrocochlear problems.) In acoustic reflex decay testing, the reflex threshold is found. A sustained tone is presented at 10 dB above the reflex threshold. The initial strength of the contraction of the muscle is measured; 5 seconds later it is measured again. If the reflex is half-strength or less, then that is termed positive reflex decay and is consistent with retrocochlear involvement. Just as some adaptation is normal, persons with normal retrocochlear system can have some reflex decay, especially at high frequencies, so reflex decay testing is typically conducted only in the low and mid-frequencies.

TEMPORARY THRESHOLD SHIFT

In contrast to auditory adaptation, temporary threshold shift occurs because of prior exposure to intense sounds. For example, a subject might be exposed to 100 dB SPL of white noise. Afterward, hearing thresholds will be worse. The amount of deterioration is the **temporary threshold shift (TTS)**.

Several factors are implicated in TTS. Short-term metabolic changes in the hair cell occur as a result of the loud noise exposure. The excessive potassium influx into the hair cells cannot be fully excreted, and the hair cell may swell as a result. This can alter the function of the cell and reduce outer hair cell motility.

As the name implies, recovery is expected. However, repeated or prolonged noise exposure can result in **permanent threshold shift**, that is, **noise-induced hearing loss**. In those cases, cells are destroyed, rather than damaged.

SUMMARY

The ear is most sensitive to mid-frequency sounds, as was shown by examining either a minimal audible field or minimal audible pressure curve. The best thresholds are obtained by measuring hearing thresholds in sound field, partially because both ears can participate in testing. Another reason for the difference, though, is how MAP or MAP-C is measured—in the ear canal or a coupler that resonates in a manner similar to the ear canal. The resonance enhanced the sound pressure level, making the threshold appear higher.

Although there is a large difference between the SPL required for threshold at low and mid-frequencies, the ear does not respond as differently when intense sounds are presented. Phon curves, which show what frequencies and intensities are equally intense, flatten as intensity increases.

An increase in 10 dB SPL at 1000 Hz is about a doubling of loudness. This is true at least for moderate intensity and louder sounds.

This chapter discussed the effect of duration and repetition rate. Once a signal is below about 200-msec duration, it requires greater intensity to reach threshold. Also, a brief tone presented at a faster repetition rate will have a lower threshold.

We also noted the ear's exquisite sensitivity to intensity change. Under the right conditions, a 1 dB change is readily audible. Difference limen testing with pure tones showed better sensitivity for high intensity tones, a deviation from Weber's law. This results from the asymmetry of the traveling wave: intense traveling waves more rapidly involve neural responses from areas toward the base of the basilar membrane. Difference limens for intensity fit Weber's law if a wide-band noise is the test signal. There is still a deviation for very low-intensity sounds, which have a larger difference limen.

REFERENCES

Green, D. M. (1988). *Profile analysis.* Oxford: Oxford University Press.

Moore, B. C. J. (2004). *An introduction to the psychology of hearing* (5th ed.). Amsterdam: Elsevier.

Robinson, D. W., & Dadson, R. S. (1956). A redetermination of the equal loudness relations for pure tones. *British Journal of Applied Physics, 7,* 166-181.

Stevens, S. S., & Davis, H. (1938). *Hearing. Its psychology and physiology.* New York: Wiley.

Watson, C. S., & Grengel, R. W. (1969). Signal duration and signal frequency in relation to auditory sensitivity. *Journal of the Acoustical Society of America, 46*(4), 989-997.

30

Calculating Loudness

Figure 29–11A showed that loudness growth changes above and below about 40 dB SPL. Loudness quickly increases as the signal goes from threshold to about 40 dB SPL, then it grows more slowly (and predictably) as intensity increases further. In this chapter, we consider some of the reasons for the rapid growth of loudness for low-intensity sounds, and explore the calculations for loudness for sounds above about 40 dB SPL.

PHYSIOLOGIC CORRELATES OF LOUDNESS AND LOUDNESS GROWTH

To predict loudness and explain loudness growth, it is helpful to review some of the physiologic factors that affect our calculations. The resonances of the ear and the active mechanism affect loudness, and as mentioned in the previous chapter, the way the ear responds to the traveling wave also affects loudness.

The Transfer Function of the Ear

Not all frequencies pass through the outer and middle ear equally well. Recall that the outer ear creates resonances that enhance the mid-frequency sounds. The

middle ear also does not transmit all sounds equally well. The mass and stiffness of the middle ear attenuate transmission of the very low- and very high-frequency sounds. This is one reason that not all frequencies, if presented at the same SPL, will be equally loud.

A graph of the measurement of how much the sound has been attenuated or amplified as it passes through a system (such as a hearing aid or the outer and middle ear) is called a **transfer function**. A transfer function tells us how the spectrum would be altered as the sound is transmitted (transferred) through the system.

Predicting loudness mathematically requires understanding of how much the ear resonates or attenuates at each frequency. We can predict that a 40 dB SPL, 2-kHz tone will be louder than a 250-Hz tone because the ear canal resonates 2 kHz, and the middle ear transmits this frequency through the middle ear efficiently.

Role of the Active Mechanism

Outer hair cells contract and elongate in response to low-intensity stimulation. The active role of the outer hair cells, as you recall, enhances the vibration of basilar membrane, and creates greater shearing of the inner hair cell cilia (Chapters 18 and 19). There is a limited range of contraction; the outer hair cells can only contract a certain amount, and further stimulation will not create greater basilar membrane movement. It is often said that this range is over about 45 dB.

The active mechanism appears then to enhance basilar membrane motion for very low-intensity sounds. This permits the rapid increase in loudness for the lowest level sounds, and agrees fairly well with the growth of loudness curve.

Spread of Activity Along the Basilar Membrane

As a pure tone signal grows louder, the traveling wave spreads out more and more on the basilar membrane. More neurons are able to encode the signal intensity, especially those located more basal-ward of the traveling wave peak (Figure 21–6). If the displacement is great enough at these additional locations along basilar membrane, then there will be shearing of the inner hair cell cilia, and release of neurotransmitter. The neurons will fire and contribute to the encoding of the signal, increasing perceived loudness.

CALCULATING LOUDNESS OF PURE TONES

In the previous chapter, the formula for loudness in sones was given as

$$L = k \times I^e \quad \textit{(Eqn. 30.1)}$$

where L is loudness level, k is a constant, and e is an exponent. For sounds in the range above 40 dB SPL, that constant is about 0.0105 for 1000 Hz. (The constant would vary with frequency because of the transfer

function of the ear.) If measuring the sound in µPa, the exponent is 0.6. When measured in watts/meter^2, the exponent is 0.3.

Let's see how this formula works. The formula requires knowing the intensity of the signal in micropascals. In the first example, let's look at a 1-sone sound. By definition, a 40 dB SPL 1-kHz tone has the loudness of 1 sone. What sound pressure level created the 40 dB SPL (1 sone) sound? To obtain the pressure level created by 40 dB SPL, use *Equation 30.2.*

$$\text{dB SPL} = 20 \times \log (\text{pressure level} / 20 \text{ µPa})$$
$$\textit{(Eqn. 30.2)}$$

In this case then,

$$40 \text{ dB SPL} = 20 \times \log (I/20 \text{ µPa})$$
$$2 \text{ dB SPL} = \log (I/20 \text{ µPa})$$

Take the inverse log of each side of the equation

$$100 = I / 20 \text{ µPa}$$
$$2000 \text{ µPa} = I$$

Using *Equation 30.1*, $L = 0.0105 \times 2000^{0.6}$

$$L = 0.0105 \times 95.6$$
$$L = 1.004, \text{ or just about 1 sone.}$$

This example then shows how the formula works for 1 sone. Next let's see what the formula calculates as the loudness of a 60 dB SPL, 1-kHz tone.

Again, first obtain the pressure of the 60 dB SPL tone.

$$60 \text{ dB SPL} = 20 \times \log I/20 \text{ µPa}$$
$$3 \text{ dB SPL} = \log (I/ 20 \text{ µPa})$$
$$1000 = I/20 \text{ µPa}$$
$$I = 20,000 \text{ µPa}$$

Now, calculate the loudness

$$L = 0.0105 \times 20,000^{0.6}$$
$$L = 0.0105 \times 380.7$$
$$L = 4.0$$

As was noted in Figures 29-9 and 29-10, using data from a very old study (Stevens & Davis, 1938) the loudness is 6 sones. The error is 2 sones, which is about 33% off from what the calculations predicted; 100 dB SPL is predicted as 63 sones, and measured at 85 sones. This shows reasonable agreement between measured and predicted results. The error of 22 sones out of the 85 measured means the calculation is off by 26%.

Now, let's try calculating the loudness of a very low-intensity sound using this formula. A 10 dB SPL sound is measured as 0.017 sones. The pressure creating 10 dB SPL is 63.2 µPa. The calculated loudness is

$$L = 0.0105 \times 63.2^{.6}$$
$$L = .0105 \times 12.03$$
$$L = .126$$

Although the absolute size of the error is small, 0.109 sones, the ratio of that error to the originally measured 0.017 sones is more than 6 to 1. There is a 641% error rate, showing that loudness calculations don't work well for very low-intensity sounds.

COMPLEX TONE LOUDNESS

Calculating the loudness of a complex sound is not necessarily so easy. If two signals are very different in frequency, then you can make a fairly simple calculation of the loudness as the summation of the loudness of the two individual signals. However, if the signals have traveling waves that overlap, then the loudness is not simply summed. Figure 30-1 illustrates. A smaller total or

overall area on basilar membrane is stimulated when the frequencies are close together, which reduces the overall loudness. This concept will be covered again as we discuss masking principles.

SUMMARY

Loudness calculations reveal the working of the basilar membrane. We can find evidence for the active mechanism, because the formula does not predict loudness accurately below about 40 dB SPL. When two sounds are present, and close together in

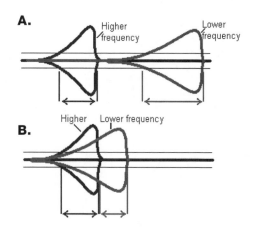

Figure 30-1. A. Two traveling waves on the basilar membrane peak at different areas. The two thin horizontal lines indicate the amount of basilar membrane movement theoretically required to create a neural impulse. The arrows show the range of area on the basilar membrane that is stimulated by each pure tone. **B.** When two tones both stimulate the same area on the basilar membrane, the neuron will either respond to one or the other. The total area of basilar membrane stimulated by the two tones is reduced because of the overlap of the traveling waves. The loudness of the tones in (**B**) is less than the loudness from the tones illustrated in (**A**).

frequency, they are less loud than if separated. This supports what we know about the traveling wave and neural encoding, and upcoming chapters on masking will delve further into this topic.

REFERENCE

Stevens, S. S., & Davis, H. (1938). *Hearing. Its psychology and physiology.* New York: Wiley.

31

Basics of Pitch Perception

In this chapter we examine the psychologic attributes related to perception of different frequency sounds. Although it's often said that the limits of human hearing extend from 20 Hz to 20,000 Hz, it is more appropriate to say that this is the limit of our ability to perceive stimuli as tonal. Sounds lower than 20 Hz can be heard, if loud enough, but aren't perceived as tonal.

As frequency increases, the perception of pitch increases. As the musical octave scale is based on doubling of frequency, it may be surprising to learn that a doubling of frequency is *not* equal to a doubling of pitch. This is particularly true for frequencies above 1000 Hz. The unit of pitch, the mel, is introduced in this chapter.

The ability of humans to detect changes in frequency (the difference limen for frequency [DL_F] or just noticeable difference for frequency) is described. Is the ear more sensitive to frequency change in the low or high frequencies? The answer to that question depends on how you choose to describe the results. If you note the frequency difference, in Hz, between two tones that are just noticeably different in pitch, you conclude that change in the frequency of low-frequency signals is easier to detect. However, if you consider what the ratio is of the just-detectable change in frequency, versus the original frequency, you would consider the difference limen for frequency to be better in the mid-frequencies. That sounds more confusing than it is. You can tell 250 Hz from 251 Hz, but 1000 Hz and 1001 Hz are indistinguishable. You could probably distinguish 1000 Hz from 1002 Hz, though. But look at these findings as ratios—1 Hz/250 Hz = .004; 2/1000 = .002. Viewed in that manner, the changes in mid-frequency sounds are easier to detect. The ear becomes less sensitive in detecting pitch change, both as a ratio and in absolute numbers, for the very high frequencies.

Combining two or more tones in the same ear creates the perception of a complex signal with more than two pitch components. The spacing between the signals, and the signal intensity, affect which distortion components are perceived. This chapter examines the "combination tones" that are produced by the inner ear, which include difference tones and summation tones.

PITCH PERCEPTION

The Limits of Tonal Perception

Although the normal hearer is aware of pressure changes (sound) at frequencies below 20 Hz, these frequencies do not produce a perception of tonality. These very low frequencies produce a complex perception which may include a rumble, slapping, or thrusting sensation. At about 20 Hz, however, tonality starts to emerge and the perception of tonality continues to about 20,000 Hz. (Some might not consider the sound as particularly tonal above 8,000 Hz, however.) At frequencies above 20,000 Hz, we are unable to perceive the sound, regardless of its intensity. This 20,000-Hz upper limit of hearing rapidly decreases with age.

Pitch Perception Is Intensity Dependent

Although the primary determiner of pitch is frequency, the intensity of the sound may influence the pitch that one perceives. There is a tendency for low-frequency tones to sound lower in pitch as intensity is increased, and for high-frequency tones to sound higher in pitch as intensity is increased. Because of this, when reviewing studies of pitch perception, one should note the intensity of the stimulus presentation.

Pitch Perception Is Duration Dependent

Brief tones don't have full tonality. A single cycle of a 1000-Hz pure tone sounds more like a pop or a click than a tone. There is a mathematical principle involved that dictates this—the shorter the duration the more spread of energy there is to adjacent frequencies. It's not surprising then that for the ear to detect a tone as tonal, some minimum duration is required. The longer the duration, the cleaner the spectrum of the signal, the more precise the location of the traveling wave on the basilar membrane, and the more tonal the sound becomes.

Very low frequencies, such as 50 to 100 Hz, require 3 to 4 full cycles before tonality is perceived, so a 100-Hz tone won't be tonal unless it is about 35 msec in duration. A 1000-Hz tone requires 12 cycles (12-msec duration), and the number of cycles required continues to increase as the frequency increases.

Recall from Chapter 22 on neural encoding that different neurons within the nerve bundle phase-lock to different wave peaks. Multiple wave cycles are needed to trigger nerve impulses that occur once per cycle, which allows the auditory nervous system to abstract the timing information.

Even after these critical durations are reached, lengthening the tone continues to improve tonality. After about 250 msec, full tonality is reached. You will see numbers like 200 msec and 250 msec many times when reading about how the ear integrates information over time—that one-fifth to one-quarter of a second is a critical time.

PITCH SCALING

The Mel Scale of Pitch

Although there is a relationship of low pitch to low frequency and high pitch to high frequency, it is not a linear function. That is, doubling the frequency does not result in the perception of the pitch being twice as high.

The unit of pitch is an arbitrary unit called the **mel**. The mel is defined as a pitch that is 1/1000th of the pitch of a 1000-Hz tone at 40 phons. That is, the pitch of a 1000-Hz, 40 dB SPL tone is 1000 mels. Five hundred mels is a tone which is perceived as one-half the pitch of 1000 mels (but that is not the same as 500 Hz) and 2000 mels is a tone perceived as having twice the pitch of 1000 mels (again, that is not the same as 2000 Hz). Figure 31–1 (based on the da-

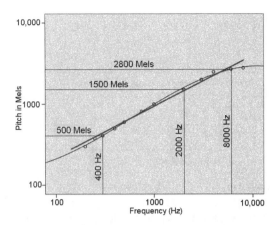

Figure 31–1. The relationship between frequency and perceived pitch. By definition, a 1000-Hz tone (at 40 dB SPL) is equal to 1000 mels. As frequency is halved, the mel value drops by less than half (or as pitch is halved, the frequency changes by more than just dividing by two). Above 1000 Hz, doubling the frequency creates less than a doubling of pitch. The thin, slightly curved line is the line of best fit. The thicker solid line shows that the data come close to fitting a straight-line function.

ta of Stevens, Volkman, & Newman, 1936 as discussed by Stevens & Volkmann, 1940) shows the relationship of frequency in hertz to pitch in mels. The frequency of 1000 Hz produces a pitch of 1000 mels as mandated by the definition of the mel, but that the farther one goes either up or down the frequency scale from 1000 Hz, the less agreement there is between frequency in hertz and pitch in mels. The figure shows data that almost fit a straight line; however, the slope of that line is not 1:1. That is, a doubling or halving of the value in Hz creates less change in the mel value.

The method used for making the pitch judgments dramatically affects the results. Figure 31-1 shows the results of fractionation—the subjects made the pitch half or twice as high. The frequency at which one starts, and the method used in conducting the experiment, influence the results; however, the trend that doubling frequency creates less than a doubling of pitch holds no matter what method is used.

Octave Scales

The musically inclined student might be puzzled to hear that a doubling in frequency is not equal to the doubling in pitch. In the **octave scale**, frequency doubles, and there is certainly a phenomenon of octave equivalence. That is, the ear recognizes the similarity between A4 (440 Hz) and A5 (880 Hz). This is not in dispute; however, the perception of sameness in doubling the frequency is not exactly the same as doubling pitch.

Bark Scale Introduced

Another method for describing the perception of pitch uses the **bark** scale. One bark is equal to the frequencies that comprise a "**critical band**." Frequencies within a critical band are close enough in frequency to mask each other. That is, the presence of one tone can keep you from detecting another tone of similar frequency. For example, frequencies from about 900 to 1060 Hz can mask 980 Hz, frequencies more distant, such as 850 Hz or 1100 Hz would not. If 1060 Hz is the edge of one critical band, and the next critical band ranges from 1060 to 1250 Hz, that range is also equal to one bark. The bark scale and its relationship to pitch will be discussed again in Chapter 33.

One of the interests in psychoacoustics is creating a "map" of the basilar membrane to reveal what area on the basilar membrane equates to what pitch. One theory is that each mel, or each bark, is an equal distance on basilar membrane. After discussing masking and critical bands, we will examine the cochlear map in more detail, and return to this concept of barks.

JUST NOTICEABLE DIFFERENCE OF FREQUENCY

The **difference limen for frequency** (**DL**$_F$) is a just noticeable difference in the quality of a tone. It is the smallest pitch change that the ear can detect 50% of the time (assuming that the experimenter is using a simple up/down "yes/no that tone is different" or method of adjustment task. If using a two-alternative forced-choice procedure, threshold, of course, is the 75% correct detection point.) Like mels and barks, the DL$_F$ has been of special interest because it may give information on how the basilar membrane is "laid out" and it may give insight as to whether the place of the traveling wave peak or the firing pattern of the neuron encodes frequency. The place theory of hearing suggested that the traveling wave must peak at a different place on the basilar membrane for tones to be discriminably different pitch. That is, for a DL$_F$ to occur, one must move the traveling wave peak some minimal distance on the basilar membrane. Thus, attempts to measure the DL$_F$ have been made for more than 100 years because of the interest in knowing if the results could explain the layout of the cochlea. However, some of the early work lacked validity due to inadequate instrumentation and the failure to use systematic psychophysical methods.

Measuring DL$_F$ is complicated by the need to avoid introducing distortions into the signal. Rapid changes in frequency or intensity can create unintended changes in the spectrum of the signal. Shower and Buddulph got around these problems, publishing their results in 1931. Rather than abruptly changing frequency, the signal gradually changed frequency, as illustrated in Figure 31–2A (which shows a much larger frequency change than a difference limen). Their signals stayed on constantly; the subject indicated when the signal was no longer perceived as one steady frequency, but rather

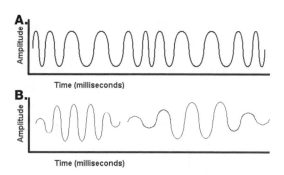

Figure 31–2. Two types of signals that can be used to establish the just noticeable difference for frequency. **A.** For a frequency modulation detection task, the period of the wave varies over time, creating a warble tone, whereas the intensity stays constant. DL$_F$ is when the period of the frequency changes enough so that the perception is no longer of a steady tone, but one that has a pitch that changes over time. **B.** A paired-comparison method (also called a two-interval forced-choice method) can also be used, where two tones, each gradually increasing in intensity to avoid distortion, are presented one after the other. The subject indicates which tone is higher in pitch. The frequency of the comparison tone is changed until the interval containing the higher frequency is correctly detected at the desired accuracy level (e.g., 75% correct in a simple two-alternative forced-choice procedure).

that a warble in frequency could be detected. Unlike what is illustrated, the rate at which the frequency changes is much slower, usually about three times per second. This is a **frequency modulation (FM) frequency difference limen task.**

Modern experimentation would use a paired-comparison method in which the signal is turned on gradually to avoid creating energy at unwanted frequencies. The subject would listen to two different frequency signals and either indicate whether they are the same or different, or tell the experimenter which one is higher in pitch. Figure 31–2B illustrates the signals used.

Changes in DL$_F$ with Frequency

The results of the frequency difference limen experiments can be shown in two different ways: the absolute change in frequency, in Hz, that can be detected (Figure 31-3A) or the ratio of that absolute frequency, divided by the frequency that the tone started out at (Figure 31-3B). In the latter case, we are discussing the relative DL$_F$, the ΔF/F ratio, also called the Weber fraction. Recall from Chapter 29 the concept of Weber's law. Weber's law holds that the change that can be detected, divided by the size of the original signal being changed, is a constant number.

Using a frequency modulation DL$_F$ task, the ear is able to detect a warble of about 3 Hz, for frequencies below 1000 Hz. As frequency increases, greater change is required to detect the signal. When viewed as a Weber fraction (the percentage of frequency change), the ear appears to be consistently able to detect a relatively small change in frequency (frequency × .002 to .005) for mid to high frequencies (Figure 31-3B). The percentage change in frequency needs to be much higher when detecting modulation of low frequencies. The data appear to indicate that the ear has a different mechanism for detecting pitch difference depending on whether the frequency is above or below about 2000 Hz.

When a paired-comparison task is used, the ear is shown to be more sensitive to low-frequency change than Shower and Biddulph's (1931) data indicated. Wier, Jesteadt, and Green's (1977) data are illustrat-

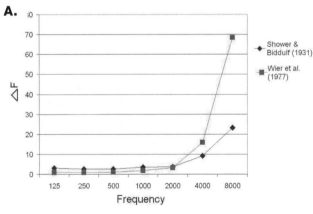

A.

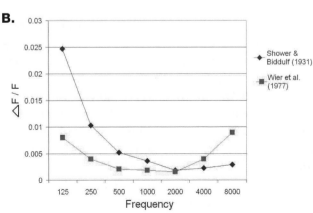

B.

Figure 31-3. Just noticeable differences for frequency. The diamonds represent data from Shower and Biddulph's (1931) study that used a warble detection task. The data from Wier et al. (1977) (*squares*) use a forced-choice procedure with pure-tone stimuli. (Data are interpolations, as the two studies used slightly different stimulus frequencies.) **A.** The DL$_F$ in Hz is shown. Viewed in this manner, ability to detect change in frequency is best in the low frequencies. **B.** The *y*-axis is then divided by the original frequency. When viewed as a Weber fraction, the best pitch detection ability is in the mid-frequencies.

ed. As shown, the paired-comparison method of measuring DL$_F$ yields generally more sensitive results except at the highest frequencies; however, the overall finding is the same in that the ear can detect change in frequency, described in Hz, best for the low frequencies.

If Weber's law fit exactly, the ratio of the just noticeable difference divided by the test frequency would always be constant. The lines in Figure 31–3B would be flat. The results of both forms of experiments show that this is not true, because the ear is most sensitive to frequency changes when the sounds are in the mid frequencies.

DL$_F$ experiments tell us something about the physiology of frequency information encoding. Consider that the ear can detect a difference between 250 and 251 Hz or 4000 and 4016 Hz. The place where these pairs of traveling waves peak would be very close together, so it seems unlikely that a strict place theory explains our phenomenally good pitch perception. Chapter 22 discussed how neurons phase-lock, with some of the neurons responding after one peak of an ongoing sound wave and others firing in response to one of the next sound wave peaks. The ear apparently uses the time between the firing of a group of neurons to encode frequency. The period of a 250 Hz tone is 4 msec, and the period of 251 Hz is 3.98 msec. The ear seems to have little trouble encoding timing differences like the difference in period of 0.02 msec. When the signal is 4000 Hz (at 40 dB SL), 16 Hz was needed to detect the pitch difference. The period of 4000 Hz is 0.25 msec; the period of 4001 Hz is 0.2499 msec, a difference of 0.0001 msec. We can't detect a change in neural timing of 0.0001-msec., but we can tell 4000 Hz from 4016 Hz, which requires neural timing precision of about 0.001-msec accuracy. There seems to be a limit to what time difference in period

the ear can detect. The poorer DL$_F$s at the highest frequencies seem to support that idea. The ear isn't terribly good at pitch encoding at the very high frequencies—for example, 8000 Hz has a 68 Hz DL$_F$. The period of 8000 Hz is 0.125 msec. The period of 8068 Hz is 0.1239 msec. Again, the ear can detect a difference in the average interspike interval (coming from the difference in the sound wave period) of about .001 msec. Differences in period less that this are not encoded reliably.

We will discuss the topic further after covering masking. The degree to which DL$_F$s agree with the bark scale, the more the place theory of pitch perception would make sense. That is—if the change in size of the DL$_F$s matches the change in size of the critical masking band, then the place theory is supported. Jumping ahead to the conclusion, the place theory and the DL$_F$ curve are similar in shape, but place theory can't explain the ear's exceptionally good ability to detect pitch change for most of the range of frequencies. There is less disagreement at the highest frequencies, so perhaps once the ear's timing detection differences are not responsible for encoding the highest frequencies, then perhaps a place theory does predict our ability to detect change in frequency.

Changes in DL$_F$ with Intensity

The higher the signal intensity, the better the difference limen for frequency (Figure 31–4). As mentioned early in this chapter, the pitch that is perceived depends partly on intensity—higher frequencies sound higher in pitch when they are louder. It's tempting to question whether that is the cause of the better DL$_F$ at high intensities, but that doesn't seem likely. We don't know of a good, simple explanation for this phenomenon.

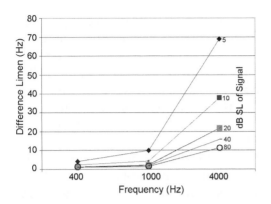

Figure 31–4. Difference limen for frequency is lower as the intensity of the reference signals increase. The data are from Wier et al. (1977).

PERCEPTION OF TWO TONES AND OF DISTORTIONS

Chapter 22 discussed some of the phenomena that happen in the cochlea when multiple tones are present simultaneously, specifically, the perception of hearing a third tone when two tones, close in frequency, are presented. A related concept, how one tone masks the other, will be discussed in the next chapter. Some of the audible tones that are created when two or more tones are heard simultaneously are discussed below.

Beats and Simple Difference Tones

When two tones are presented to the same ear, and the frequency is very close, an intensity modulation occurs. The frequency of the on and off pulsation is calculated as f2 – f1, where f2 is the higher frequency sound, and f1 the lower frequency sound. The perception is of a steady tone, intermediate in frequency between f1 and f2, that increases and decreases intensity rhythmically. The sound **beats** on and off, thus the term **aural beats**, illustrated in Figure 31-5.

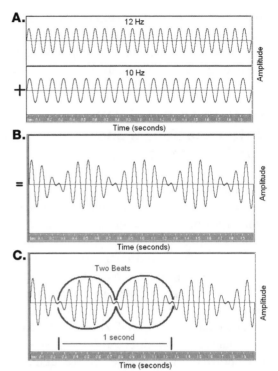

Figure 31–5. Illustration of how combination of two tones varying slightly in frequency **(A)** create a periodic cancellation **(B)** that is perceptible as a beat **(C)**. The frequencies used in this illustration are lower than audible, but provide a convenient graphic illustration. The same would be true if the signals were in the audible range, but in that case, there would be too many cycles of the sine wave in the combined, beating sound to see the individual cycles.

If the difference between the two frequencies increases to more than just several Hz apart, the perception is of one tone that is beating faster. At some point, the perception changes to that of hearing a "rough" tone in addition to the one tone with frequency intermediate between f1 and f2.

With still greater separation between the two tones (f1 and f2), you can detect the two tones as distinct from each other, and you will then also perceive a distinct third tone, the **simple difference tone.** The frequency of the simple difference tone is f2 – f1, hence the name. It is simply the difference between the two, in Hz.

Summation Tones, Other Difference Tones, and Aural Harmonics

The ear, under certain circumstances, also perceives some distortions of a single tone. A distortion is the creation of an additional spectral component, or components, that does not exist in the original signal. At high intensities, the ear produces harmonic distortion. **Aural harmonic distortion** occurs at multiples of the original frequency. For example, a 1000-Hz tone will have harmonics at 2000, 3000, 4000, and so on. The shorthand to describe the frequencies at which a single tone's distortions occur is 2f1, 3f1, 4f1, and so on. If a second, higher frequency tone were also present, its distortions would be at 2f2, 3f2, and so on. Again, by convention, f1 is the lower frequency of the tones, f2 the higher.

Harmonic aural distortion occurs when the ear is stimulated at very loud levels. However, there are other distortions, called **combination tones**, that are created by modest intensity signals, when two or more pure tones are present in the same ear. Combination tones include summation tones and difference tones. One of the combination tones is the already discussed simple difference frequency. Another is the **simple summation tone**, which occurs at the frequency f1 + f2. There are many other summation tone distortions that can occur. The listener may perceive the frequency of one of the original tones and the harmonic of the other tone. For example, one might detect a component at the frequency of f1 + 2f2 or f1 + 2f3. Likewise, one might hear the 2f1 + f2 and/or 3f1 + f2 frequency.

Just as one can hear a variety of summation tones, there are complex difference tones that can sometimes be detected. A rather prominent one is the **cubic difference tone** which occurs at the frequency 2f1 – f2. Myriad other difference tones can occur, such as f1 – 2f2, 3f1 – f2, 3f1 – 2f1, and so forth.

The **missing fundamental** is another interesting related phenomenon. If you were presented with several tones, spaced apart by some given frequency, you perceive that separation frequency. For example, if you were presented 2000 Hz, 2200 Hz, 2400 Hz, 2600 Hz, and 2800 Hz all together, you would hear the difference tone—200 Hz—quite prominently. A 200-Hz fundamental frequency tone would have harmonics spaced apart by 200 Hz, which accounts for the name of the phenomenon: the missing fundamental. The perception is that the fundamental frequency is present, even though it is not physically there.

Distortion is frequently considered undesirable, but in the case of the ear, these distortions are a normal process. The active mechanism of the inner ear creates "nonlinearities" of the ear, and distortions result. Otoacoustic emissions (Chapters 18 and 19) testing evaluates whether the nonlinearities are present, particularly the cubic difference tone. Presence of this distortion is a sign of healthy outer hair cells.

SUMMARY

The oft-quoted limits of human hearing of 20 to 20,000 Hz has been shown to actually be the limits of tonal perception, as frequencies lower than 20 Hz can be heard if loud enough, but they won't be perceived as tonal. Also, tones aren't tonal if they are too short in duration.

This chapter discussed how we perceive change in frequency—our limits of detecting the change (just noticeable difference for frequency) and our perception of the quality of pitch (the mel scale). In regard to the latter, we see that doubling frequency creates less than a doubling of pitch. The absolute just noticeable difference for frequency change is better the lower the frequency and the higher the intensity. Pitch detection described as Weber fractions shows a near-miss to Weber's law. Very low and very high pitch discrimination requires more change in the stimulus than needed for the mid-frequency range, and seems to suggest that the ear encodes these very low and very high frequencies differently.

In cases where two or more tones are present simultaneously, aural distortions occur, and we hear combination tones and, with high-intensity presentations, harmonic distortions. Aural beats are perceived when two tones, close in frequency, are presented together in the same ear.

REFERENCES

Shower, E. G., & Biddulph, R. (1931). Differential pitch sensitivity of the ear. *Journal of the Acoustical Society of America, 3,* 275–287.

Stevens, S. S., & Volkmann, J. (1940). The relations of pitch to frequency: A revised scale. *American Journal of Psychology, 53,* 329-353. As reprinted in J. D. Harris, (Ed.), 1969, *Forty germinal papers in psychoacoustics* by the Journal of Auditory Research.

Wier, C. C., Jesteadt, W., & Green, D. M. (1977). Frequency discrimination as a function of frequency and sensation level. *Journal of the Acoustical Society of America, 61*(1), 178–184.

32

Introduction to Masking

In this chapter, some of the basic concepts of masking are introduced. Masking is the process where one signal is made less audible because of another signal that is present either at the same time, or very close in time.

Two terms to introduce are the **probe** and the **masker**. The probe is a signal to be detected, which is typically a pure tone. The masker is the signal that is introduced along with the probe that causes the probe to be less audible or inaudible.

This chapter introduces **monaural simultaneous masking**. That is, the probe signal and masker are in the same ear, and both are present at the same time. Other chapters will explain how the masker can come just before or just after the probe tone and still create masking.

Chapter 18 discussed how basilar membrane moves up and down in response to sound. That basic information is required to understand this chapter. Chapter 21 provided the foundation for understanding why masking occurs, and how it is related to the traveling wave along basilar membrane. This chapter reviews this information about how one tone's traveling wave can "swamp" the traveling wave from another, softer pure tone.

First, we discuss studies of masking that used a pure tone as both the probe and the

masker. Masking of tones with white noise and narrow-band noise is more frequently used, and this chapter describes the idea that to mask a certain frequency probe, narrow-band noise with a frequency content similar to the pure tone works best. This chapter describes the bandwidth of the narrow-band noise that optimally masks a pure tone.

TONE-ON-TONE MASKING

Some of the earliest masking experiments used pure tones for both the masker and the probe. The question asked was this: "If the masker tone is at one frequency, at one intensity, how well does that tone mask probe tones at other frequencies?" When the probe frequency is close to the masker frequency, the probe must be quite loud in order to be heard, especially if the probe tone is higher in frequency than the masker. Said another way, when the probe and masker are similar in frequency, the probe tone is being masked quite efficiently. If the probe frequency is further from the masker frequency, there is less masking, and often no masking if the probe is lower frequency than the masker. The traveling wave theory explains this phenomenon.

Recall that basilar membrane changes in mass and stiffness along the length of the coiled cochlea. The area near the base of the cochlea is light and stiff; near the apex it is wide and floppy. Because of this mass/stiffness gradient, each different frequency pure tone creates maximal movement at a certain area along the basilar membrane. The traveling wave shows this movement. When a constant intensity pure tone is presented to the ear, the amount of basilar membrane movement (displacement) increases from base to apex up to the point of maximum displacement. The displacement then decreases rapidly as the wave travels up the cochlear a bit farther.

Let's take the example of a 1200-Hz tone as the masker, and suppose that it is presented at 60 dB SPL. Figure 32–1A illustrates the traveling wave from the 1200-Hz, 60 dB SPL masker. Assume that it is stimulating neurons in the shaded area on the basilar membrane. If the masker is turned off, and the 1400-Hz tone is presented at an intensity such as 30 dB SPL, it would stimulate the neurons as shown in Figure 32–1B. When both tones are present (Figure 32–1C), the 1200-Hz tone masks the 1400-Hz probe tone. Notice that the entire vibrating area on the basilar membrane that results from the 1400-Hz tone is entirely covered by the vibration from the 1200-Hz tone. The neurons are firing in response to the 1200-Hz signal, and cannot simultaneously encode information about the 1400-Hz tone. If the 1400-Hz tone intensity is increased sufficiently, as shown in Figure 32–1D, then both tones would be audible. The intensity of the 1400-Hz probe can be experimentally adjusted until the signal is "just masked." (Any further increase in intensity would allow the sound to be audible.) If this were done, one might find that the 1200-Hz, 60 dB SPL masking tone can mask a 1400-Hz probe tone of 35 dB SPL (or lower intensity).

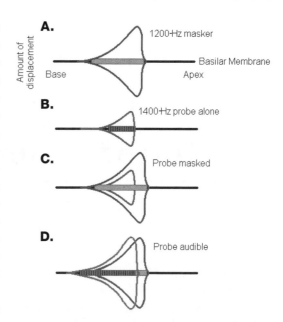

Figure 32–1. Traveling waves on the basilar membrane. The shaded area illustrates the portion of the basilar membrane where neurons are stimulated. The apex encodes low-frequency information, therefore traveling wave (**A**), from 1200 Hz, peaks more toward the apex than the 1400-Hz traveling wave illustrated in (**B**). **C.** If both signals are present simultaneously, the 1400-Hz tone would not be perceived. It is masked by the more intense 1200-Hz traveling wave. **D.** Increasing the intensity of the 1400-Hz tone, permits both signals to be heard.

As the frequency of the probe becomes further and further from the masker, there is less masking. As illustrated in Figure 32–2, it is difficult to impossible for the masker tone to mask probe frequencies that are lower than the masker frequency. The asymmetric (*right to left*) shape of the traveling wave explains this. The traveling wave dies out rapidly. It does not travel very far up the cochlea from the point of maximum displacement, and therefore is inefficient at masking low-frequency probe signals.

Figure 32–3 plots the amount of masking for each of the pure-tone probes. That is,

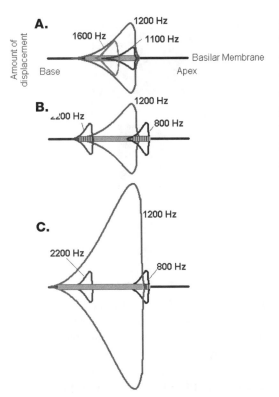

Figure 32–2. A. The 1200-Hz tone can mask a low-intensity tone that is 100 Hz lower in frequency, or one that is 400 Hz higher. **B**. This signal is unable to mask the 2200-Hz tone or 800-Hz tone. **C**. If the masker level is increased, it can mask the 2200-Hz tone (which is 1000 Hz higher in frequency), but is still unable to mask the 800-Hz tone, even though it is only 400 Hz lower in frequency.

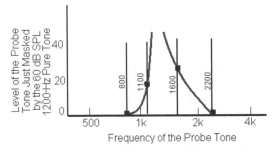

Figure 32–3. Sketch of the amount of masking for differing frequency probes from a 1200-Hz pure tone masker. The 1200-Hz tone more effectively masks probes higher in frequency.

signals any greater in intensity than shown would no longer be masked. Note that this figure has the low frequencies on the left, whereas the basilar membrane figure is drawn with the low frequencies on the right. The curve in Figure 32–3 looks something like a traveling wave that is inverted right to left. It shows that a given frequency masker is better at masking high frequencies and is largely ineffective at masking frequency probes that are significantly lower than the masker frequency.

Figure 32–3 is meant to suggest that as the probe becomes closer and closer to the masker frequency, there is more and more masking. However, recall from Chapter 31 what happens when the listener hears two tones that are similar in frequency. The listener perceives beats. For example, if listening to the 1200-Hz masker and an 1190-Hz probe, as the 1190-Hz tone increases in intensity and approaches the intensity of the 1200-Hz masker tone, a 10-Hz modulation (beating) is detected. The masker would actually be less effective for probes that are very close in frequency as the subject knows when the probe is present because of the beats that arise from the probe/masker interaction.

Chapter 31 also discussed that loud sounds create harmonic distortion within the cochlea. If the 1200-Hz masker tone were increased in intensity, it would create 2400 and 3600-Hz harmonics. These harmonics can create their own masking. However, as the probe comes very close to the harmonic frequency, there again would be aural beats. Figure 32–4 illustrates the masking patterns that would therefore result from tone-on-tone masking; it is a modified sketch of the data from Wegel and Lane's 1924 paper. (Some liberties were taken.) One of the features Figure 32–4 illustrates is that turning the masker up 20 dB creates 20 dB more masking—as long as the probe

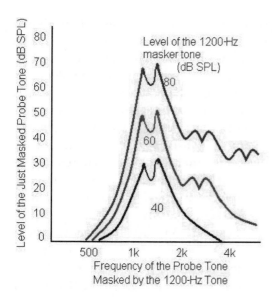

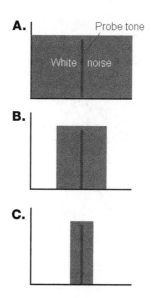

Figure 32–4. Tone-on-tone masking patterns created by 1200-Hz maskers at 80, 60, and 40 dB SPL. When the probe frequency is close to the masker frequency, or a harmonic frequency of the masker, beat frequencies are heard, which decreases the masker's effectiveness.

Figure 32–5. A. In a critical band experiment, a probe tone is first masked with white noise. The noise is band-pass filtered progressively (**B** and **C**) to find the narrowest range of frequencies that just masks the probe. The narrowest band that just masks the probe is the critical band. If the masking noise is narrower than the critical band, the probe tone is heard.

masker is near or higher in frequency than the masker tone.

CRITICAL BANDS

Because of the phenomenon of aural beats, modern masking studies typically use a masker that is a narrow band of noise. The tone-on-tone masking studies had illustrated that there is a narrow range of frequencies that best masks a probe. Therefore it will come as no surprise that, to mask a pure-tone probe, the noise does not have to contain all frequencies—it only needs to contain frequencies near the probe tone.

Studies of **critical bands** have sought to determine what range of frequencies is most important in masking a pure-tone probe signal. There are several ways to determine the width of a critical band. One of the simplest is illustrated in Figure 32–5.

First, a probe tone is masked with white noise. The noise frequencies much lower and much higher than the probe are gradually eliminated. The experimenter seeks to find the narrowest band of noise that will still mask the probe. (If the experimenter removes other frequencies closer to the probe that contributed to the masking, the probe is heard.) This is the critical band for that probe tone frequency.

As a generality, one could say that the critical band is about one-quarter to one-third of an octave wide. Thus, if you consider the number of cycles in each octave, the critical band would be wider in the high frequencies, as an octave contains more frequencies as frequency increases.

Experimentation confirmed that masking a probe with a narrow band of noise is a linear function. That is, if the noise is in-

Clinical Correlate: The Audiometer's Masking Noise

In audiometric testing, for example, when testing pure-tone thresholds using earphones, an intense sound presented to one ear can cross and be heard at the opposite (nontest) cochlea. When the audiologist wants to prevent the nontest ear from hearing the tone, masking noise is put into the nontest ear. The masking noise used is narrow-band noise, typically about one-third to one-half octave wide. A wider band of noise is not needed as it doesn't help mask the signal. Using a white noise or a wide band of noise instead of narrow-band noise wouldn't be desired, as the overall loudness of the white noise is greater, which is uncomfortable. It would be possible to mask a pure tone with a band of noise that is even narrower than one-third octave, but you wouldn't want to do that. If the noise becomes too narrow, it takes on a pronounced tonal quality. The patient would be more likely to confuse the signal tone and masker if the masker noise band is very narrow and sounds too much like a tone.

The linearity of masking is a critical finding. During clinical masking, after setting the masking noise to exclude the nontest ear "from participating," if the test ear tone is increased 10 dB, then we can increase the masking noise by 10 dB to compensate.

creased 10 dB, you can mask a 10 dB more intense probe.

SUMMARY

This chapter has discussed why the masking of a pure tone (probe) is best achieved by presenting signals that are near to the probe frequency. Noises (or pure tones) lower in frequency than the probe can travel past the probe tone's place of maximum displacement. Lower frequencies are therefore more effective maskers than noises/tones that are higher than the probe's frequency. Maskers that are higher than the probe tone frequency peak before the probe tone location on the basilar membrane and therefore do not mask the traveling wave

peaking more apically. Masking is greatest with frequencies closest to the probe. Tone-on-tone masking studies are helpful in validating the traveling wave theory; however, the presence of aural beats complicates interpretation. Most modern experiments and all clinical test procedures use narrow bands of noise to mask a pure tone. A critical band of noise includes those frequencies that are near enough to the probe to assist in masking the probe.

REFERENCE

Wegel, R. L., & Lane, C. E. (1924). The auditory masking of one pure tone by another and its probable relation to the dynamics of the inner ear. *Physics Review, 23,* 266–285.

33

More About Masking and Cochlear Frequency Distribution

Chapter 32 discussed the basics of masking and how masking is consistent with what we know about the traveling wave. This chapter covers some of the more advanced concepts in simultaneous mon-aural masking, starting with a discussion of some of the earliest work in masking, which was conducted by Harvey Fletcher, published in 1940. Fletcher and others interested in masking were attempting to understand the layout of the cochlea, and the limits of the place theory of hearing. We relate masking experiment results to the results of pitch perception experiments and examine what these findings suggest about how the cochlea is arranged.

Additionally, this chapter covers some more modern concepts in masking. One of these concepts, comodulation release from masking, lets us understand that what happens on basilar membrane is not all there is to masking. The central nervous system uses cues from across different auditory "bands" or areas on the basilar membrane.

MASKING PURE TONES WITH WHITE NOISE AND NARROW-BAND NOISE: CRITICAL BANDS AND CRITICAL RATIOS

The previous chapter discussed tone-on-tone masking, work published in 1924 by Wegel and Lane. Another very early type of masking experiment was one that used white noise to mask a pure tone. White noise, of course, has all the frequencies in it. Fletcher theorized that there was a narrow range of frequencies that contribute to the masking phenomenon. His **critical ratio theory** was that if you sum the energy in this narrow range of frequencies, it will equal the energy of the tone that it is masking. To understand Fletcher's work, the reader has to understand the concepts of levels per cycle and decibel addition.

Level per Cycle Calculations

Before further discussing masking with white noise, we need to understand how a white noise can be described both as being X dB SPL, and also how that same noise's intensity can be described in **level per cycle**. And before defining and describing calculations for level per cycle, it is helpful to review a few concepts about white noise and decibel addition.

First, recall that by definition white noise has a flat spectrum. That is, if you could detect just the amount of energy at 1000 Hz (not 999 Hz or 1001 Hz, just 1000 Hz) it would be the same as the amount of energy at 2000 Hz (or at 321 Hz or 4987 Hz, etc.) (The energy per frequency in white noise does fluctuate somewhat over time, but will be the same at every frequency on average.) Although you can't readily measure the energy at just one single frequency, we know that each frequency will have the same energy because of the definition of white noise.

Once a speaker or earphone transduces white noise, it is no longer precisely white. Most transducers are designed to send a wide range of frequencies through without altering intensity too much. Typically, the variation in intensity from one frequency to another is less than 3 dB across the range the transducer can produce. However, there will be an upper and a lower frequency limit to what the transducer can transmit. For example, Hawkins and Stevens (1950), in studying white noise masking, had earphones that efficiently transmitted frequencies above 100 Hz and below 9000 Hz. The bandwidth of the earphone is that range between the lower and upper cutoffs, 8900 Hz in this case.

The next basic concept to review is decibel addition. If you have one pure tone that is 40 dB SPL, and then present a different frequency tone at 40 dB SPL, you now have 43 dB SPL of sound present. Why? First, remember that dB SPL is equivalent to dB IL. The 3 dB increase occurs when you add the power of two pure tones of the same frequency and phase, and it is just as valid to say that when you present two different frequency pure tones of the same intensity, the sum of those two 40 dB IL sounds has an intensity of 43 dB IL. When presenting two tones simultaneously, you have double the power. That is not the same thing as having twice the pressure (see Chapter 2). So, when you double the power, you calculate the decibel increase with the equation: dB increase = 10 log 2/1. (The ratio of two cycles versus 1 cycle.) This is equal to 10 log 0.3, or 3 dB. If there is a 3 dB increase in power, there is also a 3 dB increase in pressure. (If you turn the sound up 3 dB IL, you have also increased the sound by 3 dB SPL.)

If 10 pure tones are present rather than just one pure tone, how much more intensity is present? The general formula is 10 log (number of cycles / one cycle as reference). In this example of adding the power of 10 tones, this would be 10 log 10, or 10 dB. Ten simultaneous pure tones of equal energy produce an overall sound that is 10 dB more intense than the level coming from just one of those tones. As 10 log 20 is 13 dB, you can see that doubling the number of pure tones from 10 to 20 gives 3 dB more sound intensity than when 10 tones were present. You could have calculated this by considering how much more intense 10 tones are than 20 tones, (10 log 20/10 = 3 dB), to discover that it is a 3 dB increase relative to the level from 10 simultaneous tones.

If 8900 tones are present, how much more intense is that than if one tone were present? As 10 log 8900 = 39.5 dB, it provides an increased sound intensity of 39.5 dB. That is, the total sound power created by presenting 8900 tones is 39.5 dB higher than the level of just one of the pure tones present alone.

The same concept holds true for noise. The intensity present at each individual frequency is some given level, and this is termed the noise's **level per cycle (LPC).**

The intensity that sums from having energy at each frequency throughout the bandwidth is higher than the level per cycle, and can be calculated. The formula is overall level (OA) is equal to LPC + bandwidth expressed in dB. Bandwidth in dB is certainly a foreign concept, but all we are saying is how many more Hz are present than 1 Hz, then put that in the 10 log formula. The bandwidth of 8900 Hz, in dB, is equal to 10 log 8900 (39.5 dB). Now, back to the formula for overall level. In this example, if the level per cycle of the noise is 10 dB SPL, and the bandwidth is 8900 Hz which equals 39.5 dB, then the overall level would be 49.5 dB SPL.

Generally, though, we think in terms of going from the overall noise to the noise intensity at each cycle (the LPC), because it is easier to measure the overall level, and fairly easy to measure the bandwidth of the earphone. For example, if the noise were 79.5 dB overall, and had a bandwidth of 100 to 9000 Hz (8900 Hz), the level of noise at each single frequency (the LPC) is equal to Overall Level—Bandwidth in dB: The general formula is the same:

Overall Level (OA) = Level per cycle (LPC)
+ 10 log [bandwidth in Hz] (BW in dB)

Or the equivalent
LPC = OA – 10 log BW in Hz

In summary, white noise can be described in two ways: the overall level and the level per cycle. The level per cycle is fairly easy to calculate if you know the range of frequencies the transducer can produce. Fletcher's masking theory used the level per cycle information, and we can use this information to further explore the experimental critical bands as well. In an upcoming section we will return to Fletcher's critical ratio theory and examine whether it agrees with the critical band experimental data. First,

we will use our knowledge of LPC calculations to further examine critical band experimental data.

Critical Bands in Hz and in dB

The previous chapter introduced the idea that the typical critical band experiment used band-limited white noise (a "narrow-band" noise) as the masker. Recall from the previous chapter that in one form of critical band experiment, a white noise overall SPL is adjusted to just mask the probe tone. The white noise is then progressively filtered to reject the highest and lowest frequencies. The task is to find the narrowest noise band that still masks the probe. That experiment showed us which frequencies were outside the critical band—removing them from the masking signal didn't alter the masking of the probe tone.

In critical band experiments, the level of the noise at each frequency within the pass-band is equal in intensity. The noise closest to the probe frequency is not made louder to reflect its greater importance in masking.

Let's take an example. In a critical band experiment, the probe tone is 980 Hz. The white noise has an overall level of 60 dB SPL, and the earphone has a bandwidth of 8900 Hz. Converting the bandwidth to dB (10 log 8900) we find the bandwidth to be 39.5 dB.

The level per cycle is the overall level minus the bandwidth. In this example, the level per cycle would be 20.5 dB SPL (60 – 39.5).

In this critical band experiment, let's assume that for this subject, the 60 dB SPL white noise masks a 1000-Hz pure tone that is 38 dB SPL. Experimentally, the white noise is narrowed. The narrowest band of noise that masks the signal ranges from 900 to 1060 Hz. This is the critical band (in Hz). How intense is the noise in this band? It could be measured with a sound level meter, but we can calculate it as well. The bandwidth can be converted to dB. The bandwidth from 900 to 1060 Hz is 160 Hz; 10 log 160 = 22 dB. The noise level per cycle was 20.5 dB SPL, so the overall level of the narrow-band noise, obtained using the formula OA = LPC + 10 log BW, is 42.5 dB (20.5 LPC + 22 dB BW).

For this experimental subject, the narrow band of noise from 900 to 1060 (the 160-Hz-wide critical band) at 42.5 dB SPL just masked the 38 dB SPL, 1-kHz tone. The noise was 4.5 dB above the level of the tone intensity. As thresholds vary from test to retest, using half-decibel steps is more precise than experimentation really permits, so it would be appropriate to round to 4 dB. That is, in this experiment, the critical band of noise was 4 dB more intense than the probe. So, in summary, the noise that masks a pure tone can be described in Hz, and we can find out how much louder the narrow-band noise is than the tone.

A Critical Band Is Also Called a Bark

You may occasionally hear the term **bark** in psychoacoustics, a term introduced in Chapter 31. A bark is equal to a critical band. You could create a series of these critical bands where the highest frequency of one becomes the lowest frequency of the next highest critical band or bark. If you put the critical bands side to side (e.g., the band from 20 Hz to 110 Hz, then the band from 110 Hz to 200 Hz, etc.), the human ear has about 24 to 25 critical bands, and thus 24 to 25 barks.

How Critical Bands Vary with Frequency

Figure 33–1 illustrates the results of Zwicker, Flottorp, and Stevens (1957) of the size of the critical band across frequencies. Figures 33-1A shows that the critical band in Hz stays relatively the same below 1000 Hz, then increases above 1000 Hz. This means that masking a high-frequency sound (e.g., 8000 Hz) takes a wider range of frequencies. Another way to think about the critical band is as a ratio—how large is the critical band divided by the center frequency of the critical band. In Figure 33–1B these results are shown. Sometimes critical bands are thought of in octave terms. The formula for the octave scale is: New frequency = original frequency $\times 2^{\text{octave change}}$. Using Zwicker et al.'s data, a critical band (a bark) starts at 250 Hz and ends at 345 Hz. $345 = 250 \times 2^{0.55}$—the 250-Hz critical band is a little more than a half-octave wide. The band nearest 1000 Hz is about 0.24 octaves, as is the 4000-Hz band, but the 8000-Hz band is about 0.30 octaves. A generalization is that the Zwicker et al. study put the critical band at about one-quarter to one-third octaves wide, but as you see, that is a rather gross generalization.

Fletcher's Theory of Critical Ratio

Before critical band studies were conducted, Fletcher (1940) theorized that masking would occur when the frequencies, in what we now call a critical band, would sum to the intensity of the pure tone to be masked. He masked tones with white noise. In his experimentation, he found that 60 dB SPL white noise masked a 1000-Hz tone if the pure tone was 38 dB SPL or less. He thought that if the tone is 38 dB SPL, that meant that there is an important region of frequencies where the LPCs sum to an overall level of 38 dB SPL. He believed that would be the range of frequencies responsible for the masking.

As in the above critical band experiment, assume the earphone's bandwidth is 8900 Hz, so the level per cycle of a 60 dB SPL white noise is 20.5 dB. According to Fletch-

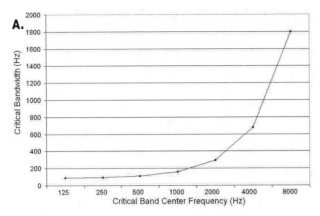

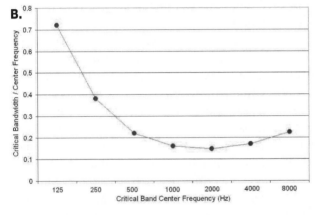

Figure 33–1. A. The size of the critical band for masking increases as the center band of the frequency increases. Here, the y-axis scale is Hz. **B.** We often think of ratios of change. The data in this part of the figure are treated more as a Weber ratio—the y-axis is size of the critical band divided by the center frequency.

er's theory, the critical-for-masking noise bandwidth should sum up to 38 dB SPL, the level of the tone that was just masked. Fletcher would have calculated the **critical ratio** (as a bandwidth in dB) as the masked pure tone level minus the level per cycle. Here, that is the 38 dB SPL probe tone level minus the 20 dB noise LPC, which equals 18 dB (or 18.5 dB if you want to retain the decimal number). That would be the critical ratio in dB. We can turn critical band in dB back to Hz. As 18.5 dB = 10 log 71, this gives a critical ratio of 71 Hz. Note that Fletcher's theoretical critical ratio in Hz is smaller than the actual 160-Hz critical band.

Fletcher made a critical assumption that later was proven incorrect. In actuality, if you sum the noise in a critical band it will be about 4 dB more intense than the probe tone. A wider range of frequencies is in the actual critical band. We still honor Fletcher's

conceptual work, though. He realized the importance of finding the frequencies that are important for masking as a tool for understanding the layout of the cochlea, a concept to be discussed later in this chapter.

EQUIVALENT RECTANGULAR BANDWIDTHS

Tone-on-tone masking experiments reveal to us that not all frequencies within a critical band are equally important. You already can surmise that frequencies in a narrow-band noise that are closest to the probe tone frequency are most effective in masking.

The bell-shaped curve in Figure 33–2 shows what is called an **auditory filter**. It represents how different frequencies within a masking band contribute to the masking phenomenon differently. Those closest to the center frequency are the most important. This model is more realistic than assuming that all frequencies within a certain range are equally important to masking. How this filter is experimentally obtained is a bit more advanced than the intended scope of this book. It is another masking experiment, so it too describes which frequencies are important in masking the pure-tone probe. The rectangle superimposed on this figure gives a convenient way to describe the outer bounds of the filter. The area of the rectangle is the same as the area under the curved auditory filter, but, as it's a rectangle, it's easy to define the lower and upper bandwidth frequencies—which gives us the reason for the name **equivalent rectangular bandwidth** (ERB). If you multiply the center frequency by about 15% you have an approximation of the bandwidth of the ERB for probes 500 Hz and higher. For example, the 1000-Hz bandwidth is approximately 150 Hz, spanning from 925 to 1075 Hz.

Studies of ERBs have shown that, as intensity increases, the ERB widens. The traveling wave created by the probe tone is apparently broadening out as intensity increases, which means that noise that is farther away on the basilar membrane will be important in the masking of the probe tone.

OTHER WAYS TO EVALUATE CRITICAL BANDS

Although critical bands can be investigated with masking studies, that is not the only way to experimentally derive the critical band. Critical bands are also areas that are interrelated in terms of encoding loudness. If several pure tones are present within a narrow area (a critical band), and their traveling waves overlap closely, the perception will be of a less intense sound than if one or more of the pure tones fell outside the critical band. Critical band experiments

have been conducted using this experimental method. Several tones are initially spaced close together in frequency, and then they are spaced wider and wider apart. If all the tones are in the same critical band, the changes in frequency don't create changes in loudness. When one of the tones is outside the critical band, then the perception is that the signal is louder, even though the overall SPL of the combined tones has stayed the same. Once one of the tones is outside a critical band, it stimulates a different group of neurons, and that increases the perceived loudness.

Loudness perception of narrow-band noise also sheds light on this issue. If the overall level of the noise is kept constant while bandwidth increases (and as a result, level per cycle decreases), at some point the noise is perceived as increasing in loudness. This increased loudness perception comes when some of the noise frequencies are outside the critical band. New auditory filters or "channels" are stimulated. When the noise is no longer confined to one critical band, loudness increases.

THE RELATIONSHIP BETWEEN DL$_F$, CRITICAL BANDS, CRITICAL RATIOS, AND EQUIVALENT RECTANGULAR BANDWIDTHS

One of the reasons that masking studies and difference limen for frequency studies are interesting is that they may explain the layout of the basilar membrane. Figure 33–3 shows several different experimental results together. In Figure 33–3A, the y-axis is absolute frequency, and in Figure 33–3B, it is the result divided by the center frequency or reference frequency, creating a Weber fraction. In both of these views, it appears that the ear handles low and high frequencies some-

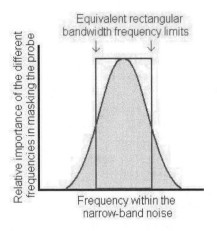

Figure 33–2. The curve shows the relative importance of different frequencies that comprise the narrow-band noise in the masking a probe tone. The frequency components nearest the center (which is the frequency of the probe) are most important. If a rectangle is superimposed over the curve so the rectangle has the same area as under the curve, and its top is at the tallest point of the curve, that shows the equivalent rectangular bandwidth (*ERB*). The ERB width is about 15% of the center frequency for most frequencies.

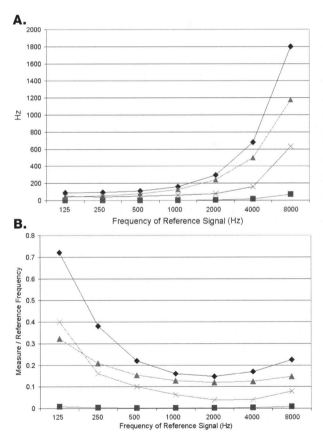

Figure 33–3. Comparison of different methods of studying the ear's place specificity. **A.** Data on the size of the critical band (*diamond*), equivalent rectangular bandwidth (*triangle*), critical ratio (*X*), and difference limen for frequency (*square*). **B.** These same data, plotted as Weber fractions. Although the results differ, there is a trend for a basal (high-frequency) place on the cochlea to have more frequencies (in Hz). The apex has areas that span a greater fraction of an octave.

what differently. The general trend is that if a given distance on the basilar membrane represents some unit—the size of the criti-

cal band, the size of the ERB or a DL_F—then that given area has more frequencies in it at the base of the cochlea.

Clinical Correlate: Acoustic Reflexes to Pure Tones and Broadband Noise

It is more accurate to say that the middle acoustic reflex occurs when a loud sound is present than to say they occur in response to intense sounds. It is the perception of loudness (reflexively, at a brainstem level) that creates the stapedial contraction.

When using pure-tone stimuli, only one critical band is stimulated. If using a white or wide-band noise, many critical bands are stimulated. The stimulus in each individual band creates some of the perception of loudness. For this reason, the threshold for a reflex elicited by broadband noise is lower than for pure tones. For example, a reflex might occur at 65 dB HL for broadband noise, and 85 dB HL for individual pure-tone signals. The energy in the broadband noise is sensed across a large number of critical bands and sounds louder, permitting a lower acoustic reflex threshold.

Cochlear hearing loss does more than just change the threshold of hearing. It also creates recruitment, the phenomenon where loud sounds are still perceived as loud. As Chapter 38 will discuss further, an additional change with cochlear loss is that the critical band limits are made wider. If a normal hearer has 24 or 25 critical bands, then perhaps a person with cochlear loss might have 10 critical bands. With fewer critical bands to summate loudness, the threshold for the broadband acoustic reflex becomes higher. Because of recruitment, patients with mild to moderate cochlear loss typically have pure-tone acoustic reflexes that are near normal levels. Said another way, the acoustic reflex thresholds coming from the perception of loud pure tones, presented to a single critical band, are about the same for those with mild/moderate cochlear loss and normal hearers. However, the patient with cochlear loss is not as sensitive to the noise across critical bands as the normal hearer, because she or he has fewer critical bands. The cochlear loss ear does not have as reduced a reflex threshold for the broadband noise. This is the basis for the **sensitivity prediction by the acoustic reflex** (SPAR) test. When the noise and tone thresholds are similar, that finding predicts cochlear loss.

COMODULATION RELEASE FROM MASKING

This chapter has discussed masking studies that tell us about the way the cochlea responds. However, some masking phenomena are the result of what happens within the central nervous system. Chapter 36 will examine how masking occurs when stimuli are spaced close in time, and Chapter 37 will describe the binaural masking phenomena. Those are examples of the involvement of the central nervous system in the phenomenon of masking. There is a simultaneous, monaural masking phenomenon that also reveals that masking is not just about what happens on basilar membrane. The phenomenon is called **comodulation release from masking (CMRM)**. We'll need to define some terms first.

The "envelope" of a signal is the broad, relatively gradual increases and decreases in intensity of the signal across time. In Figure 33–4A, the time waveform for the word "comodulation" is illustrated. The different phonemes of course have different spectral content. Figure 33–4B illustrates the fine detail of one portion of the time waveform. Noise has less of an envelope, though it has some, and this is shown in Figure 33–4C. It is possible to change the overall envelope of the noise waveform. In Figure 33–4D, the noise has its envelope now shaped the same as the speech signal; however, the perception of this signal is still of hearing noise. This is illustrated in Figure 33–4E which shows a small time segment enlarged. This is a long introduction to what one hopes will be a simple idea. A narrow band of noise can be modulated, and have a distinct time waveform, but yet still have the frequency content that is narrow-band. Comodulation release from masking experiments use this type of signal.

Release from masking means that adding another signal to the combination of masker and probe reduces the amount of masking. In a comodulation release from masking experiment, the probe could be a pure tone. The masker could be a narrow band of noise that has some form of modulated envelope. In the first part of the experiment, we determine how loud the probe has to be to be just audible in the presence of modulated narrow-band noise, and then just barely masked. For example, the thresh-

old for a 2000-Hz probe alone without the noise might be 25 dB SPL. Add in the modulated 2000-Hz narrow-band masking noise and the threshold for the probe becomes 45 dB SPL. We have 20 dB of masking. Now,

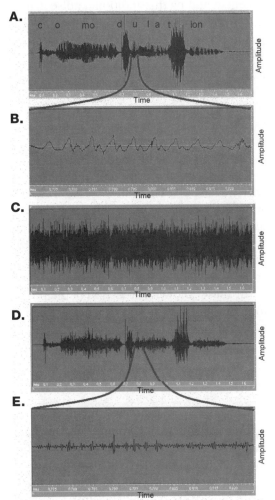

Figure 33–4. Figures showing the amplitude of waveforms across time. **A.** Illustration of the envelope of speech, the word "comodulation." **B.** Note that the temporal components and thus frequency content changes depending on the phoneme. **C.** A narrow band of noise **D.** The envelope of the noise has been modulated by the shape of the speech waveform. **E.** The content is still just noise, not speech.

add a third noise. Make this noise of a different frequency altogether, one that should not create any masking given what we know about the traveling wave. For example, it might be a 250-Hz noise. Here's the important part. Have that noise modulate with the same envelope as the 2000-Hz noise. Surprisingly, adding this additional noise makes the probe tone more audible. The 2000-Hz probe threshold might be 35 dB SPL now. We have 10 dB less masking—a 10 dB "release from masking".

This release from masking only happens if the two noises have the same envelope, that is, if they are comodulated. If the 250-Hz noise were modulated differently, then there would be no release from masking.

At present, there are only theories as to why we have release from masking. Perhaps adding the second, comodulated noise (modulated the same way as the original masking noise) allows the neural system to recognize when the noise fluctuates up and down. It could then "pay attention" during the dips in the noise, allowing detection of the probe tone during those moments when the noise is a little quieter.

REMOTE MASKING

Can an intense high-frequency sound mask a low-frequency tone? The mechanics of the basilar membrane don't allow for this to happen, but there is a small amount of masking of this type, which is called **remote masking,** so named because the place of the masker is remote from the place of the peak of the traveling wave of the probe. There are two possible explanations for this type of tone-on-tone masking, and a third mechanism if the masker is a narrow-band noise signal.

The acoustic reflex may be a part of remote masking. Intense high-frequency signals trigger the stapedial reflex, and the increased stiffness of the middle ear system

attenuates low-frequency sound transmission. However, remote masking is a larger effect when the signal and masker are in the same ear, rather than in opposite ears. If the effect were just from the acoustic reflex, which creates bilateral middle ear stiffness and reduced sound transmission, then we would expect the remote masking effect to be the same when the high-frequency sound is presented either ipsilaterally or contralaterally.

The second partial explanation is that the loud sound triggers the efferent system. Although efferent suppression of afferent neural encoding happens to the largest degree when the signal and masker are of the same frequency, there may be some suppression even at the remote frequencies.

If the masker is a band of noise, that band of noise has an envelope to it. (Figure 33–5). The content of the noise may be high frequency, but if the amplitude in general

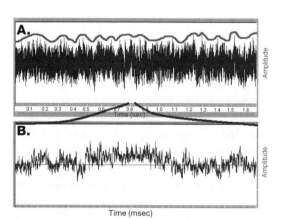

Figure 33–5. A. Illustration that a band of noise can have a temporal envelope (highlight above the time waveform in the upper part of the figure). **B.** A small segment of the noise is shown, illustrating that the content of the noise is high frequency. Remote masking occurs when this high-frequency noise masks a low-frequency tone, a phenomenon that cannot be explained based on basilar membrane mechanics.

fluctuates, then the neural response, which increases and decreases, may mask the audibility of the low-frequency neural response.

Whatever mechanisms are responsible for remote masking, the phenomenon is another illustration that masking is more than just a result of waves on basilar membrane. Masking may be partially a central phenomenon.

SUMMARY AND SOME FURTHER ANALYSIS

In the previous chapter we saw how much of the masking phenomenon is explained by understanding the spread of excitation of the traveling wave on basilar membrane. This chapter focused on the range of frequencies that mask a probe, and how that range changes with frequency. Fletcher's critical ratio theory hypothesized that we could determine the range of frequencies mathematically once we knew how loud a white noise needed to be to mask a given pure tone. His theory held that the pure-tone probe was masked when the energy in the surrounding critical range of frequencies summed to the level of the pure tone. When later experimentation permitted varying the noise band frequency range, Fletcher's assumption was found to be slightly wrong. A wider band of noise is actually responsible for masking the pure tone than Fletcher assumed. The wider band's individual levels per cycle sum to a greater level than the SPL of the probe tone, so Fletcher's assumption didn't hold, but his general theory did: there is a range of frequencies near the pure tone that masks the pure tone. The measured critical band is just wider than Fletcher's theoretical critical ratio.

It's convenient to think that there is a set region on basilar membrane that con-tributes to masking of the probe and that there is no effect once that region is widened. The truth is that the closer the noise component is to the frequency of the probe, the more that noise component contributes to the masking of the tone. The importance gradually drops off as the frequency of the noise component becomes further and further from the probe frequency. Nonetheless, we can set arbitrary limits on the frequency ranges that are important for masking. Equivalent rectangular bandwidths (ERBs) are just such limits. So are critical bands—the two are obtained using different experimental techniques.

Masking studies show that there are more frequencies within a critical band, critical ratio, or ERB when the center of that band is in the high frequencies. Similarly, we had seen in Chapter 31 that the difference limen for frequency is higher in the high frequencies. This provides evidence that the ear may be using different mechanisms for pitch encoding and masking depending on frequency.

REFERENCES

Fletcher, H. (1940). Auditory patterns. *Review of Modern Physics, 12,* 47–65.

Hawkins, J. E., & Stevens, S. S. (1950). The masking of pure tones and of speech by white noise. *Journal of the Acoustical Society of America, 22,* 6–13.

Wegel, R. L., & Lane, C. E. (1924). The auditory masking of one pure tone by another and its probable relation to the dynamics of the inner ear. *Physics Review, 23,* 266–285.

Zwicker, E., Flottorp, G., & Stevens, S. S. (1957). Critical bandwidth in loudness summation. *Journal of the Acoustical Society of America, 29,* 548–557.

34

Psychophysical Tuning Curves

This chapter returns to the masking of pure tones by narrow-band noise. Figures that show how different levels and frequencies of noise mask a given pure tone probe are called psychophysical tuning curves. This chapter's goal is to show how the psychophysical tuning curve relates to the neural tuning curve, and explain how both are consistent with the traveling wave theory.

PSYCHOPHYSICAL TUNING CURVES (PTCS)

How PTCs Are Obtained and Interpreted

In an experiment to obtain a **psychophysical tuning curve (PTC)**, a pure tone signal is used as the probe. The shorthand F_p, would mean frequency of the probe and L_p, the level of the probe. To obtain a PTC, the probe stays constant at that F_p and L_p. Narrow-band noises at different center frequencies are used to mask the probe. The frequency of the masker (F_m) varies systematically during the experiment. The level of the masker noise (L_m) that just masks the probe is noted. Figure 34–1 shows an idealized hypothetical curve. In actuality, there might be 20 or more separate frequencies of masker used, and the results would

be connected with a smooth line. Here those actual data are omitted and just the outline of the curve is shown. In a PTC figure, the axes show both the masker and probe intensity and frequency. In reading Figure 34–1, you can see from the location of the dot that the probe is a

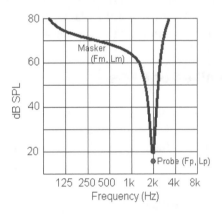

Figure 34–1. Example psychophysical tuning curve. The dot tells the frequency of the probe (F_p) and the level of the probe (L_p). The solid line shows the combinations of narrow-band masking noise frequency (F_m) and levels (L_m) that would prevent the probe from being audible. This figure illustrates that, as the masker frequency becomes lower than the probe, the intensity of the masker increases. Narrow-band maskers with center frequencies significantly above the probe frequency are not effective maskers.

2000-Hz pure tone, at 15 dB SPL. It looks like about 19 dB SPL of 2000-Hz masker noise is required to mask that probe. When the masker frequency is centered at 1500 Hz, the masker has to be about 55 dB SPL to mask that same 15 dB SPL, 2000-Hz pure tone. A 250-Hz, 71 dB SPL masker noise can also mask the probe. Maskers with center frequencies higher than the probe are not effective maskers, as we discussed in Chapter 32.

Correlation to Traveling Wave Locations

Figure 34–2 shows how this finding is consistent with what we know about the traveling wave on basilar membrane. Maskers close in frequency need not be very intense to mask the probe. More intense maskers that are lower in frequency and peak farther up basilar membrane toward the apex can mask the probe; maskers that peak toward the base never reach the place of excitation of the probe and can't create masking.

Families of PTCs

Figure 34–3 illustrates what a series, or family, of psychophysical tuning curves might look like. The probe intensities vary

slightly as might happen if the experimenter wants all the probes to be the same sensation level. (Recall that hearing threshold in dB SPL varies across frequency.) The tuning curves for lower frequencies are wider than those for the high frequencies.

Tips, Tails and Q_{10}s

The narrow portion of the tuning curve is its tip, which points toward the probe tone frequency (Figure 34–4). To describe how narrow or wide the tip is, you can examine the PTC's Q_{10dB}. Find the point of the tip and go up 10 dB. Draw a horizontal line

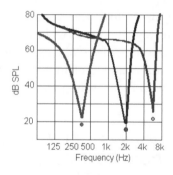

Figure 34–3. Family of psychophysical tuning curves, illustrating that the PTC curves are wider in the low frequencies.

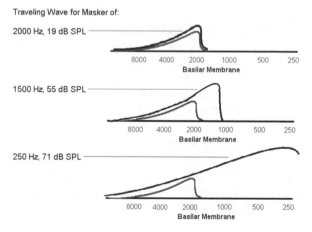

Figure 34–2. Illustration of how different frequency maskers (*annotated, darker, more ragged lines*) would prevent encoding of the traveling wave from the 2000-Hz probe tone (*lighter curve*). Hypothetical characteristic frequency locations along basilar membrane are noted. The more toward the apex the traveling wave peaks, the louder the masker needed to mask the 2000-Hz probe.

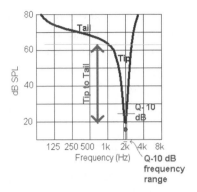

Figure 34–4. Tuning curves can be described by the shape of the tip and the shape of the tail. The width of the tip 10 dB above the curve's tip point is used to calculate the Q_{10dB}. The tip-to-tail range can also be used to describe the PTC.

at this intensity, and find the frequencies that intersect the line. The probe tone frequency divided by the range of frequencies that Q_{10} line intersected gives you the Q_{10dB} of the psychophysical tuning curve.

The tail of the tuning curve is the region on the left (low-frequency) side. It illustrates the masking ability of intense low-frequency stimuli—that is, it shows upward spread of masking. Sometimes the tip to tail intensity is reported.

NEURAL TUNING CURVES REVISITED

One hopes that reading this elicits a feeling of déjà vu, if not an outright recollection that neural tuning curves are very similar. Chapter 21 may warrant review. Recall that a neural tuning curve shows what combinations of frequency and intensity cause one single neuron to fire above its spontaneous firing rate (Figures 21-10 through 21-12). Which stimuli cause the neural firing, as shown by the neural tuning curve, is directly related to the amplitude of the traveling waves on basilar membrane (Figure 21-9).

THE LINK BETWEEN PTCS AND NEURAL TUNING CURVES

PTCs tell us what masker frequency/intensity combinations mask a probe tone. Masking of that pure tone occurs if the traveling wave of the masker "swamps" the traveling wave for the probe.

Neural tuning curves tell us what pure tone frequency/intensity combinations cause a neuron, located at one location of basilar membrane, to fire above its spontaneous rate. That increase in firing rate occurs if the traveling wave of the stimulus vibrates basilar membrane at the location of that neuron.

PTCs and neural tuning curves both tell us about the traveling wave. The asymmetry of the curves—the sharp rise of the curve as frequency is exceeded—agrees with what we know about the shape of the traveling wave, which grows gradually to its maximum, then rapidly falls.

SUMMARY AND A CONFESSION

Neural tuning curves have a direct psychophysical equivalent—the psychophysical tuning curve. Both provide evidence that the traveling wave grows in amplitude gradually as it reaches the place where the membrane will vibrate best for that frequency. Because basilar membrane grows more massive as it courses apically, a given pure tone cannot vibrate basilar membrane well at a location that is more apical than the place where vibration peaks. The steep slope on the high-frequency side of these tuning curves illustrates this.

This chapter has conveniently neglected to mention one fact. Tuning curves obtained using a simultaneous masking paradigm—where the probe and masker are presented contemporaneously—actually are broader than illustrated, and not entirely in agreement with the neural tuning curve.

Chapter 36 will touch on this and show that a properly conducted experiment where the masker and tone are separated a bit in time does reveal the marvels of the traveling wave, and agrees with data obtained from animal neural tuning curve experiments.

35

Temporal Processing

Temporal processing studies investigate how humans use time information that is present in the acoustic signal. One aspect of temporal processing is how the auditory system takes advantage of longer duration signals (temporal integration), a concept previously introduced when we examined how threshold and pitch perception change as the signal duration is lengthened. This chapter revisits these issues.

We can also study the ability of the ear to use very fine details of the auditory signal. We have already examined that issue in studying pitch perception when we noted how small a change in a pure tone's period is detectable. Studies of difference limen for frequency (DL_F) showed the remarkable time-processing ability of the ear. For example, a 2000-Hz tone can be differentiated from a 2004-Hz tone. The neural interspike interval difference between the two is 0.001 msec—a remarkably small difference in time.

Having already studied the ear's ability to make use of fine changes in the signal, this chapter describes how the ear responds to general changes in the overall envelope of waves—how waveform fluctuations are perceived when the signal is amplitude modulated or turned on and off. Temporal integration issues are reviewed first.

REVIEW OF TEMPORAL INTEGRATION FOR THRESHOLD-LEVEL STIMULI

As discussed in Chapter 29, the ear can detect brief stimuli, but the threshold increases (worsens) when the total duration shortens. For example, a pure tone of 16-msec duration had a threshold that was elevated by about 10 dB. As the signal lengthens to about 200 to 250 msec, further increase in duration doesn't improve threshold.

This **temporal integration** indicated that having multiple neural impulses created in response to successive cycles of a pure tone aids in signal detection. The brain integrates the signal over time; that is, it uses successive parts of the neural signal, from successive action potentials, in detecting the presence of the signal.

REVIEW OF DURATION EFFECTS ON PITCH PERCEPTION

Just as a given duration of time is required to have a low threshold, full pitch perception requires that the signal not be too brief. Chapter 31 mentioned that very brief signals (even if it is a part of a pure tone) are actually wide-band stimuli, and sound like clicks. Perceiving tonality requires several cycles of the tone to be present. Low-frequency pure tones aren't perceived as tonal until there are 3 to 4 cycles of the wave, and at least 12-msec duration was needed for mid- to high-frequency tonality to develop. Full tonality developed over the same period of time as the temporal integration phenomenon—about 200 or 250 msec.

The ear uses the interspike interval of firing of different nerves in the bundle to encode period, and thus permit pitch perception. The central nervous system needs to have a long enough duration tone to use that interspike interval effectively—firing of a nerve just once or twice would not fully encode periodicity, even though the location of the neuron that fires provides some information on pitch.

Duration effects and temporal integration reflects neural function; however, other temporal processing aspects also give insight into the function of the cochlea, as discussed below.

GAP DETECTION

Gap Detection Ability Is a Function of Frequency

A gap detection task asks the listener to determine if an ongoing sound has a silent interval in it. Gap detection ability depends on the frequency content of the signal—the ear is better at detecting gaps in high-frequency signals than in low-frequency signals. Figure 35–1 illustrates.

Gap Detection Ability Is Related to the Auditory Filter Bandwidth

You may have expected this next finding, given what you know about the ear's ability to detect pitch, and thus timing, dif-

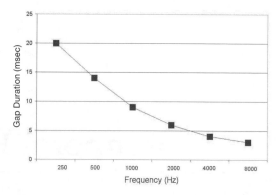

Figure 35–1. Illustration of gap detection ability for band-pass noise stimuli. (Data adapted from Shailer & Moore, 1983.)

ferences. We can detect smaller time changes for high-frequency signals, so it makes sense we can detect smaller gaps as well. The reason for experiencing the better gap detection in the high frequencies is related to the characteristics of the "auditory filter," that is, gap detection ability is related to the psychophysical tuning curve or equivalent rectangular bandwidth characteristics of low- versus high-frequency areas of basilar membrane. First though, let's examine a couple of real-world "filters."

When you strike an object suddenly, it will (if it doesn't break!) resonate. Take, for instance, a partially filled wine glass. If you tap it with your fingernail, the wine glass produces a musical note that dies off slowly—that is, the glass has a lot of "ring" to it. If you were to give the same fingernail tap to a partially filled soda can, a dull thud is heard, and that sound dies off quickly. Figure 35–2A shows the time waveforms of the soda can thud and then the wine glass ping. Note how short duration the thud is relative to the wine glass ping. Figures 35–2B and C show the spectrum of each; notice that the thud (*B*) is wide-band, and the ring (*C*) is narrow-band. A physical principle is that objects with narrow resonant peaks will ring longer.

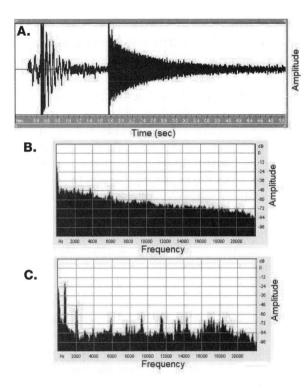

Figure 35–2. A. Time waveforms of the sound produced when a soda can is thumped with a fingernail and then the waveform resulting when a wineglass is thumped. **B.** The spectrum of the soda can sound is wide-band. **C.** The wineglass produces a complex series of tones, but has its primary energy in a narrow frequency range. The bandwidth of the wineglass sound is narrow in comparison to the soda can. Objects with narrow bandwidths will have pronounced ringing. (The very lowest frequency energy is room noise.)

A potentially confusing point is that the wine glass ping tends to be a higher pitch sound—the fundamental frequency in this example is about 700 Hz. The principle is *NOT* specific to high frequencies. A large metal bell struck to produce a low-pitch "bong" sound would also ring for a long time—it, too, has a narrow bandwidth.

In acoustics, we can test the bandwidth of an electrical filter by sending a brief duration pulse of energy—a click—to that filter. The sound that comes out of the filter is no longer a click—it is a ringing tone whose frequency is centered at the frequency of the filter band. In Figure 35–3, the click (*A*) is sent first to a relatively wide filter, a 3000-Hz center frequency filter that is four-octaves wide (*B*), then to a narrower 3000-Hz filter, one that is two octaves wide (*C*). The overall amplitudes were equalized, and as shown, the narrower filtering created a tone that "rings" longer.

Think back to the masking critical band width in Hz. Recall that a critical band, in

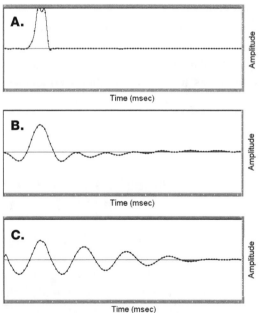

Figure 35–3. The time waveforms of the unfiltered click (**A**) and that same click first filtered by a 4-octave wide filter (**B**), then by a 2-octave wide filter (**C**). Note that the narrower filtering created a longer duration signal—it "rings" more.

Hz, spans a narrow range of frequencies when centered at the lower frequencies. Critical bandwidth increases in the high frequencies. The auditory filter (Figure 33-1) is wider for high frequencies than low frequencies. If a low- and high-frequency auditory filter were each to be "hit" with a brief pulse of energy, the filter—the basilar membrane at that location—would continue to vibrate for a longer time at the apex, because those filters are narrower. Or, said in reverse, the base of the basilar membrane will stop vibrating more quickly than does the apex.

Think, then, of what would happen if a white noise is turned off suddenly, then restarted abruptly 10 msec later, as may happen in a gap detection experiment. The wider tuned base of the cochlea would stop vibrating while the apical area is still in the process of slowly coming to a stop when the gap in the noise ends and the noise comes on again.

This relates to gap detection. In a gap detection task, the signal is turned off briefly. If basilar membrane can come to a stop quickly, as it does for higher frequencies, then the gap can be more easily detected.

Detection of Gaps in White Noise Uses the High-Frequency Cochlear Filters

If presented with a white noise that has a gap in it, typical performance is as good as for listening to high-frequency stimuli. A gap of about 2 msec can be detected if the noise contains energy up to 12 kHz. The theory is that the high-frequency auditory filters are better at gap detection, and those are the filters used to "listen for" the gap. This theory can be tested by adding in a second noise that does not have a gap. That second noise could be a continuous high-pass noise, which prevents the ear from recognizing the white-noise gap using the high-frequency filters. When that high-frequency noise is present, gap detection performance is poorer, as predicted. The ear then uses lower frequency channels to detect the gap, and the gap needs to be longer to be detected.

TEMPORAL SUCCESSIVENESS

What are the limits on detecting differences in the starting time of two signals? Of

Clinical Correlate: Auditory Processing Testing of Gap Detection

Some individuals with normal hearing sensitivity have inordinate difficulty with speech perception. Tests of auditory processing ability explore which auditory processes are affected. There are tests for gap detection that can be used clinically. One example is Musiek et al.'s (2005) *Gaps-in-Noise* test. Where normal hearing and processing individuals can detect a 5-msec gap, those with lesions in the auditory nervous system require more than a 7-msec gap. Cochlear loss would also affect gap detection test performance.

Clinical Correlate: Auditory Processing Testing of Temporal Successiveness

Some clinicians test auditory temporal processing using a form of temporal successiveness testing. Two tones are presented, one low-frequency and one high-frequency, and the patient is asked if the tones came on at the same time or different times. Most normal listeners can detect a couple milliseconds difference in the onsets. If the patient can't detect a 20-msec difference in the onsets, then that is considered abnormal processing of time information. Note that this is a test of temporal successiveness, not discrimination. The patient only has to determine if there were one or two sounds; the patient does not need to determine which came first. Clinical results won't show as good performance as seen in controlled experimental studies, because the patients are not trained in the task, the procedures are less rigorous, and the environment is probably not as free of distraction and noise.

---

course, it depends on the signal, and these experiments are complicated by the distortion of turning tones on quickly. Studies of this sort might use a click signal to get around that problem (although that won't tell us about how frequency might affect perception, as a click is a wide-band signal).

As a generality, the ear can detect 1 to 2-msec difference in the starting time of two clicks. That is—a trained subject can tell the difference between two clicks that are presented 1 to 2 msec apart versus two clicks presented simultaneously.

TEMPORAL DISCRIMINATION

Knowing that there were two stimuli present is not the same as knowing which stimulus came first. For example, if presented with two clicks that differ in intensity, with one presented a couple milliseconds later than the first, you would be able to tell there were two stimuli, but you couldn't reliably determine if the more or less intense click came first. To do that task, or tell if a low- or high-frequency tone burst started first, takes about a 20-msec interstimulus interval.

Temporal Discrimination Relates to Distinguishing Voiced from Unvoiced Consonants

Those who have had a course in acoustic phonetics or read Chapter 9 may recall that consonant sounds can be grouped as "voiced" or "unvoiced." For example, the phoneme /p/ is unvoiced, whereas /b/ is voiced, meaning that the latter sound is created with vocal fold vibration. This can be demonstrated by resting ones fingers on the neck at the larynx (voice box) and saying each sound.

When produced in a syllable (e.g., "pea" and "bee"), a better way to think of the difference is the time between the burst of energy coming from the start of the consonant and the start of the low-frequency energy from the vocal cords vibrating as the vowel begins. Figure 35–4 illustrates that there is a larger gap between the burst and the vowel for "pea" than "bee." To differentiate these words, the listener has to be sensitive to the difference in the time of the burst and the vowel onset. We would expect, then, that grossly abnormal timing detection would relate to speech perception problems. In the case of discriminating voiced and unvoiced sounds in this example, there is about a 25-msec longer pause between the burst and the voicing for the syllable with the unvoiced /p/ sound.

TEMPORAL MODULATION TRANSFER FUNCTIONS

Another class of studies about the ear's ability to use time information are studies of **temporal modulation transfer functions (TMTFs)**. In these studies, the amplitudes of signals are modulated (increased and decreased in amplitude) at different rates. The amount of modulation required to detect the signal as modulating (rather than being a steady tone) is determined. If the rate is very slow, then this is really a difference limen for intensity task. As rate increases, then we are assessing how the ear uses rapidly changing waveform information. As illustrated in Figure 35–5, the faster the rate of modulation, the more (deeper) modulation is required for detection to occur. If the modulation occurs very rapidly, above 1000 times per second (once per millisecond) then the amplitude fluctuation isn't noted at all.

SUMMARY

One can view the time-detection ability of the ear in many ways. In terms of fine changes of the signal—a difference limen for frequency task—the ear is incredibly

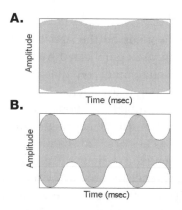

Figure 35–5. Illustration of the temporal modulation transfer function (TMTF) task stimuli. The envelopes of the pure tones are shown. The individual cycles of the waves are spaced too close together to be visualized. In a TMTF task, the stimuli are amplitude modulated at different rates, and the amount of amplitude modulation that is needed for the subject to detect that the tone is modulating, rather than being a steady amplitude, is noted. **A.** When the modulation rate is slow, a small modulation can be detected. **B.** Faster modulation rates require greater modulation depth for detection.

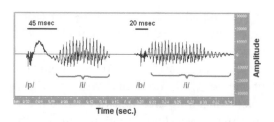

Figure 35–4. The spectral waveform (frequency on the *y*-axis, time on the *x*-axis) for the syllables /pi/ (*pea*) and /bi/ (*bee*). The primary difference between the two words is the time between the burst of energy from the consonant and the vowel's start.

sensitive. The detectably different 2000 and 2004-Hz sine waves have periods that differ only by 0.001 msec.

Fine discrimination of the content of signals is different from examining how the overall envelope of the waveform is analyzed. Temporal modulation transfer functions show that the ear is unable to differentiate amplitude fluctuations in the waveform envelope that occur more rapidly than about once per millisecond. Similarly, the ear can't detect signal onset differences that are less than a millisecond apart.

Gap detection ability depends on the frequency of the stimulus. Under the best circumstances, gaps of about 2 msec can be detected. Gap detection is best if the signal has high-frequency energy, because the auditory "filters" are wider in the high frequencies. Wide filters are associated with less

"ringing"—the filter dies down quickly. Neurons at the apex of the cochlea would continue to fire for a longer period of time after the signal stops because basilar membrane continues to vibrate for a longer time, which relates to the narrow filter bandwidth.

REFERENCES

Musiek, F., Shinn, J. B., Jirsa, R., Bamiou, D. E., Baran, J. A., & Zaidan, E. (2005). GIN (Gap-in-Noise) test performance in subjects with confirmed central auditory nervous system involvement. *Ear and Hearing, 26,* 608-618.

Shailer, M. J., & Moore, B. C. J. (1983). Gap detection as a function of frequency, bandwidth, and level. *Journal of the Acoustical Society of America, 74,* 467-473.

36

Temporal Masking

Forward and backward masking occur when there is a brief silent time between the presentation of masker and signal (forward masking) or between signal and masker (backward masking). Forward and backward masking may also be called **temporal masking** or **nonsimultaneous masking**. In both these cases, the presence of one sound alters perception of another. This brief chapter discusses the phenomenon of temporal masking.

FORWARD MASKING—MASKER PRECEDES PROBE SIGNAL

Magnitude of the Effect

In forward masking, a masker, usually a noise, is presented briefly. After the noise is turned off, the probe tone is presented. The presence of the noise that precedes the probe tone elevates the threshold for the probe signal. The amount of elevation depends on just how brief the silent interval is between noise and probe. The exact results depend on the stimulus and noise characteristics; here data using a click as the probe and white noise as masker are discussed. If the delay is just a millisecond or so, it is possible to have up to 40 dB of threshold elevation. With 50 msec of separation, the mask-

ing effect is down to 10 dB, and by 200 to 250 msec, there is no effect.

Physiologic Explanations

How is it that a noise heard previously can affect threshold for a probe that occurs later? Just because the noise has stopped does not mean that the basilar membrane has ceased vibration. If the vibration continues—if the cochlea is still ringing (moving)—then it is harder to encode a low-intensity sound that comes afterward. The efferent system may also play a role. If the masker is relatively intense, a suppression of cochlear sensitivity may result, and may remain briefly even after the loud signal is turned off.

Forward Masking Psychophysical Tuning Curves Are Sharper

If a psychophysical tuning curve is obtained using a forward-masking paradigm, the tuning curve is sharper than if tested using a simultaneous masking paradigm. The forward masking results agree more closely to those from neural tuning curves. Discussion of the cause of the phenomenon is outside the intended scope of this book. The reader should be aware, though, that this is the preferred method of obtaining psychophysical tuning curves.

BACKWARD MASKING—MASKER FOLLOWS PROBE SIGNAL

Magnitude of the Effect

Backward masking may be simply confusion by the listener as to the task, rather than a physiologic phenomenon. The more you train the listener, the less the effect. In backward masking, the presence of a masker just a few milliseconds after the probe blocks probe perception. Backward masking is present to a meaningful degree only if the probe to noise silent interval is less than about 20 msec. The size of the effect varies with experiments, but it can be quite sizable—up to 40 dB—if the interstimulus interval is very short.

Physiologic Explanation

Those who have theorized that backward masking is a real effect speculate that the perception of the less intense probe is blocked by the following louder signal, which "overruns" the weaker signal. As neural conduction times are not vastly different dependent on stimulus intensity, this theory has some weakness.

SUMMARY

Masking occurs not just when the masker and probe are present at the same time—it can occur with time separation. The most widely discussed effect is forward masking—where the noise occurs before the probe tone. This technique is often used when obtaining psychophysical tuning curves.

37

Binaural Hearing

There are a number of listening situations in which the two ears perform in a manner different from how each would perform alone. In this chapter we look at some of the effects of listening with two ears simultaneously. As discussed in Chapter 29, threshold is better binaurally. Also, the just noticeable difference for intensity and frequency are lower if using both ears.

This chapter also examines how we **localize** (find the origin of sound in the world around us) and **lateralize** (determine if sound from headphones is in one ear or the other, or somewhere inside our head). Finally, masking level differences are introduced, which is a phenomenon where hearing the signal and the noise somewhat differently in the two ears enhances hearing and understanding. It relates to the cocktail party effect. If listening in a situation with considerable background noise, try closing one ear. You probably will understand less of what is said. You can improve your ability to understand the speaker by turning your head this way and that, creating differences in the signal and noise at the two ears. This chapter introduces this phenomenon.

BINAURAL SUMMATION

When a sound is presented to the two ears simultaneously there is a summation of the acoustic energy reaching the two ears. This **binaural summation** probably occurs in the brainstem and is reflected in binaural thresholds for pure tones and complex stimuli being lower (better hearing) than monaural thresholds. This summation is also evident in loudness perception. As discussed in Chapter 29, the average binaural threshold is 2 dB better and the equated binaural threshold is 3 dB lower. A suprathreshold monaural tone must be 3 dB to 6 dB more intense to be judged equally loud to a binaural tone of the same frequency. There is about a 3 dB difference at threshold and at low sensation levels, increasing to about 6 dB at high sensation levels.

IMPROVED DL_I AND DL_F ABILITY BINAURALLY

The binaural advantage extends beyond thresholds of audibility. Both DL_I and DL_F measures are more sensitive when testing is conducted binaurally. Although it's possible some of the advantage is just because the signals are louder binaurally, the effect is much larger than attributable to a 3 to 6 dB signal intensity increase. For example, the difference limen for intensity (expressed as a Weber fraction of $\Delta I / I$), is about half the size binaurally.

Clinical Correlate: Monaural Versus Binaural Amplification

If a person is fit with two hearing aids, that person needs less amplification in each ear. Not all hearing aid fitting systems take this into account, and the audiologist must remember to lower the overall amplification (gain) of the hearing aids when fitting two aids.

The reader who remembers the phenomenon of recruitment might see a potential disadvantage to binaural summation. Do we want moderate- to high-intensity sounds to be louder for a person with cochlear loss, who may have normal perception of loud sounds? Actually, it's not a disadvantage after all. David Hawkins and his colleagues (1987) have shown that loud sounds, although perceived as louder binaurally, are also better tolerated when presented binaurally. In essence, they are less obnoxious when heard binaurally.

BINAURAL BEATS

Chapter 31 on pitch perception described how two tones of similar frequency, presented together, are perceived as one sound that pulses (beats) on and off. A related phenomenon is that of **binaural beats**. If a 1000-Hz tone is presented to the left ear, and a 1004-Hz tone is presented to the right ear, the listener hears a tone of about 1002 Hz that pulses off and on four times per second. This illustrates that the central nervous system is combining information from the two ears.

CENTRAL MASKING

Another illustration of the integration of information from the two ears is the **central masking effect**. Noise put into one ear elevates the threshold of the other ear. The effect is not large; it is about 5 dB (though it varies with the intensity of the masker). Unlike monaural masking, it is not a linear phenomenon. Recall that when you increase a monaural masker intensity by 10 dB, you obtain a 10 dB threshold shift. Increasing the contralateral ear's masking level creates a slight elevation in threshold, but it is not the 1:1 increase seen with monaural masking.

BINAURAL FUSION

In everyday listening, the sounds reaching the two ears are similar, but not quite identical. Yet, we typically hear one sound, not two. This phenomenon, one sound heard from two separate ears, is called **binaural fusion**. An example of binaural fusion is a person listening to music under earphones. Even though the music may be slightly different at the two ears, the listener hears it as a unified or fused sound; not as something in the right ear and something else in the left. If the music is equally loud in the two ears, the fused image appears to be in the center of the head.

LOCALIZATION

The term **localization** refers to the process of locating the source or direction of a sound in space. **Lateralization** is the term used for study of perception under earphones. Our ability to localize and lateralize depends on a complex interaction of temporal (time) and intensity cues.

The signal's **azimuth**, that is, the angle at which it arrives, relates to how the listener localizes the sound. As Figure 37–1 shows, sound that is directly in front of the listener originates from 0-degrees azimuth. The azimuth is described in portion of the 360-degree circle around the listener.

Temporal Cues to Localization

There are two aspects of temporal or time phenomena that play a part in localization. First, there is the actual difference in the time of arrival of a sound at the two ears. A particular sound traveling through space will reach one ear before it reaches the other ear, except in those cases where the two ears are the same distance from the sound sources. This latter condition occurs when the sound source is in the median plane; that is, an imaginary plane that proceeds

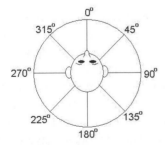

Figure 37–1. Azimuth, the location of the sound source, is expressed in degrees, in the horizontal plane, circling to the listener's right.

from directly in front to directly overhead to directly behind to directly underneath to back in front of the listener. The time of arrival at the two ears is not dependant on the nature of the sound as neither frequency nor intensity affects the speed of sound.

A sound arriving from 90-degrees azimuth travels the distance between ears in about 0.66 milliseconds. That is then the maximum difference in arrival time. A sound from 45-degrees azimuth arrives 0.36 msec earlier at the nearer ear, and one at 30-degrees comes in 0.25 msec earlier.

A second aspect of the temporal phenomena is related to phase difference at the two ears. Because the sounds not originating in the median plane will arrive at the two ears at different times, they also arrive out of phase. It is actually the phase difference at the ears, rather than the time of arrival, that appears to be the relevant signal feature for localization.

The phase difference between ears depends on the distance between the two ears at the sound's azimuth and the period of the sound. For example, a 250-Hz pure tone has a period of 4 msec. The sound travels at about 1100 feet per second. If the sound source was at 30-degrees azimuth, it arrives about 0.25 msec earlier at the right ear; 0.25 msec is one-eighth of 4 msec (that is, the wave is 45-degrees out of phase at the two ears [$1/8 \times 360^0 = 45^0$]).

Only low-frequency sounds (where one-half the distance of the wavelength is longer than the interaural distance) provide unambiguous phase cues. This is because when there is a phase difference of 180 degrees or more, there is a problem in telling which ear is leading and which is lagging. Furthermore, 360 degrees of phase shift puts the signal back in phase and is identical to zero degrees of difference. Could you use a concrete example of that? Let's take a 4000-Hz tone, with its 0.25-msec period. If the sound comes from 30-degrees azimuth, it reaches the right ear 0.25 msec earlier than the left ear. Because the period of the wave is 0.25 msec, both ears receive the sound wave at the same phase. The phase difference is not meaningful for high-frequency sounds, but is the cue for low-frequency sound localization. Figure 37–2A further illustrates. Low-frequency sounds, with their long wavelengths, arrive at the two ears at different phases. In Figure 37–2B we see that if the sound has a wavelength shorter than the diameter of the head, the phase can be the same as it reaches both ears. The phase information would not be helpful. The cutoff point for when the phase information is no longer helpful is about 1500 Hz.

Intensity Differences

Intensity differences at the two ears are due largely to head shadow, which occurs only for high-frequency sounds. Low-frequency sound waves, with wavelengths longer than the width of the head, tend to wrap around the head and reach the "far" ear without much reduction in intensity. Frequencies whose wavelengths are shorter than the width of the head do not to wrap and a "shadow" effect results. Figure 37–2C illustrates this effect. Thus, higher frequencies will have less intensity at the ear opposite the sound source. This difference can be 10 to 20 dB. In addition, the pinna may produce a small shadow effect for high frequencies originating behind the head.

Combined Effect of Intensity and Phase Differences

We tend to perceive sound as coming from the direction of the ear in which the sounds are louder and the ear which the sound reaches first, either thought of as the initial time of arrival or the phase relation-

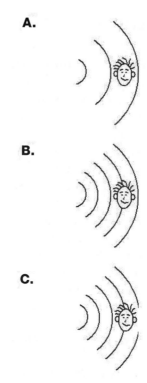

Figure 37–2. Sound wave compression phases are illustrated with semicircles. **A.** A low-frequency sound arrives at different phases at the two ears. **B.** A high-frequency sound could have signals that are in phase at the two ears, which would not give a cue for localization. **C.** The head shadow will reduce the intensity of the sound at the opposite ear. This occurs for high-frequency sounds, creating a difference in intensity of the sound at each ear, which provides a cue for localization.

ship. Phase differences are most important in the low frequencies where the wavelength is longer than the width of the head. Intensity differences play a more important role for higher frequencies where the head shadow in more pronounced. Our localization ability appears worst at about 3000 Hz where the cues related to phase have dropped off and the cues related to intensity have not become fully effective.

One way to think of localization ability is to determine the average error in sound localization. For example, a blindfolded listener could point to the perceived position of a sound speaker that rotates around him or her. The listener will generally have an average **localization error** of at least 10 degrees. At around 3000 Hz, the error rate reaches 25 degrees. It improves for the very highest frequencies, approaching 10 degrees average error by 10,000 Hz.

Another way to gauge a listener's ability to localize is to find that listener's **minimum audible angle**, that is, the smallest change in sound azimuth that is detectable. Both the sound source azimuth and the sound frequency affect the results. We do best with low-frequency (below 1500 Hz) sounds that are located directly in front and worse when the sounds are to the side.

Central Nervous System Cells Are Responsive to Phase or Intensity Differences

There are cells in the brainstem that receive input from each ear. Some of those cells are excited when the phase of signals is *different* by a given amount at the two ears. These cells would be ones that tell the nervous system about sound localization using phase differences at the two ears. These cells have low characteristic frequencies. There are other cells, with high characteristic frequency, which only respond at given intensity differences between the two ears, and obviously those too help to encode localization information.

LATERALIZATION

Lateralization is a term used to discuss the perceived lateral position of a fused sound within the head. It is experienced only when listening under earphones. When two sounds of identical frequency, loudness, and phase are introduced to the two ears simultaneously, the listener perceives the sound as being in the middle of the head. The same parameters that affect localization (i.e., intensity and time of arrival/phase) are responsible for whether the sound lateralizes to one ear, the other ear, or is somewhere in between. Next time you are listening to a stereo under headphones, give this a try. Adjust the left/right loudness balance, and you will experience the shift in lateralization from one ear to the other. That demonstrates the intensity difference effect, but as with localization, the time of arrival can also alter the perception of the location of the sound.

Interaural Time Difference

While listening under earphones, if we start with the condition that produced a midline lateralization and successively delayed the time of arrival of the sound to one ear, we find that the sound begins to move from midline toward the "leading" ear. Time differences as small as 10 μsec create a shift in the perceived location of the sound. If we continue to increase the time difference, the sound will continue to move until it is lateralized to the leading ear.

Interaural Intensity Differences

Interaural intensity differences also produce a change in the apparent lateral position of the sound image. It only takes about 1 dB difference to produce a detectable movement from midline. As with time difference, however, the larger the intensity difference, the greater the degree of laterality, and when the intensity difference becomes sufficiently large (about 10 dB or less depending on the stimulus) the signal is perceived only in the louder ear. This per-

> **Clinical Correlate: Stenger Test for Nonorganic Unilateral Hearing Loss**
>
> Persons feigning a hearing loss (presenting with nonorganic hearing impairment) often decide to report the loss as being only in one ear. The patient may feel this is easier to simulate, and less likely to be detected than if bilateral loss is reported. (With bilateral loss, the feigning patient may be tripped up into accidentally hearing something and be discovered.) These malingering patients aren't able to beat the Stenger test, however. Simultaneously, a soft sound is put into the ear that is reported as normal, and a loud sound that is below the admitted threshold is put into the "bad" ear. The perception is that the sound is just in the "bad" ear, because it is so much louder in that ear. The patient won't admit to hearing the tone in the "bad" ear and fails to respond to the bilaterally presented tones. The patient cannot detect the tone in the "good" ear. The patient's failure to respond actually indicates that the louder sound was heard! (If there had been a true hearing loss, the sound presented to the "good" ear would have been detected and the patient would respond to it.)

ception of the sound in the ear in which it is louder without any awareness that it is also being presented to the ear where it is softer is sometimes referred to as the **Stenger effect**.

Combined Effects of Intensity and Phase

As lateralization occurs only when listening under earphones, it is possible to vary the time and intensity functions independently. That is, one could simultaneously increase the loudness to the right ear while leading the stimulus to the left ear. This, of course, would result in contradictory information being sent to the brain and the effects are that the two would offset each other to some degree. However, the tradeoff is not a simple predictable phenomenon and it holds for only a small range of times and intensities.

Why Is Lateralization a Different Phenomenon from Localization?

Sounds presented via headphones merge in the head; sounds heard in sound field are perceived as "out there." Why the difference? The acoustics of the head and head movement. If you make careful measurement of how the subject's head and pinna accentuate and attenuate sound from different angles, and process the sound delivered to the two ears by headphone to mimic these sound changes, you can create a recording that sounds "out there" rather than "in your head."

In listening to sounds in sound field, one thing we all do naturally is move our heads a bit. This changes the spectrum of the sound from ear to ear, and allows better localization. While the first author of this text was a postdoctoral student circa 1987, psychoacoustician Frederick Wightman, who worked in a nearby lab, related the results of this little experiment.

An anatomic manikin (Knowles Electronic Manikin for Acoustic Research, KEMAR) was used to pick up sounds at the dummy's "eardrums." When the manikin was "seated" on a desk, the listener hearing the sounds presented in sound field to the dummy perceived the sounds as inside his or her head. The manikin was then mounted atop the listener's head, and the listener was instructed to hold still. Even though there was no visible movement of the dummy, the listener then heard the sounds as at their proper location in the sound field. The small head movements made unconsciously created the difference.

MASKING LEVEL DIFFERENCES

Hearing in noise has long been an area of interest. Pilots in the World Wars faced this problem acutely when they attempted to listen to commands over their airplanes headphones with the high-level engine noise in the background. The earphones used were TDH style, the same used in audiometry (see Figure 8–2D). These earphones are not very effective at excluding ambient noise. Licklider (1948) made an interesting discovery about hearing in noise: changing the phase of the speech signal in one earphone improved listening. This had application for our pilots. If one of the earphones was hooked up "wrong," so that the negative lead was connected to the positive lead, and

vice versa, causing the signal to be reversed in phase 180 degrees, then the pilots heard better in noise. This is the principle behind **masking level differences**, or "release from masking" when the signal and noise differ between ears. That is, there are conditions that allow better hearing than having both the signal and the noise arrive at the same phase and same intensity at each ear.

Shorthand has been used to describe the ways we can manipulate the signal and the noise. S stands for signal, and N refers to the noise. Subscripts follow to describe the signal and noise conditions. The letter m means that the stimulus is monaural, "o" indicates it is present binaurally but at the same phase. The symbol for pi, π, means the stimulus is present binaurally but differs in phase between ears by 180 degrees. The noise signals can also be generated separately though they are of the same type (e.g., both ears hearing white noise) in which case the symbol would be N_u, for uncorrelated noise. The noise could be the same in each ear, but time delayed to create a phase shift, which is noted as N_t.

The standard or reference condition is S_oN_o—identical binaural signal and binaural noise. The amount of advantage to the different conditions is termed the amount of release from masking. There is no release from masking for S_mN_m. Table 37–1 shows the amount of release from masking in the other conditions.

Table 37–1. The Different Masking Level Difference Test Conditions and the Approximate Amount of Threshold Improvement from Either the S_oN_o or S_mN_m Conditions

Condition	Amount of Release from Masking
S_oN_t	3-10 dB, depending on time delay
S_mN_o	9 dB
S_oN_π	13 dB
$S_\pi N_o$	15 dB

> ## Clinical Correlate: Binaural Advantage to Hearing Aids
>
> The single greatest complaint of hearing-impaired patients is difficulty understanding speech in noise. If the patient has a normal central nervous system, and has bilateral hearing loss, the patient will be expected to function better with two hearing aids. Those who use just one hearing aid will not have the masking level difference advantage working for them.

Release from masking studies can be conducted with pure tone signals, and also with speech signals. You can find a speech threshold advantage, or you could note how much the percent correct identification of the speech material improves in these noise conditions. The latter case relates to the **cocktail party effect**. Next time you are in an adverse noise event, where you want to understand a speaker in noise, notice that you will tend to angle your head this way and that. You are unconsciously trying to create a difference in the relative signal and noise between ears. Cocking the head to hear the speaker more from the right ear than the left, for example, is an S_mN_o condition. Listening has just become easier.

Masking level difference studies show that the brainstem is appropriately integrating sound, and indicates function of the lower brainstem, at the level of the superior olivary complex and above.

SUMMARY

Humans are designed to use information from two ears. Our hearing sensitivity is better; our tolerance for loud sound is equal or better. Our ability to detect difference in signal intensity and frequency is better. Having two ears allows us to localize sound, generally with only a 10 to 15-degree error. Most importantly, two ears working together lets one take advantage of differences in the signal and noise at the two ears, improving ability to hear and understand in background noise, as was shown by masking level difference studies. A healthy brainstem is key to utilizing this information, as there are specialized neural units that react differently to binaural stimulation conditions.

REFERENCES

Hawkins, D. B., Prosek, R. A., Walden, B. E., & Montgomery, R. A. (1987). Binaural loudness summation in the hearing impaired. *Journal of Speech and Hearing Research, 30*(1), 37–43.

Licklider, J. C. R. (1948). The influence of interaural phase relations upon the masking of speech by white noise. *Journal of the Acoustical Society of America, 20*, 150–159.

38

Introduction to Results of Psychoacoustical Assessment of the Hearing-Impaired

One of the most commonly heard complaints of the hearing-impaired is "I can hear, but I can't understand. Words aren't clear." This statement is typically accompanied by the observation "I do OK in quiet, but I can't hear if there is background noise."

This chapter explores some of the reasons for this problem that the hearing-impaired face when the cochlea is damaged. Lack of audibility can be frequency specific, and may impair hearing for some speech sounds more than others. Speech is heard because the typical patient has the ability to detect some sounds of speech with residual hearing, with loss of hearing for speech sounds containing certain frequencies causing problems with speech understanding. However, there is more to explaining why cochlear loss creates problems with speech audibility. This chapter highlights a few of the changes in perception that typify cochlear loss: rapidly increasing loudness once sound reaches an audible level, somewhat poorer ability to analyze frequency information, increased susceptibility to the effects of masking, and variable performance on tests of temporal processing.

Chapter 3 contained some information on understanding audiograms. If you have not had a course in basic audiology, a review of that material (e.g., Figure 3–8) will help in understanding this chapter.

THE EFFECT OF HEARING LOSS ON AUDIBILITY OF TONES AND SPEECH

Effect of Loss Type and Severity

Hearing loss can occur from damage to the outer or middle ear—the parts of the ear that conduct sound into the cochlea—in which case there is a **conductive hearing loss. Cochlear hearing loss** occurs when the inner ear is the site of the damage. Damage to the nerves of hearing, either in the internal auditory canal or in the central nervous system, causes **retrocochlear hearing loss.** When there has not been a thorough determination of whether the site of lesion (location of the damage) is cochlear or retrocochlear, the term used is **sensorineural hearing loss.** Retrocochlear

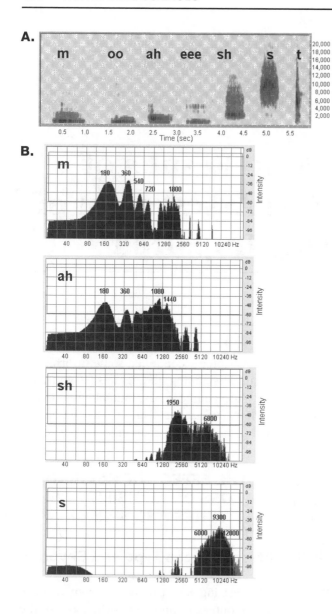

Figure 38–1. A. The spectrogram shows the frequency content (*y*-axis) of select speech sounds. The *x*-axis is time, and intensity is shown by the shading. **B.** Frequency analyses of several of these speech sounds. The major energy regions (in Hz) are identified. If a person had hearing loss below 2000 Hz, the sounds "m" and "ah" would probably not be heard. If a person with high-frequency hearing loss had hearing loss at about 1500 to 2000 Hz and above, the "sh" and "s" sounds would not be heard. The "s" sound shown here is very high frequency with its major energy above 6000 Hz.

loss is relatively rare, so this chapter will not cover the ramifications of this form of damage to the ear.

Conductive loss, such as coming from fluid in the middle ear or a fixation of the stapes in oval window, adds stiffness to the middle ear system. Although there is not much extra mass added when a bony growth fixates the stapes in the oval window, there would be added mass in the case of middle ear infections, accompanied by fluid accumulation. The added stiffness reduces the sound transmission especially for the low frequencies, and the additional mass reduces high-frequency transmission. Conductive loss, therefore, typically has worse hearing in the low frequencies or a fairly flat audiometric shape (equal loss across the frequency range).

Cochlear loss, coming from loss of inner and/or outer hair cells, most commonly creates worse hearing in the high frequencies. That general rule has many exceptions, but discussion of that topic falls within the bounds of a course in diagnostic audiology, rather than hearing science. The fact that cochlear loss severity changes across frequency has important implications. The typical person with cochlear loss is able to hear sounds with low-frequency energy better than sounds such as many of the consonants (e.g., "p" and "s") that contain mostly high-frequency energy.

Loss of Sensitivity for Pure Tones Predicts Loss of Speech Perception Ability

As discussed in Chapter 10, we can analyze the frequency content of various speech sounds to make some inference about how hearing loss will affect audibility. Vowel sounds and nasal consonants like /m/ and /n/, have mostly low-frequency energy. Consonant sounds, especially those that are unvoiced, that is, not produced with vibration of the vocal folds, tend to have mid- to high-frequency energy. Figure 38–1 illustrates the spectra of several speech sounds. The spectrogram (Figure 38-1A) provides an overview of the frequency content of seven select phonemes, but doesn't show much detail. Figure 38-1B shows frequency analysis of some of these speech sounds. The intensity scale in this picture is in arbitrary decibel units, so it only illustrates how intense the sound energy peaks are relative to each other.

If a person had a conductive loss with preserved high-frequency hearing, he or she might be able to hear "sh," "s," and "t," but may have difficulty hearing the "m" and the vowel sounds. Cochlear loss tends to start at the highest frequencies, so this "s" sound would be inaudible if a patient had loss of hearing above 4000 Hz, as the peak energy is from 6000 to 12,000 Hz. The "sh" sound would become indistinct with high-frequency hearing loss above 1500 Hz.

Of course, different speakers produce sounds differently, which affects the speech spectrum. French and Steinberg (1947) were interested in determining the approximate percentage of speech that would be understood with different amounts of hearing loss. They created a calculation called the **articulation index**. Despite the name, which makes one think it has something to do with speech production, this index predicts how well a person would hear speech. The number, which can range from 0 (no speech understood) to 1.0 (100% of speech is understood), was based on knowing what the hearing thresholds are at different frequencies, and determining how much speech is audible. These calculations did not treat all the frequencies as equally important. In general, it is more important to understand consonant sounds than vowel sounds. Speech has about half the information below 1600 Hz and about half above that frequency.

Mueller and Killion (1990) simplified the articulation index calculations using the "count the dot" audiogram. A sample is shown in Figure 38-2. The dots on the audiogram represent the frequencies and intensities important for hearing speech. Note that the dots are spread out both in the frequency range and on the intensity scale. At each frequency, the dots span a range in intensity of about 20 to 30 decibels, indicating that not all speech sounds, even having the same frequency content, are the same loudness. The dots are more densely packed together in the high frequencies because those frequencies are more important to speech understanding. There are 100 dots on the audiogram.

If a person has thresholds at 0 dB HL at all frequencies (or even 10 dB HL thresholds), then all the dots are above threshold, which shows that all the sounds of speech would be heard. If a person had hearing thresholds at 50 dB HL at all frequencies, none of the dots are above threshold, and we would predict

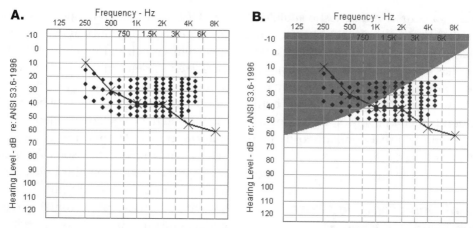

Figure 38–2. The Mueller and Killion (1990) count-the-dot audiograms based on the articulation index. The audiogram shows the thresholds of hearing on the vertical axis for the frequencies shown across the top. Unlike most scientific graphs, the farther down, the louder the sound (see Chapter 3). In (**A**), the left ear's thresholds are shown. They range from 10 dB HL (no hearing loss) at 250 Hz to 60 dB HL (a moderately severe loss) at 8000 Hz. On the audiogram are 100 dots. Counting the audible dots, those that fall below the threshold line, predicts the percentage of words that should be heard. Here about 32 dots are below the line, so the person is expected to understand 32% of the test words. **B.** Background noise is often predominantly low frequency. It may further mask speech perception. As shown, this background noise would predict that audibility is reduced to about 20% when this noise is present. Audiogram generated with AuDSim software, used and reproduced with permission courtesy of www.audstudent.com .

that no speech would be understood. In Figure 38-2A, thresholds of hearing (for a left ear, but let's assume both ears have the same hearing) are shown. There are 32 dots that are above threshold (farther down on the graph), so we would infer that the patient would understand about 32% words if given a test of speech understanding. Background noise, which tends to be low frequency, can further reduce speech understanding by masking speech sounds (Figure 38-2B). This shows that the noise masks additional speech information, and it would be predicted that in the noise, the word understanding score would fall to 20%. In reality, for most with cochlear loss, speech understanding would be even worse than what is predicted. We will return to this point shortly.

Articulation Index Predictions of Speech Understanding Are Imperfect

The articulation index concept is that lack of hearing for speech sounds is what creates the loss of speech understanding. Although this simple concept is unquestionably true, it doesn't tell us the complete story. Two patients with the exact same audiogram, both having cochlear hearing loss, may have different speech understanding abilities. Many factors may contribute to these between-patient differences in speech understanding. Age, and presumably some associated changes in the central nervous system function, should be considered. Surprisingly, intelligence in general is also a small factor. (Perhaps those with higher intelligence are a little better at mentally filling in the missing pieces of information.) Those factors aren't enough to explain all the between-patient differences.

Studies that compare the performance of normal hearers, deprived of auditory information by presenting masking noise, to the performance of the hearing-impaired help to reveal that lack of audibility is not the only issue facing the hearing-impaired. Studies that examine this issue present carefully frequency-adjusted noise to the normal hearer. The noise elevates hearing thresholds. In this way, normal-hearing listeners can have simulated hearing loss. When these studies are conducted, the speech understanding errors made by a normal hearer whose thresholds are elevated by masking noise are different from the speech errors made by those with hearing loss. And, to reiterate, not all hearing impaired with the same audiogram have the same errors either. The nature of the damage, and how it affects the cochlea and the central nervous system, seems to differ between patients. That is, the different pathologies of the ear create varying psychoacoustic profiles, which affects speech understanding.

There are two other ways we can demonstrate that hearing loss is more than just loss of audibility. First, those with conductive loss typically understand speech better than those with cochlear loss. The conductive loss does not create changes to the processing of speech, other than simply attenuating the speech signal. In contrast, cochlear loss creates internal signal distortions and reduced speech understanding, even when the signal is raised in intensity to be made audible. Additionally, we know that hearing aids, which can bring speech into the range of audibility, do not provide for perfect speech understanding. Even though speech is audible, it is not perfectly "clear."

This chapter continues by evaluating how the cochlear processes are changed as a result of cochlear hearing loss.

COCHLEAR LOSS CAUSES RECRUITMENT

Although cochlear loss prevents low-intensity sounds from being detected, once sound is above threshold, loudness quickly increases. For example, a normal hearer might have threshold for a 1000-Hz tone of 10 dB SPL. Perception of this 1000-Hz tone at 50 dB SPL might be that the tone is comfortably loud; at 75 dB SPL, loud but OK; and at 100 dB SPL, loud. A person with cochlear loss may have a threshold of hearing at 50 dB SPL, consider an 80 dB SPL as comfortably loud, and 100 dB SPL as loud. This is known as **recruitment**. Loud sounds are perceived as loud, even though quiet sounds are inaudible.

Another way of thinking about recruitment is to say that it is an abnormally rapid growth of loudness. Recall from Chapter 29 that the sone is the unit of loudness. A 1-sone sound is a 40 dB SPL, 1000-Hz tone, or any other sound that is equal in loudness. A 2-sone sound is twice that loudness. Four sones is four times as loud as one sone, and so forth. For normal hearers, a 10 dB increase is close to a doubling of loudness. We cannot ask a hearing-impaired subject to complete exactly the same task if the 40 dB SPL, 1-kHz tone is inaudible, but we could take our knowledge of loud sounds being loud to the hearing-impaired person and work backward, for example, assuming that the 100 dB SPL, 1-kHz tone is 85 sones, as it is for a normal hearer. The hearing-impaired person could then be asked to determine what sound is half as loud, and so forth. Another way this could be done is to test subjects with unilateral hearing loss. After establishing the sone curve in the normal ear, the subject could then be asked to adjust the intensity of the sound in the impaired ear until it was equal in loudness. That is, the subject would balance loudness back and forth between the two ears, adjusting the intensity of the sound presented to the impaired ear until it is equally loud as the sound in the unimpaired ear. Figure 38–3 shows what these results might look like. The curve of loudness in the impaired ear quickly increases, showing the rapid growth of loudness that is known as the phenomenon of recruitment.

Dynamic range is the difference between the intensity of the loudest sound tolerable and the softest sound that is audible. A normal hearer's dynamic range typically falls between 70 and 100 dB. For example, a threshold of 10 dB HL, and perception that 95

dB HL is uncomfortably loud, provides a dynamic range of 85 dB. Recruitment reduces the dynamic range. Although threshold is elevated (e.g., 50 dB HL), the sound perceived as uncomfortably loud may be equal to what the normal hearer perceived as loud (e.g., 95 dB HL, giving a 45 dB dynamic range).

Recruitment is thought to be related to the loss of the active mechanism of the inner ear, and the presence of some inner hair cells that respond normally with enough stimulation. Recall that the outer hair cell motility increases basilar membrane vibration size when low-intensity sounds are present. If all the outer hair cells in one region of the cochlea are lost, but there is no damage to the inner hair cells, about 50 dB of hearing loss occurs. Once sound is above 50 dB HL, the motion of basilar membrane, even without the active mechanism, is enough to shear the inner hair cell cilia. Further increase in intensity creates more shearing of the cilia, more release of neurotransmitter, and the perception of increased loudness. When sound is very loud, the outer hair cell motility does not boost the movement of basilar membrane.

Equal loudness curves could also be constructed for a hearing-impaired subject, and would also show recruitment. Figure 38–4 illustrates what a phon curve might look like for a patient with normal hearing through 1500 Hz, and a sloping loss above.

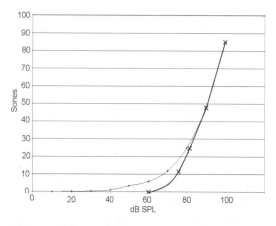

Figure 38–3. Recruitment, which occurs with cochlear loss, is often described as an abnormal growth of loudness. The normal relationship between loudness in sones and 1000-Hz signal intensity is shown with the dots. The X symbols shows the results that might be found if a person with unilateral hearing loss balanced the loudness of the sound in the unimpaired ear (e.g., 70 dB SPL, 12-sone sound) to the sound in the impaired ear (e.g., 77 dB SPL sounds equal in loudness). Loudness quickly grows for cochlear loss patients due to recruitment.

DIFFERENCE LIMENS FOR INTENSITY

Chapter 29 described how normal hearers have smaller **difference limens for intensity** for pure tones as the signal intensity increases. Hearing-impaired people have better sensitivity for detecting changes in intensity if we reference the signal intensity in terms of how close it is to threshold. For example,

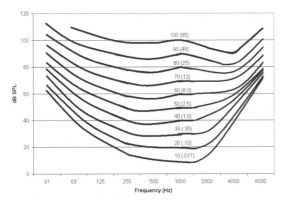

Figure 38–4. Hypothetical phon curves for a subject with cochlear hearing loss above 1500 Hz. The phon level is noted above the curve and the sone level is in parentheses. Thresholds are elevated, and with it the 10-phon curve. Because loudness grows quickly above threshold, the phon curves are more closely spaced in the high frequencies where the hearing loss is most severe.

a person with a 60 dB hearing loss would do better at detecting small intensity increases in a 70 dB HL tone (10 dB above threshold) than the normal hearer does listening to a tone that is 10 dB above threshold. (This was the basis for the Short Increment Sensitivity Index [SISI] test discussed in Chapter 29.) However, if you compare the sensitivity of normal-hearing and hearing-impaired listeners at the same intensity levels in dB SPL or HL, the results are similar. In this example, the normal hearer and hearing-impaired listener would have about the same JND_I for detecting changes to the intensity of the 70 dB HL stimulus.

THRESHOLD TEMPORAL SUMMATION EFFECTS

When stimulus duration is less than about 200 to 250 msec, the normal hearer requires greater intensity to detect the tone. For example, if the threshold for a 1000-Hz, 200-msec tone is 10 dB SPL, if the tone dura-

tion is decreased to 20 msec, threshold might increase to 20 dB SPL. The normal hearer summates the neural signal energy over time, and as a result, threshold improves.

A hypothetical hearing-impaired listener has a threshold for the 200-msec tone at 60 dB SPL. The threshold for the same tone with a duration of 20 msec is 64 dB SPL. (This is an example: there is variability among hearing-impaired in their temporal summation results.) How should these **temporal integration** results be viewed? You can interpret the results as saying that this patient does not take advantage of the increased information available as duration increases. On the other hand, one could say that this hearing-impaired patient is not as handicapped by tone durations that are shortened.

Not all hearing-impaired have altered temporal integration, though that is the general trend. When it is affected, it is most so for the high frequencies.

The phenomenon of reduced temporal integration could be thought of as related to recruitment. The change in perceived loudness when the sound increases from 60 to 64 dB SPL, as processed by an ear with recruitment, may be as large as the loudness change that the normal hearer experienced as the signal went from 10 to 20 dB SPL.

Nonetheless, the repercussion is that if the person with cochlear loss and altered temporal summation is presented with low-intensity, brief-duration signals, the hearing loss doesn't permit detection. Many consonants (e.g., plosives like /p/ or /t/) are relatively short duration and low intensity.

WIDENED PSYCHOPHYSICAL TUNING CURVES

One of the most significant effects of cochlear hearing loss is that the person listens through wider **critical bands**. Figure

38-5 illustrates this. The probe tones must be elevated because of the loss of hearing and of course, the masking noises must be louder too. Normal hearers have wider **tuning curves** when the probe tone is louder. Hearing-impaired persons vary in whether their tuning curves are similar to those of normal hearers listening to loud sounds, or even wider than that.

Wide tuning curves mean that a given neuron can be stimulated rather easily by frequencies farther away from characteristic frequency, if they are loud enough (as probably happens when wearing hearing aids). Examine the tuning curves in Figure 38-5. For this listener, if the background noise were a loud air conditioner, with 500-Hz peak energy, amplified by the hearing aid to 70 dB SPL, that sound would stimulate not just the 500-Hz auditory filter (neuron), but it would stimulate the 1000 and 2000-Hz filters as well. This phenomenon is known as **upward spread of masking**. A given signal's influence spreads to higher frequencies, and potentially can mask processing within those higher frequency channels. The widened tuning curves make the hearing-impaired listener have greater upward spread of masking.

COCHLEAR DEAD REGIONS

A cochlear dead region is an area on basilar membrane that has no inner or outer hair cells. Typically, just a part of basilar membrane is affected. If presented with sounds that fall in the dead frequency region, it is possible that the person will detect the sound using hair cells of other characteristic frequencies located in an area of the cochlea that has residual hair cells. This is called off-frequency listening, a phenomenon described in greater detail before discussing how cochlear dead regions are diagnosed.

Off-Frequency Listening

Off-frequency listening occurs when a signal is processed by an auditory filter that is not "tuned" to the frequency of the signal: the neurons are not within that critical band. Off-frequency listening can occur for normally hearing people in some experimental conditions, as well as occurring when there is a cochlear dead region. For example, if a 1000-Hz sine wave is present in the cochlea along with a sufficiently more intense 800-Hz narrow band of mask-

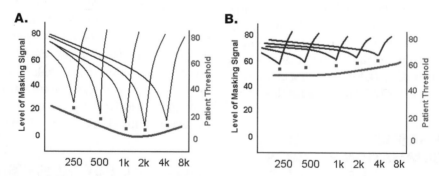

Figure 38–5. Example tuning curves for a hypothetical normal hearer (**A**) and patient with hearing loss (**B**). The lower curves show the listener's thresholds and are read on the scale on the right of the graphs. The squares mark the probe tones. The combinations of frequency and intensity of the narrow-band masking noise that masks the various probes are shown. Whereas the normal hearer has relatively narrow tuning curve tips, the hearing-impaired listener does not.

ing noise that is one-third octave wide, the place on the basilar membrane that normally encodes the 1000-Hz tone is unable to encode the sound. However, as the pure tone's traveling wave passed higher frequency hair cells as the traveling wave moved base to apex, those higher frequency cells may be able to encode the presence of the 1000-Hz tone. If so, then "off-frequency" listening is occurring.

If a person has no inner hair cells in one region of the cochlea, it is possible that the person will be able to detect pure tone signals by using off-frequency listening. Figure 38–6 shows how the traveling wave mechanics work. It is possible to have lower characteristic frequency hair cells detect a higher frequency sound (Figure 38–6A), but it is much easier for residual high-frequency hair cells to encode low-frequency sound, should the apical area of the cochlea be dead (Figure 38–6B).

Audiometric Characteristics of Dead Regions

Although one might guess that the absence of hair cells would cause profound hearing loss, that is not always the case. Off-frequency listening can create thresholds that are as low as 50 to 80 dB HL. If the dead region is in the high frequencies, then a very steeply sloping audiogram would be typical. An audiometeric slope of 35 dB per octave or more (e.g., a 1000-Hz threshold of 40 and a 2000-Hz threshold of 75 dB HL or worse) is an indication of a possible dead region.

If the apex of the cochlea has the dead region, then less loss of sensitivity would be measured when conducting pure tone testing. The low-frequency pure tone travels past the mid- and high-frequency hair cells, which, if intact, can encode the presence of the sound.

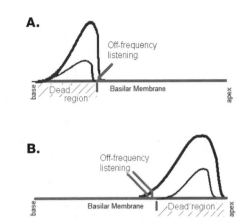

Figure 38–6. A patient with cochlear loss may have areas of the basilar membrane that are devoid of inner hair cells, called cochlear dead regions. In some cases, an area of basilar membrane that has functional hair cells may respond, a process called off-frequency listening. **A.** If a high-frequency sound is present at a loud enough level, the sound may be detected by areas of the basilar membrane more apical, but the shape of the traveling wave limits that ability. **B.** In the more unusual cases where low-frequency regions of the cochlear are dead, it is relatively easy to create off-frequency listening using regions more basal-ward.

What Is Perceived When Off-Frequency Listening Occurs?

In Chapter 22 neural encoding was discussed. It was mentioned that nearby hair cells can respond to pure tones that are not exactly at their characteristic frequency. If the signal is near in frequency, the neural excitation will still be in phase with, or time-locked to, the stimulus. As a rule of thumb, a neuron can phase-lock to a sound that is 1 octave lower than its characteristic frequency or one-half octave higher in frequency than that neuron's characteristic frequency. If the stimulus has a frequency that is outside that range, then the neuron may be stimulated, but the neuron does not fire "in synch"

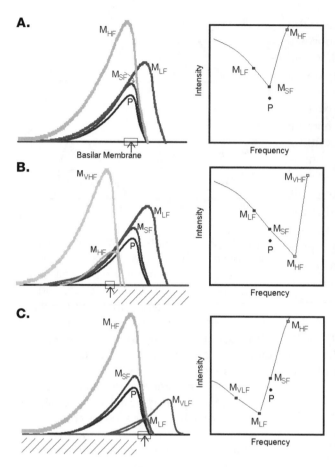

Figure 38–7. A. In a cochlea without a dead region, the probe (*P*) (if alone, without a masker) is detected at the expected place, denoted with the arrow. The probe tone is most readily masked by a masker of the same frequency (M_{SF}). It can be masked by a lower frequency masker (M_{LF}) or a very intense high-frequency masker (M_{HF}). The tuning curve on the right illustrates that it takes less intensity for the masker of lower frequency to alter threshold than if the masker is higher in frequency. **B.** If the basilar membrane has dead regions in the low frequencies (*hatched portion of basilar membrane*) and a higher frequency area is detecting the presence of the probe tone (*area with arrow*) the masker that best masks the tone is one of the same frequency as the area encoding the response, in this case the high-frequency masker (M_{HF}). A masker of the same frequency as the probe is not as effective in masking the probe as was the higher frequency masker. (It took a greater intensity M_{SF} than M_{HF} to mask the probe.) To complete the tuning curve, a masker with lower frequency (M_{LF}) and a masker of very high frequency (M_{VHF}) are also shown. **C.** If the high-frequency region of basilar membrane is dead, the tuning curve tip shifts to a lower frequency, and a masker of very low frequency (M_{VLF}) is the next most effective masker.

with the stimulus peaks—it doesn't phase-lock, and as a result, the sound is not heard as a pure tone. The tone might be perceived as a noise, as static, or as distorted. One imperfect means of determining whether the signal is being processed by off-frequency listening is to ask the patient about the quality of the signal. If it is perceived as a pure, clean, musical tone, then it is unlikely that there is a dead region at that stimulus frequency.

Psychophysical Tuning Curves for Dead Regions

Dead regions can be detected using clinically administered psychophysical tuning curves. When there is a dead region, a pure tone (with a frequency in the dead region) is not masked best by narrow-band noise that is centered at the probe tone frequency, as would normally be the case. When a pure tone is being detected by an off-frequency place on the cochlea, hearing for the pure tone is most readily masked by presenting masking noise with a center frequency that is the same as the characteristic frequency of the neuron that is responding to the pure tone. Figure 38–7 illustrates. If a psychophysical tuning curve is obtained, the tuning curve points to the edge of the dead region.

The Threshold Equalizing Noise Test

The **Threshold Equalizing Noise (TEN) test** is a clinical procedure that tests for cochlear dead regions. It involves putting a noise into the test ear (ipsilateral ear) while retesting the pure-tone thresholds. It is a clever test, devised by B. C. J. Moore and his colleagues in England (Moore, Glasberg & Stone, 2004). Understanding the premise of the test requires some mental agility, so be prepared to study this closely!

By definition, threshold equalizing noise is a broadband noise signal with a spectrum shaped so that it will elevate thresholds of normal hearers to the same level at all frequencies. For example, if 50 dB TEN is put into the ear of the normal hearer, then thresholds in that ear will be elevated to 55 dB HL (the 50 dB TEN would mask tones to 50 dB HL),. Something different happens with cochlear dead region hearing loss—the TEN disrupts hearing when that finding is not expected. In Figure 38–8A we see traveling waves that illustrate the relative thresholds at 1000 and 1500 Hz. In Figure 38–8B, we assume that the cochlea does *not* have any dead regions. The TEN noise would mask the 40 dB HL, 1000-Hz tone, and raise

that threshold to 55 dB HL, but it would not alter the 80 dB HL threshold at 1500 Hz. In Figure 38–8C, we examine what would happen if there is cochlear dead region extending from about 1400 Hz and upward to the higher frequencies. Note the area of basilar membrane with the arrow pointing to it, which is the area responsible for detecting the 1500-Hz tone. The person is using off-frequency listening. The 50 dB TEN prevents this off-frequency listening. The 80 dB HL, 1500-Hz tone should not have been masked by the 50 dB TEN, but it was, because a different place on basilar membrane was responding.

For a threshold shift to be considered clinically significant, indicating a dead region, the threshold shift would have to be 10 dB or greater. Smaller threshold shifts may be due to test/retest variation.

There is reasonably good agreement between PTC diagnosis of dead regions and TEN test diagnosis. At this writing, the TEN test has not been normed for use with insert earphones, only the supra-aural TDH earphones that were commonly used decades ago in the United States, which are still the earphone of choice in Europe. Therefore, at present in the United States, audiologists may resort to asking the patient if the tone is perceived as a clean musical note versus a noise, because it's generally not feasible to obtain tuning curves clinically, and it is time consuming to retest with different earphones in order to do the TEN test.

Enhanced DL$_F$s Near Dead Regions?

If a region of the cochlea is not stimulated, as with a dead region, the neurons located near the edge of the dead region might develop extra dendritic branching, so that neurons connect to hair cells in the remaining nearby "live" region. Perhaps it is that

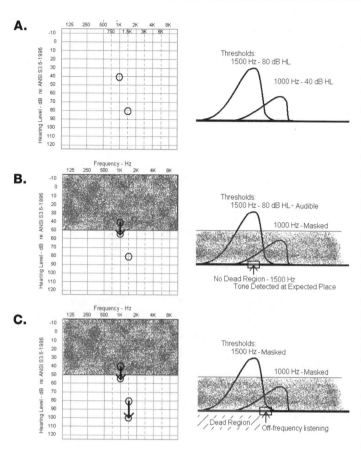

Figure 38–8. Basis for the Threshold Equalizing Noise (TEN) test. **A.** The patient has a precipitously sloping audiogram, with thresholds of 40 dB HL at 1000 Hz and 80 dB HL at 1500 Hz. The traveling waves creating these thresholds are illustrated. **B.** If there are no cochlear dead regions, if 50 dB of threshold equalizing noise is presented, the 1000-Hz threshold would be raised to 55 dB HL; however, the 1500-Hz threshold would remain unchanged. **C.** If the 1500-Hz tone was detected at a lower frequency place on basilar membrane (*see arrow*) because of a dead region at and above 1500 Hz, the 50 dB TEN masks the 1500 Hz tone – threshold for 1500 Hz is elevated. The TEN prevented the off-frequency listening from occurring. Because a threshold above 50 dB HL was shifted by 50 dB of TEN, the dead region was detected. Audiogram generated with AuDSim software, used and reproduced with permission courtesy of www.aud-student.com .

extra neural activity that permits those with dead regions to have somewhat better **difference limens for frequency** right at the "living edge" of the dead region.

Amplification for Those with Dead Regions

A general principle, articulated succinctly by audiologist Ted Venema (2006, p. 36), is "you can help the dying, but you cannot help the dead." Stimulating dead regions of the cochlea won't permit the dead hair cells to create neural impulses, so the rule of thumb is that there is no reason to amplify those frequencies using a conventional hearing aid.

There is, though, a notable exception to that rule. Because a neuron can phase-lock to pure tones that are one octave lower than the neuron's characteristic frequency, or one-half octave above characteristic frequency, it makes sense that the hearing aid provide some amplification above the frequency cutoff for the dead region. Providing amplification more than one octave above a dead region wouldn't, however, be prudent.

Clinical Correlate: Frequency Compression Hearing Aids and Short-Electrode Cochlear Implants

Patients with extensive cochlear dead regions may not be good candidates for traditional hearing aids. If a patient has high-frequency dead regions, the hearing aid may not allow for detection of high-frequency consonant sounds, which are critical for speech understanding. Two options are the use of a frequency-compression hearing aid and a partial cochlear implant.

Frequency compression (sometimes called frequency transposition) hearing aids are digital devices that shift the frequency of the sound. For example, if there was a dead region above 1500 Hz, sounds above 1500 Hz would be transformed into lower frequency sounds. The resulting sound doesn't sound "normal," but the listener can learn to recognize the frequency-transposed/compressed speech sounds.

Another alternative is a combination of a cochlear implant and a hearing aid. A cochlear implant has electrodes inserted in the cochlea. Activating the electrodes stimulates the nerves directly, by-passing the hair cells entirely. There is one version of a cochlear implant that only goes a short distance up basilar membrane, and can help those with high-frequency dead regions. A traditional hearing aid can be used to amplify sounds to be sent to the damaged, but not dead, lower frequency regions.

GAP DETECTION THRESHOLDS

Results with White Noise Stimuli

Chapter 35 discussed that **gap detection** thresholds are better for high-frequency stimuli than for low-frequency sounds, and when presented with white noise, the normal hearer detects the gap with the high-frequency areas (filters) on basilar membrane. Those stop ringing (moving) most quickly and can detect smaller duration silent intervals. Most cochlear loss creates greater high-frequency hearing loss than low-frequency loss, so the person with cochlear loss must rely on a low-

er frequency range to detect the gap. As a result, the gap detection results for wide-band signals would be worse for the person with high-frequency cochlear hearing loss.

Gap Detection Results for Pure Tones Depend on Stimulus Intensity Levels

Normal hearers have improved gap detection ability as the sound levels increase to about 60 dB SPL. Whether you consider hearing-impaired patients as having abnormal gap detection thresholds depends on the signal intensity.

A hearing-impaired patient doing gap detection while listening to a near-threshold-level pure tone (e.g., perhaps 50 dB HL for someone with 40 dB of hearing loss) needs a larger gap than a normal-hearing person does listening to that same 50 dB HL pure tone. But if you have those same two persons listen to a loud pure tone, perhaps 85 dB HL, then the gap detection results look more similar, with some studies concluding that the hearing-impaired require a still greater gap to detect the silent interval in the signal.

Without amplification, the poorer gap detection ability may interfere with speech intelligibility. Pauses in speech, such as the time between the energy burst of a plosive consonant like /k/, and the onset of the vowel that follows, may be more difficult to detect, or the person might be more likely to confuse /k/ with the voiced /g/ sound, which has a shorter time delay between the burst and vowel energy. With amplification, we expect the gap detection ability to be more normal, and it may be that the timing information becomes a crucial clue, as the ear has more difficulty processing the details of the spectral content of speech because of the widened critical bands.

Gap Detection Levels Should Theoretically Be Better in Hearing-Impaired

Gap detection ability is related to how quickly basilar membrane stops vibrating once the sound has stopped. Auditory filters are wider at the base of the cochlea, and wider filters are related to less ringing. Cochlear loss patients have wider filters (tuning curves/critical bands). That would lead one to think that the gap detection thresholds would actually be better than normal. However, remember that if you compare the tuning curves (which show the filter width)

of normal hearers listening to loud probes and maskers, the results aren't all that different from the results for the hearing-impaired. The poorer gap detection thresholds of some hearing-impaired listeners may reflect a problem with their ability to encode timing information—a problem unrelated to the width of the auditory filter.

TEMPORAL MODULATION DETECTION ABILITY IS GOOD IF THE SIGNAL IS FULLY AUDIBLE

In temporal modulation transfer function testing, the signal varies in amplitude at some warble rate (e.g., if the signal increases and decreases in intensity 20 times per second, then it is said to be modulated, or warbled, at 20 Hz). Recruitment should give the hearing-impaired enhanced ability to detect changes in amplitude, as long as the signal is fully audible. Figure 38–9 illustrates results in a case of hypothetical unilateral cochlear hearing impairment. The impaired ear is presented with a signal with a minor amplitude variation, but because of recruitment, the perception is that the amplitude chang-

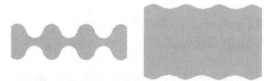

Figure 38–9. Theoretical results of a balancing of stimulus qualities of temporally modulated signals in the normal ear (*left*) and impaired ear (*right*) of a listener with unilateral cochlear hearing loss. The signal must be more intense in the impaired ear, but the relatively small intensity variation is equated to a much larger amplitude variation in the unimpaired ear. The impaired ear is more sensitive to the loudness changes.

es are quite dramatic. The signal would be matched (to one presented to the normal hearing ear) to a sound with much more variation in amplitude. The recruitment accompanying the cochlear loss creates an advantage, and a smaller amplitude fluctuation can be detected. However, that is true only if the signal is fully audible in each ear.

If a hearing-impaired person with a sloping high-frequency hearing loss listens to white noise that amplitude modulates, the hearing loss prevents use of the information from the high frequencies. The high-frequency channels are normally the best at detecting how the signal changes over time. With those channels not participating because of the high-frequency hearing loss, the hearing-impaired person's performance is degraded.

POORER PITCH PERCEPTION ABILITIES

The **frequency difference limen** is typically higher (poorer) for those with cochlear loss, and the greater the loss, generally the poorer the pitch change discrimination. There is a good bit of intersubject variability, though. Another general finding is that the difference between hearing-impaired and normal hearers' DL_Fs is greatest at the high frequencies. In the low frequencies, the DL_F may be entirely normal even with significant hearing loss, although there still is a trend toward somewhat worse pitch perception, even for the low frequencies.

The impaired pitch perception may be related to the widening of the critical bands that occurs with cochlear loss. We usually discriminate pitch when slightly different areas of basilar membrane are stimulated, and the neurons carefully encode the periodicity of the signal by firing in synchrony with the peaks of the cycles of the pure tone. The tuning curves being wider means

that various neurons, including those that encode other frequencies, are stimulated. If those neurons not near the signal peak send a signal that does not help encode frequency, that may make pitch detection more difficult. Another possibility is that the poor pitch perception comes from problems with the ear's temporal integration ability—that is, the timing coding of the ear is impaired.

SUMMARY

Cochlear hearing loss reduces speech audibility, impairing speech understanding. However, not all hearing-impaired have equal speech detection impairment, and the differences may result from different underlying perception abilities.

Psychoacousticians and audiologists recognize recruitment as a fundamental characteristic of cochlear hearing impairment. Sound quickly increases from barely audible to loud. The recruitment may be an advantage in certain ways. If listening to well above threshold-level sounds, some perceptual abilities become fairly normal and may be better than normal. Difference limens for intensity are good—the ear detects changes in amplitude well, including changes such as the amplitude modulation used in temporal modulation detection tasks.

Generally, the ear's ability to detect timing differences is not impaired too dramatically, although results vary between patients. Gap detection tests are one way to evaluate timing detection ability. If the patient is presented with a fully audible signal, the results approximate normal for many.

Difference limens for frequency may be larger for the hearing-impaired and, if so, that may be related to the ear's loss of some ability to use timing information—in this case, not the slowly changing time waveform information, but the fine detail timing information that encodes frequency information.

One of the best understood concepts is that hearing-impaired are listening through widened critical bands. They are more susceptible to one sound masking another because a given auditory filter is not terribly restricted in which high-intensity sound it will respond to. Problems with speech understanding in noise are an anticipated result.

Although there are correlations between poorer psychoacoustic tests and impaired speech understanding, our understanding of just how perceptual abilities relate to speech recognition is far from perfect. Understanding some of the principles involved is helpful in working with the hearing-impaired. Hearing aids can restore audibility, but will not "correct" cochlear hearing loss. Understanding the reasons why can help when counseling the hearing-impaired patient.

REFERENCES

French, N. R., & Steinberg, J. C. (1947). Factors governing the intelligibility of speech sounds. *Journal of the Acoustical Society of America, 19,* 90–119.

Moore, B. C. J., Glasberg, B. R., & Stone, M. A. (2004). New version of the TEN test with calibrations in dB HL. *Ear and Hearing, 188,* 478–487.

Mueller, H. G., & Killion, M. C. (1990). An easy method for calculating the articulation index. *Hearing Journal, 9,* 14–17.

Venema, T. (2006). *Compression for clinicians* (2nd ed). Clifton-Park, NY: Thompson-Delmar.

APPENDIX A

The Math Needed to Succeed In Hearing Science

Some students haven't had math recently. Some wish they could forget having ever had math! Basic hearing science doesn't require heavy mathematical computations, but it is important that you know the basic rules of math and algebra or, at very least, know where to find them when you need them. Basic math skills are needed to understand how to calculate decibels, which is the topic of Chapter 2. You'll also need basic math to understand acoustics, so that you can calculate a sound wave's wavelength or period. Understanding sine waves is enhanced by knowing a little trigonometry.

MATHEMATICAL NOTATION

- In math, we can let letters stand for a numerical value.
- If I say "a = b + c," you can come up with an infinite number of numbers that you can fill in, like if a = 12, then b could = 10.23 and c would = 1.77.
- Sometimes letters are used not to stand for a number, but a unit of measurement, such as sec stands for seconds, or t stands for time.

Common examples are shown in Table A–1.

- So, when we create an equation like F = mA:
  - In these equations, if two letters are next to each other without any sign, it means multiply. A dot ($\cdot$) also means multiply, as does an asterisk ($*$) or $\times$.
  - Here, force equals mass times acceleration.
- When you see "d," the italicized d, it is a special notation meaning derivative, which deals with calculus. You will see this notation in research literature.

FRACTIONS

The number on the top part of the equation is called the **numerator**, and the one on the bottom is the **denominator**.

- Any number divided by 1 is still that original number: 23/1 = 23
- When you convert from a fraction (also called a ratio of 2 numbers), such as 4/7, to a decimal number, such as 0.571428, here are some rules to use.

Table A–1. The Symbols for Common Concepts in Acoustics, Along with the Equations and the Units and Symbols for the Units That You Will Commonly See

Concept	Symbol in Equation	Equation	Unit Used and Symbol for Unit
Acceleration	a	= v/t	cm/sec^2 or m/sec^2 (velocity / time) (centimeters per second squared or meters per second squared)
Area	A	= width × length for a rectangle = 3.14 × radius^2 for a circle	cm^2 or m^2 (centimeters or meters squared)
Displacement	X	= distance moved	cm or m (centimeters or meters)
What you are solving for in an equation	x (or any letter)		*Note*: in an algebraic equation, the letter x is commonly used to mean what you are solving for, so x will not always mean displacement.
Force	F	= m * a (mass × acceleration)	N/m^2 or Pa or d (newtons per meter squared or pascals or dynes) *Note:* 1 N/m^2 = 1 pascal = 10 d/cm/m^2 = 1 × 10^{-6} µPa
Intensity	I	= P/A (power divided by area)	W/m^2 or W/cm^2 (watts per meter squared or watts per centimeter squared)
Power	P	= w/t (work divided by time)	W (watts)
Pressure	p	= F/A (force divided by area)	Pa (pascal) or µPa (micropascal) or d/cm^2 (dynes/cm^2). See also Force above.
Work	w	= F/X (force divided by displacement)	N × m (newton times meter) or Joule *Note:* 1 Nm = 1 Joule

- You may want to round when the number doesn't come up even. We usually leave at least two "significant digits," that is, numbers other than 0.
- Example: 0.0000012 has two significant digits.
- Round "up or down"—numbers higher than 5 are rounded up, round them down if it is lower than 5.

- Example: Round 0.571428 to two significant digits. The third digit, 1, is rounded down, so the rounded number is 0.57.
- Example: The number 0.579 would be rounded up to 0.58.
- If the last digit omitted number to be rounded is a 5, then round so the resulting last digit is an even number.

- Example, if leaving three significant digits when rounding 1.245, it rounds to 1.24. 1.255 would round to 1.26.

Manipulating Math Equations That Involve Fractions

Let's review some of the rules that apply to solving simple math equations.

- When you multiply both the numerator and denominator by the same number, the fraction remains the same. (Below, remember the asterisk means multiply.)

$$\frac{A}{B} = \frac{A * C}{B * C}$$

$$\frac{1}{2} = \frac{1 * 10}{2 * 10}$$

- Another example: the fraction 5/7 is the same as 10/14. Both the numerator and denominator were multiplied by 2.

Cross-Products and Equality of Equations

Cross-products are when you multiply the numerator on one side of an equation with the denominator on the other side of the equation to check that the equation is true. We use this principle in solving equations as well.

$$\frac{A}{B} = \frac{C}{D}$$

Only if A * D = B * C
That is,

$$\frac{10}{20} = \frac{20}{40}$$

because 10 * 40 is equal to 20 * 20.

We use this principle to solve equations quite often. If 1/x = 16/32, what does x equal? As

$$\frac{1}{x} = \frac{16}{32}$$

Then x * 16 = 32 * 1.

As we now have x * 16 = 32, we can take both sides of the equation and divide by 16 (or if you prefer you can think of it as multiplying by 1/16), and we solve x = 32/16, or x = 2.

You could have also chosen to multiply both sides of the original equation

$$\frac{1}{x} = \frac{16}{32}$$

by x/ 1.

$$\frac{1 * x}{x * 1} = \frac{16 * x}{32 * 1}$$

That will cause the x on the left hand side to cancel out, leaving you with

$$\frac{1}{1} = \frac{16x}{32}$$

You can then multiply each side of the equation by 32/16 to find that

$$\frac{32}{16} = \frac{x}{1}$$

You arrive at the same answer, of course. As they say, there is more than one way to skin a cat (although I've never been quite sure about why you would want to). There are reasons to solve basic algebra equations, however!

Reducing Fractions to the Simplest Value—The Lowest Common Denominator

When you see something like

$$\frac{4}{2} * \frac{2}{1}$$

You can cancel out the 2's, because you are multiplying by 2 on both the numerator side of the equation and the denominator side. This would simplify to 4/1 or 4.

We will often want to get an equation to be as simple as possible. For example,

$$\frac{10000}{20000} \, \frac{10000}{20000} = \frac{1}{2}$$

Here we cross off the zeros that are both on the top and bottom.

If the equation had had one more zero on the denominator side, we'd be careful not to get rid of it.

$$\frac{10000}{200000} = \frac{1}{20}$$

If the number were

$$\frac{2}{4}$$

We could simplify it to 1/2. How did we do that? Well, what we really did was multiply both the numerator and denominator by 1/2.

$$\frac{2 * \frac{1}{2}}{4 * \frac{1}{2}} = \frac{1}{2}$$

(Because 2 in the numerator can be thought of as 2/1 and then when you multiply that by ½ the 2's cancel out, so it is just 1 left over.) But the conceptually simpler way to think about it would be "2 goes into 2 once and 2 goes into 4 twice, so I'll make that ½." Using this same logic, 3/9 = 1/3.

Multiplication of Fractions

Next, we review the rules for multiplication of fractions.

$$\frac{a}{b} * \frac{c}{d} = \frac{a * c}{b * d}$$

For example:

$$\frac{2}{4} * \frac{1}{2} = \frac{2 * 1}{4 * 2} = \frac{2}{8} = \frac{1}{4}$$

What Is a "Reciprocal"?

When you have a fraction, and flip the numerator and denominator, that is called a reciprocal.

3/4 is the reciprocal of 4/3.

Reciprocals are directly related to division of fractions.

Division of Fractions

Division Rule: Multiply the dividend (the number to be divided) by the reciprocal of the divisor.

So, if you want to divide

$$\frac{4}{5}$$

by 2 (which could be written $\frac{4/5}{2}$)

it is the same as multiplying 4/5 * 1/2, which gives you 4/10.

And if you were to divide

$$\frac{4}{5}$$

by ½

It is the same as multiplying 4/5 * 2 (the reciprocal of ½), which gives you 8/5.

Adding Fractions

Let's review the rules for adding fractions without the aid of a calculator.

Adding fractions is easy if the denominators are the same, such as

2/24 + 5/24 = 7/24

But what do you do if the denominators aren't the same?

3/4 + 1/2 = ?

First you need to make the denominators the same. Here you see that you can multiply the 1/2 by 2/2 so it becomes 2/4, then you can do the addition.

It's not always easy to figure out how to make the denominators the same. You can always ask yourself "What number is the result of multiplying both denominators together?" In this case it is 8.

Next, consider what you need to do to get each denominator to equal that product, 8 in this example.

You would multiply the 3/4 by 2/2, to obtain 6/8, and multiply 1/2 by 4/4 and so that it is now 4/8.

Now you can add, and find the answer as 10/8.

Simplify the result to 5/4, which you recognize as the same as 1¼.

Yes, you can also just punch both into the calculator, get the decimal number, and add them. However, sometimes these rules are required to solve an equation, rather than just to achieve the end product.

Subtracting Fractions

The same principles apply to subtracting fractions as adding them. It is easy when the denominators are the same, otherwise, first make them the same or use your calculator.

WHAT YOU NEED TO REMEMBER FROM ALGEBRA

When you are multiplying, dividing, subtracting, and adding, the order doesn't matter **IF** there is only one type of math going on in the equation (you're not both adding and multiplying in the same equation.)

- Example: 2 + 4 is the same as 4 + 2, and – 2 + 4 is equal to 4 + –2, which is simpler when expressed as 4 – 2.
- 8 * 2 = 2 * 8

However, if you were combining adding and multiplying in an equation, it **does** matter which you do first. You have to do the multiplying and dividing first, then the adding and subtracting. If the equation wants you to do it in another order, they will put parenthesis in to tell you "do this first."

3 + 4 * 8 means multiply 4 * 8 first then add 3, so this equals 3 + 32 or 35.
But (3 + 4) * 8 means add first, then multiply, so this is 7 * 8 or 56.

By the way, if you type this into your calculator, it will know what to do first. And if an equation has parentheses, you can enter those in and the calculator will handle them! (Isn't technology wonderful?)

The Distributive Law

Solving equations may entail a sequence of steps. One of the steps may be to use the Distributive Law.

$$a(b + c) = ab + ac$$

Remember that? Multiply the part outside the parentheses by each of the things you are adding.

Absolute Values

Occasionally you will come across the concept of absolute value, which means the value without the plus or minus sign. The symbol for absolute value is the vertical slashes around the number or symbol, such as

$|-5|$, which equals 5.

Because the straight up and down slash is easy to mistake for the letter I or number 1, you may see diagonal slashes, such as /-5/.

What an "Exponent" Means

What is the notation for saying $2 * 2 * 2$? It's 2^3. It's often convenient to express numbers in scientific notation, that is, using exponents. For example, the area of a cube that has equal sized sides is the size of one side, raised to the power of 3. So when you see some "base" number, raised to an exponent, like

$$B^n$$

it means take B and multiply it by itself n times.

DIMENSIONAL ANALYSIS

Dimensional analysis, meaning converting from one measurement system to another, really is all about multiplying by one. This review section is an easy one. As you know, there are different measurement systems. For example, you can measure height in inches or in feet. If something is 2 feet long, how many inches is it? You know intuitively to multiply by 12, but what's the math principle?

$$2 \text{ feet} \times \frac{12 \text{ inches}}{1 \text{ foot}} = 24 \text{ inches}$$

(You can do that because 12 inches = 1 foot, so you have in effect multiplied by one, which doesn't change the value of the equation.)

You cancel out the feet/foot and you have inches in the answer.

Most of the unit analysis we will be doing is relative to the metric system, for example, putting inches into centimeters. 1 inch is equal to 2.54 centimeters, or 25.4 millimeters.

$$1.5 \text{ inches} * \frac{2.54 \text{ cm}}{1 \text{ inch}} = 3.81 \text{ cm}$$

Dimensional analysis may also involve conversion from one unit within the mks (**mass kilogram second**) **system** to another. Table A–2 may help with those conversions.

DECIBELS, SCIENTIFIC NOTATION, LOGARITHMS, EXPONENTS, AND SQUARE ROOTS

You should be ready to read Chapter 2 now. It covers scientific notation, exponents, and logs. This next section includes a few additional concepts as a reference.

Table A–2. Prefixes for the MKS (mass kilogram second). System abbreviations and values are shown, along with an example of how to convert from those units to meters.

Prefix	Abbreviation	Exponential Value	Decimal Value	Example
giga-	G	10^9	1,000,000,000	1 Gm = 1 X 10^9 m
mega-	M	10^6	1,000,000	1 Mm = 1 X 10^6 m
kilo-	k	10^3	1,000	1 km = 1 X 10^3 m
hecto-	H	10^2	100	1 Hm = 1 X 10^2 m
deca- (or deka-)	da	10^1	10	1 dam = 1 X 10^1 m
deci-	D	10^{-1}	.1	1 dm = 1 X 10^{-1} m
centi-	c	10^{-2}	.01	1 cm = 1 X 10^{-2} m
milli-	m	10^{-3}	.001	1 mm = 1 X 10^{-3} m
micro-	μ	10^{-6}	.000 001	1 μm = 1 X 10^{-6} m
nano-	n	10^{-9}	.000 000 001	1 nm = 1 X 10^{-9} m
pico-	p	10^{-12}	.000 000 000 001	1 nm = 1 X 10^{-12} m

Multiplying and Dividing Numbers with Exponents

A 9-year-old would probably not believe you, but multiplying can be easier than adding and subtracting. That's the case with exponents, anyhow. Here you don't have to get the numbers into the same base, so it really is easier.

If you were multiplying

$(A * 10^B) * (C * 10^D)$, this would be the same as $(A * C) * 10^{B+D}$

That is, multiply the digit term and add the exponents.

■ For example
$5.0 * 10^2 * 6.0 * 10^5 = 30 * 10^7$
(which should be written $3.0 * 10^8$).

When you are dividing, you divide the digit terms and subtract the exponent on the bottom of the equation from the one on the top of the equation.

■ For example

$$\frac{5.0 * 10^2}{6.0 * 10^5} = .833 * 10^{-3}$$

Raising an Exponent to an Exponent

What is $(5.0 * 10^2)^2 = ?$
Raise both the digit term to that exponent and also multiply the exponent by that exponent:

$$(5.0 * 10^3)^2 = 5.0^2 * 10^{3 \times 2} = 5.0^2 * 10^6$$

Remember that 5 squared is 5 * 5, or 25, so the simplified equation then becomes 25 * 10^6 which should be written as 2.5 * 10^7.

Square Roots

When you square something, you say "x times itself equals what?" When you obtain a square root, you are asking "what times itself equals x?"

- So 5 squared, or $(5^2) = 5 * 5 = 25$.

On the calculator, that would be 5, and then hit the button that says x^2.

- The square root of 25 = 5.

On a calculator, you would enter the number, like 25, then find the button that looks like this:

$$\sqrt{x}$$

Other Powers on the Calculator

What if you want to find x * x * x, which is of course x^3? Let's say you want to find out what 34^3 is. Enter 34, then the key that says y^x then enter 3.

You calculator may have a cubic root and cubic function also, if so they look like

$$x^3 \text{ and } \sqrt[3]{x}$$

and probably are "second function" buttons on your calculator.

Index